CRITICAL CARE
MEDICINE
THE ESSENTIALS

CRITICAL CARE MEDICINE
THE ESSENTIALS

JOHN J. MARINI, M.D.

Professor of Medicine
University of Minnesota
Director of Pulmonary/Critical Care Medicine
St. Paul-Ramsey Medical Center
Minneapolis-St. Paul, Minnesota

ARTHUR P. WHEELER, M.D.

Vanderbilt University
Nashville, Tennessee

WILLIAMS & WILKINS
BALTIMORE · HONG KONG · LONDON · MUNICH
PHILADELPHIA · SYDNEY · TOKYO

Editor: Timothy Grayson
Associate Editor: Carol Eckhart
Copy Editor: Bill Cady, Susan Vaupel
Design: Dan Pfisterer
Illustration Planning: Lorraine Wrzosek
Production: Theda Harris

Copyright © 1989
Williams & Wilkins
428 East Preston Street
Baltimore, MD 21202, U.S.A

Accurate indications, adverse reactions, and dosage schedules for drugs are provided in this
book, but it is possible that they may change. The reader is urged to review the package
information data of the manufacturers of the medications mentioned.

Printed in the United States of America

Library of Congress Cataloging-in-Publication Data

Marini, John J.
   Critical care medicine: the essentials / John J. Marini, Arthur Wheeler.
      p.   cm.
   Includes index.
   ISBN 0-683-05554-2
   1. Critical care medicine—Handbooks, manuals, etc. 2. Surgical intensive care—Handbooks,
manuals, etc. I. Wheeler, Arthur. II. Title.
   [DNLM: 1. Critical Care. 2. Emergencies. 3. Life Support Care. WX 218 M339c]
RC86.7.M368 1989   616'.028—dc19
DNLM/DLC for Library of Congress   88-26190
                                                                                CIP

10 9 8 7 6 5 4

DEDICATIONS

To Peggy, with love and admiration.
John J. Marini

To my wife and parents for their assurance that I
can accomplish anything, and to my sons, Aaron
and Eric, for reminding me that I can't.
Arthur P. Wheeler

PREFACE

Almost by definition, critically ill patients present life-threatening problems that must be solved quickly with little margin for error. To practice effectively in this setting, the clinician must be firmly grounded in the pathophysiology of critical illness and life support. This book is our attempt to simplify the complexity that permeates the intensive care unit, threatening to overwhelm the clinician who must make urgent decisions under the stress of this environment.

Acting alone, no single physician can care optimally for all types of critically ill patients. Yet, although critical care is inherently a multi-specialty discipline, the physician who assumes primary responsibility must be familiar with a wide range of problems and possess a good working knowledge of specialized techniques of diagnosis and life support.

Almost 10 years ago, one of us (JM) undertook to write a succinct manual of vital information needed by the house officer to manage common respiratory problems and cardio-pulmonary aspects of intensive care. In the time since the first printing of that book—*Respiratory Medicine and Intensive Care for the House Officer*—the field of respiratory medicine has redefined its scope to include the rapidly maturing discipline of critical care. As a result, present day specialists must have substantial knowledge of the acute hematologic, gastrointestinal, neurologic, renal, infectious, and cardiovascular problems considered outside their purview a short time ago. In revising the original work for a second edition, two things were clear. First, a single manual of reasonable length cannot address both critical care and non-intensive pulmonary medicine. Therefore, only pulmonary physiology and the non-critical aspects of respiratory medicine were addressed in the revised second edition of *Respiratory Medicine for the House Officer*, which serves as a companion to the current volume. Second, many physicians, nurses, and allied health professionals have need for a succinct

text in critical care geared toward maximal practical value in daily practice—regardless of their primary specialty, experience, or stage of training. The current volume recognizes that broader audience.

Critical Care Medicine—The Essentials was written with special attention to the needs of house officers and advanced students. However, it should also help others who deal frequently with patients in this arena—e.g., nurses, respiratory therapists, and fellows in pulmonary disease, cardiology, anesthesiology, and intensive care medicine.

Our collaboration combines the knowledge of an experienced intensivist 10 years out of fellowship (JM) with that of a physician (AW) who is just now completing his training in pulmonary and critical care medicine. From these different but complementary perspectives we have carefully sifted through our joint experience for information of maximal practical value and interest—a fair amount of which is difficult to find elsewhere. We deliberately excluded much that is either commonly known or easily accessed in more comprehensive sources. A good deal of the material chosen for inclusion originated in discussions with housestaff and other physicians on the "front lines". Although no pretense is made as to comprehensive coverage or evenness of presentation, we believe that this book forms an appropriate core text with which to prepare for Certification Examinations in Critical Care. We do not apologize for the strong cardiopulmonary emphasis, because in a real sense cardiopulmonary crises define the need for intensive care. Chapter length and depth of treatment vary with our perceptions of frequency or importance of the topic, as well as the knowledge base of our intended audience.

Many aspects of critical care cannot be learned from a book, however comprehensive and well written. Consequently, we have emphasized approaches and principles wherever possible, omitting technical discussion of procedures that must be learned at the bedside. To maximize utility we have organized the text into three major sections dealing with techniques of life support, medical problems, and surgical crises. The illustrations are composite diagrams and line drawings, a format that effectively transmits conceptual information. For the most part, suggested readings are important references and scholarly reviews that expand upon the points summarized in the text.

The content of this book reflects our shared background as internists who focus on adult intensive care. No attempt has been made to address problems in pediatrics or neonatology, nor will the reader find information relevant to specific emergencies in obstetrics, gynecology, or the surgical subspecialties. The reader should clearly understand that we are not surgeons; therefore, we have omitted specific details of surgical technique and management.

We have tried our best to ensure that our descriptions, recommendations, and medication dosages are accurate. However, the pace of change in this discipline is very rapid, and there is often more than one "correct" option. Whereas specific details of management change quickly, management principles rooted in physiology do not. We, therefore, present concepts and principles which guide our thinking in critical care in the hope that they will give insight to others.

John J. Marini
Arthur P. Wheeler

ACKNOWLEDGMENT

It is difficult to adequately express our appreciation and thanks to Brenda Plunkett, to whom we are indebted for her assistance, advice, and friendship during the preparation of this text. Without her dedicated help, completion of this project might not have been possible.

CONTENTS

SECTION 1

Life Support Techniques

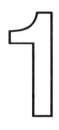

Hemodynamics

CHARACTERISTICS OF THE NORMAL CIRCULATION

Cardiac Anatomy

The circulatory and respiratory systems are tightly interdependent in their primary function of delivering appropriate quantities of oxygenated blood to metabolizing tissues. The physician's ability to deal with hemodynamic dysfunction requires a well-developed understanding of the structure and control of the circulation under normal and abnormal conditions.

From a functional viewpoint, there are two distinct circulations—right and left. Except during congestive failure, *the atria* serve primarily as reservoirs for blood collection, rather than as key pumping elements. The *right ventricle* (RV) is structured differently than its left sided counterpart. Because of the enormous gas exchanging surface of the lungs, the RV normally needs to generate mean pressures only 1/7 as great as those of the left side in driving the same output. Consequently, the free wall of the RV is normally thin and poorly adapted to acutely increased afterload.

The thicker *left ventricle* (LV) must generate sufficient pressure to drive flow through much higher, widely fluctuating vascular resistance. The RV and LV share the interventricular septum, circumferential muscle fibers, and the pericardial space—features which tend to link them in a functional sense. For example, when the RV swells in response to increased afterload, the LV is made functionally less distensible, and left sided filling pressures tend to increase. Ventricular interdependence is enhanced by processes that crowd their shared pericardial fossa: high lung volumes, high heart volumes, pericardial effusion, and constriction (see p. 10).

Coronary Circulation

The heart is nourished by the *coronary circulation*. The right coronary artery emerges from the anterior aorta, and in the great majority of persons distributes to the RV, to the atrioventricular (AV) and sinus nodes, and to the posterior and inferior surfaces of the LV. The left coronary system (circumflex and left anterior descending arteries) nourishes the interventricular septum, the conduction system below the AV node, and the anterior and lateral walls of the LV. Were the heart totally relaxed, flow through the coronary circulation would be driven by the difference between mean arterial pressure (MAP) and coronary sinus pressure. However, because the wall tension that surrounds the coronary vessels determines the effective downstream pressure, perfusion varies phasically with the cardiac cycle. The LV is perfused mainly in early diastole, when tissue pressure is least. Because the RV generates a much lower compressive force, right coronary flow is less phasic. The LV myocardial pressure is highest close to the endocardium and lowest near the epicardium. Hence, under stress, the endocardium is more likely to experience ischemia.

Myocardial blood flow normally parallels metabolic activity. Locally active neural and humoral stimuli cause the coronary circulation to dilate under stress; however, the precise mediators of this linkage are incompletely known. Tachycardia and bradycardia have dual effects on coronary blood flow. Because changes in heart rate are accomplished chiefly by shortening or lengthening diastole, tachycardia shortens the time available for diastolic perfusion while increasing the heart's need for oxygen. Normally, this reduction in mean coronary flow is overridden by coronary dilatation. However, coronary disease prevents full expression of this compensation. During bradycardia longer periods of time are available for diastolic perfusion, and metabolic needs are less. However, diastolic myocardial fiber tension rises as the heart expands, and marked bradycardia may lower MAP and coronary perfusion pressure.

Vascular Anatomy

Between beats continuous flow of blood from the *heart to the periphery* is maintained by the recoil of elastic vessels distended during systole. Although the aorta is predominately an elastic structure, the peripheral arteries are muscular in character. Thus, the arterioles serve as the main resistive units of the vascular tree. By adjusting caliber, these small vessels regulate tissue blood flow and aid in the control of arterial pressure. The capillaries downstream from the arterioles are so numerous that flow through them is slow. These vessels are short and narrow, however, so that the capillary network contains relatively little of the total circulating blood volume—the true capacitance vessels of the circulation are the venules and small veins. At any time, only a small percentage of the total capacitance bed is recruited. The precise distribution of the circulatory volume is gated by arteriolar vasoconstriction.

In the low-pressure *pulmonary circuit* the central vessels are thinner and there is normally little anatomic difference between arteries and veins. The capillary network, however, is even more luxuriant than in the periphery. Flow distribution is highly gravity dependent and influenced by alveolar pressure, oxygen tension, and chemical stimuli (see p. 17).

CIRCULATORY CONTROL

Determinants of Cardiac Output

Pump Function

When averaged over time, cardiac output (CO), the product of heart rate (HR) and stroke volume (SV), must be matched to metabolic requirements. Although the precise mechanism which links output to metabolism remains uncertain, the primary determinants of SV are well defined: precontractile fiber stretch (*preload*), the tension developed by the muscle fibers during contraction (*afterload*), and the forcefulness of muscular contraction under constant loading conditions (*contractility*). These characteristics determine the stroke volume—the volume of blood ejected from the heart during each beat. Because the SV of both ventricles must be equal despite differing end-diastolic volumes, the fraction of end-diastolic blood volume ejected dur-

ing systole (ejection fraction, EF) differs between them. The product of SV and HR is CO.

Stroke Volume Determinants

Preload.   According to the Frank-Starling principle, the vigor of cardiac contraction is influenced by muscle fiber length at end-diastole. The tendency of ejected volume to increase as filling pressure rises normally constitutes an important adaptive mechanism that enables moment-by-moment adjustment to changing venous return. During heart failure the Starling curve is flattened, and the ventricle is "preload insensitive"—high filling pressures are needed for modest outputs.

For a specific heart, preload changes proportionally to acute changes in end-diastolic ventricular volume. It should be understood, however, that the relationship between absolute chamber volume and preload varies over time—muscle fiber stretch within a chronically dilated heart may not differ significantly from normal. End-diastolic volume is determined by ventricular distensibility (compliance) and by the pressure distending the ventricle (the transmural pressure). Transmural pressure is the difference between the intracavitary and juxtacardiac pressures. A poorly compliant ventricle, or one surrounded by increased intrathoracic pressure, requires higher intracavitary pressure to achieve any specified end-diastolic volume and fiber stretch. The cost of higher filling pressure may be pulmonary edema.

Functional ventricular stiffening can result from myocardial disease, pericardial tethering, or extrinsic compression of the heart (Table 1.1).

The precise position of the ventricle on the Starling curve is difficult to determine. However, animal studies suggest that in the supine position there is little preload reserve, and that further increases in CO are met primarily by increases in HR. Thus, the Starling mechanism may be of most importance during hypovolemia.

Diastolic Dysfunction.   Diastole is usually considered a passive process in which elastic heart

Table 1.1
Reduced Diastolic Compliance

Myocardial Disease	Pericardial Disease	Extrinsic Compression
Ischemia/ Infarction	Tamponade	PEEP
Hypertrophy	Constriction	Tension pneumothorax
Infiltration		RV Dilation

muscle is distended by a transmural pressure. In normal individuals and many patients with heart disease, this approximation is more or less accurate. However, in recent years it has become clear that in some patients diastole is more properly considered an energy-dependent, active process (see Ref. 5). Failure of the heart muscle to relax at a normal rate (secondary to ischemia, longstanding hypertension, or hypertrophic myopathy) can cause sufficient *functional stiffening* to produce pulmonary edema despite preserved systolic function. Although diastolic and systolic dysfunction often co-exist, a diastolic dysfunction syndrome (DDS) is especially likely when congestive symptoms predominate over defects in systolic performance (as gauged by organ perfusion).

In all patients with DDS, the early rapid filling phase of ventricular diastole is slowed, and the extent of ventricular filling becomes more heavily influenced by terminal-phase atrial contraction. (Sudden loss of the atrial "kick" often precipitates congestive symptoms.)

The DDS can be strongly suspected when congestive symptoms develop despite normal systolic function in patients predisposed by coronary disease, hypertension, or hypertrophic cardiomyopathy. Confirmation, however, requires ancillary testing by M-mode or 2-D echocardiography, Doppler ultrasound, radionuclide angiography, or contrast ventriculography. The most important factor in technique selection is local expertise. With all techniques, attention must be focused on diastole, particularly during the phase of rapid filling. Regarding treatment, calcium channel blockers (verapamil, diltiazem, nifedipine) have been demonstrated to be useful in animal studies and in humans with hypertrophic cardiomyopathy. Beta-blockers can also be helpful in selected patients, but only when significant systolic dysfunction (or asthma) does not co-exist. Predictably, inotropes (such as digitalis) do not improve diastolic function.

Afterload.   Moderate changes in afterload are usually countered by increases in contractility, preload, or HR, so that the CO of the normal heart is usually little affected. Heart size remains normal and filling pressures do not rise excessively. However, heightening afterload can profoundly depress CO once preload reserves have been exhausted. Thus, the dilated chambers of a failing heart are inherently afterload sensitive (Fig. 1.1). Cardiomegaly and mitral regurgitation are clinical signs that identify patients as potential candidates for afterload reduction if impedance to ejection is high.

A practical quantitative assessment of ventricular impedance can be made by determining pulmonary (PVR) and systemic vascular resistance (SVR). These indices, the quotients of driving pressure and cardiac output across their respective beds, are calculated as if the blood and vessels fulfilled the assumptions of Poiseuille's law (see p. 23). Because CO must be interpreted relative to body size, both indices have a wide range of normal values. Although SVR may rise to support blood pressure in compensation for a reduced CO, elevations in SVR can prove detrimental to a failing heart when the increased impedance itself compromises CO. In this latter setting, judicious reduction of arterial vessel tone may allow CO to improve, and vital organ perfusion to increase, at an acceptable blood pressure.

Chamber diameter also impacts afterload. Higher systolic fiber tension must be generated to produce a given intracavitary pressure *in a dilated chamber*, especially in fibers on the periphery. Thus, diuretics as well as vasodilators may reduce afterload as well as preload.

Apart from the length and the diameter of the vessels, the blood viscosity is an important determinant of afterload. The rheology of blood flow in the peripheral circulation is complex. As hematocrit rises, so does viscosity, so that erythrocytes tend to pass more sluggishly through tissues. Effective O_2 transport eventually reaches a maximum, the value of which depends on circulating blood volume. Individual tissues appear to have different tolerances to changes in hematocrit and different optimal values of oxygen extraction.

Contractility.   Many stimuli compete to affect the contractile state of the myocardium. Sympathetic impulses, circulating catecholamines, acid-base and electrolyte disturbances, ischemia, anoxia, and chemodepressants (drugs or toxins) may all influence ventricular performance, independent of changes in preload or afterload. Contractility is sometimes impaired after blunt cardiac trauma, or when ischemic myocardium is reperfused (e.g., after cardiopulmonary resuscitation (CPR), or after coronary occlusion). Such "stunned myocardium" may stage a complete recovery after several days of transient dysfunction.

No physical sign unambiguously reflects altered contractility. An S3 gallop, narrow pulse pressure, and poorly audible heart tones suggest impaired contractility but are difficult to quantify and are influenced by myocardial compliance, intravascular volume status, and vascular tone. Radionuclide ventriculograms and 2–D echocardiography

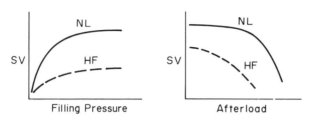

Figure 1.1 Stroke volume (SV) response of normal (NL) and failing heart (HF) to loading conditions. Impaired hearts are abnormally sensitive to afterload, but show blunted response to preload augmentation.

provide excellent non-invasive means of determining ventricular size and basal contractile properties of the LV but are not well suited to continuous monitoring.

Heart Rate

In normal resting adults the average HR is approximately 70 beats/min. Changes in HR usually involve reciprocal action of the two divisions of the autonomic nervous system. Ordinarily, parasympathetic tone predominates. When both divisions of the autonomic nervous system are blocked, the intrinsic HR of young adults has been found to average $\simeq$ 105 beats/min. The ability of a patient to cope with a demand for increased CO (increased $\dot{V}O_2$, hypoxemia, anemia) is largely determined by the ability to increase HR. Furthermore, pathological bradycardias often depress CO and O_2 delivery, especially when a diseased or failing ventricle is unable to call upon preload reserve. Because two key determinants of oxygen delivery are affected, bradycardia induced by hypoxemia profoundly depresses O_2 delivery and rapidly precipitates circulatory collapse. Marked increases in HR may also lead to circulatory depression when they cause myocardial ischemia, or when reduced diastolic filling time or loss of atrial "kick" prevent adequate ventricular preload. As a general rule, heart rates exceeding (220-age)/min reduce CO and myocardial perfusion. For example, heart rates should not exceed 150/min in a 70-year-old patient.

Peripheral Circulation

Vascular characteristics are extremely important in control of the CO—the heart cannot pump what it does not receive in venous return and may not be able to generate sufficient force to overcome massive elevations in afterload. In fact, CO may also be viewed strictly from a vascular perspective (Fig. 1.2). Under steady state conditions, venous return (VR) is proportional to the quotient of driving pressure for VR and venous resistance. The downstream pressure for VR under most circumstances is right atrial pressure (P_{RA}). The upstream pressure driving VR, the mean systemic pressure (MSP), is the average pressure existing in the vascular network. Because a much larger fraction of the circulating volume is contained in the venous side of the circulation, MSP is much closer to P_{RA} than to MAP. Were the P_{RA} to rise suddenly to equal the MSP, all blood flow would stop. Indeed, in an experimental setting, MSP can be determined by clamping the aorta and vena cava to stop flow, and opening a widebore communication between them. MSP is influenced by intravascular volume and vascular capacitance. Thus, MSP rises under conditions of hypervolemia, polycythemia, and right-sided congestive heart failure; it diminishes under conditions of abrupt vasodilation, sepsis, hemorrhage, and diuresis. Up to a certain point, lowering P_{RA} while preserving MSP improves VR. However, when P_{RA} becomes subatmospheric, the thin-walled vena cava collapses at the thoracic inlet. Effective downstream pressure for VR then becomes the pressure just upstream to the point of collapse, rather than the P_{RA}.

At any given moment, the CO selected for the organism is determined by the intersection of venous return and Starling curves. In the analysis of a depressed CO, both aspects of circulatory control must be scrutinized (see p. 30).

When positive end-expiratory pressure (PEEP) is applied, P_{RA} rises, inhibiting VR. However, MSP rises simultaneously, and compensatory vascular reflexes are called into action to reduce venous capacitance and expand circulating volume. Therefore, unlike patients with depressed vascular reflexes or hypovolemia, most healthy individuals do not experience a reduction of CO under the influence of PEEP. Although an increase in venous resistance can also reduce VR, it is uncommon for venous resistance to increase without causing an offsetting change in MSP.

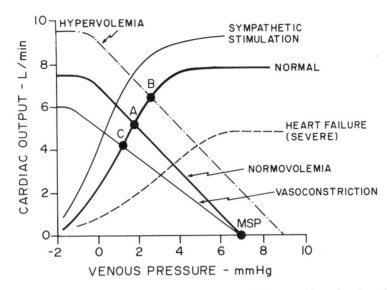

Figure 1.2. Interaction of Starling and venous return (VR) curves. With normal heart function, observed cardiac output is determined by such vascular factors as filling status (A, B), and vasoconstriction (C). Sympathetic stimulation and heart failure have opposite effects on the Starling curve and cardiac output. The mean systemic pressure driving venous return (MSP) is the hypothetical point determined by extrapolating the VR curve to the venous pressure axis. Note that VR improves as venous pressure falls—up to the point of vessel collapse.

CHARACTERISTICS OF THE DISEASED CIRCULATION

Left-Sided Congestive Failure

The term heart failure (CHF) is often loosely applied to conditions in which left heart filling pressures are increased sufficiently to cause symptoms at rest or mild exertion. However, congestive symptoms can develop when systolic cardiac function is unimpaired (volume overload, diastolic dysfunction, right ventricular encroachment, etc.) as well as during myocardial failure itself. Unlike the normal LV, which is relatively sensitive to changes in its preload and insensitive to changes in its afterload, the *failing* LV has the opposite characteristics (see Fig. 1.1). Changes in afterload can make a major difference in LV systolic performance, whereas preload manipulation usually elicits little benefit, unless it reduces afterload indirectly by shrinking chamber volume.

When faced with a patient who appears to have pulmonary venous congestion, a number of key questions should be asked in the attempt to determine its etiology.

1. **Is forward output adequate to perfuse vital tissues?**

When perfusion is severely impaired in the setting of pulmonary venous congestion, im-

mediate consideration should be given to mechanical ventilation and invasive hemodynamic monitoring. Correction of disturbances in O_2, pH, electrolytes, and loading conditions are of prime importance. If hypotension is present, temporary empirical inotropic therapy may be indicated, whereas hypertensive patients and those with an elevated SVR may benefit from vasodilators.

2. **Is there evidence of systolic dysfunction?**

If perfusion is adequate and systolic function of valves and myocardium is intact, the patient may simply be volume overloaded or manifesting the DDS (see p. 4). Echocardiography helps greatly in this assessment. Adequate perfusion does not guarantee intact systolic function—forward output may be maintained at the cost of high preloading pressures and pulmonary vascular congestion.

3. **What is the LV size?**

LV chamber dilation evident on physical examination usually indicates a chronic process—most commonly long-standing ischemic heart disease or LV diastolic overload (aortic or mitral valvular insufficiency). Therapy in such cases should be directed at optimizing afterload (with vasodilators) or at improving myocardial oxygen supply (e.g., nitrates, calcium channel blockers). The clinician should remain alert to the possibility of pericardial effusion as a cause of an enlarged heart. If LV cavity size is normal, mitral stenosis, tamponade, constrictive pericarditis, or diastolic dysfunction should be suspected. The impaired LV compliance of ischemia or DDS may severely limit CO, despite normal contractility. Likewise, LV wall hypertrophy or infiltration may limit SV and CO, despite normal contractility.

4. **Does the LV show global or regional hypokinesis?**

Regional hypokinesis/dyskinesis suggests a localized insult (e.g., coronary occlusion). Global hypokinesis in a dilated LV suggests diffuse coronary obstruction or advanced and prolonged volume overload. Diffuse hypokinesis in a heart with normal chamber size often reflects the stunned myocardium of trauma, diffuse ischemia, or toxin ingestion.

5. **Is there evidence for valvular dysfunction?**

Aortic stenosis may depress CO by causing excessive afterload or hypertrophic impairment of ventricular filling. Mitral regurgitation impairs forward output and produces congestive symptoms by allowing retrograde venting of the ejected volume. Acute chamber enlargement of whatever cause may worsen congestive symptoms by producing transient mitral regurgitation due to papillary muscle dysfunction or mitral ring dilation.

6. **Is there evidence for increased pulmonary vascular permeability?**

The tendency for pulmonary edema formation not only relates to hydrostatic forces (e.g., pulmonary venous pressure), but also to the serum oncotic pressure and pulmonary capillary permeability. Hence, pulmonary edema may form at a relatively low venous pressure if oncotic pressure is reduced or the microvascular endothelium is leaky. Conversely, the lungs may remain dry despite high left heart filling pressures when adequate lymphatic drainage has had time to develop (e.g., mitral stenosis).

The physical examination should be directed toward hypoperfusion (reduced mental status, oliguria) and compensatory vasoconstriction (reduced skin temperature, prolonged capillary filling time, etc.). Rales are often difficult to appreciate. The chest x-ray provides key information regarding heart size, vascular distribution, pulmonary infiltrates, and pleural effusions (see p. 101). Echocardiography and radionuclide ventriculography provide important information regarding chamber size, contractility, diastolic filling, valvular function, P_{RA}, pericardial volume, and filling status of the central pulmonary veins.

As a general rule, the therapy of CHF should be geared to documented pathophysiology. Whereas diuretics are helpful in most cases, inotropic agents should be reserved for documented disorders of myocardial function refractory to manipulation of filling pressure, pH, and electrolytes (see p. 34).

Systemic vasodilators should be used when an elevated SVR is documented in the setting of an adequate blood pressure. Nitrates may aid ischemia but can be detrimental in patients with borderline filling pressures. New onset atrial or ventricular arrhythmias or conduction disturbances (e.g., atrial fibrillation, atrial flutter, heart block) should be treated aggressively if they contribute to reduced forward output, see p. 37).

Hemodynamic Performance During Acute Respiratory Failure

Mechanisms of Circulatory Impairment in ARDS

Although CO may increase in the early stage of adult respiratory distress syndrome (ARDS) to compensate for hypoxemia, such compensation is often lost in advanced illness. In the latter stages, many patients with acute respiratory failure develop superimposed cardiovascular insufficiency. In such cases, the performance of one or both ventricles may deteriorate as lung disease worsens, compounding the problem of inadequate tissue O_2 delivery. Unfortunately, the cause of the cardiac dysfunction that accompanies advanced respiratory failure is incompletely understood.

One mechanism of cardiac dysfunction relates to increased pulmonary vascular resistance (PVR). Compression or obliteration of vascular channels, hypoxic vasoconstriction, and intraluminal occlusion of the vasculature impede ejection of the RV, a low pressure-high capacity pump sensitive to afterloading. The acutely afterloaded RV may also become ischemic, as increased wall tension decreases myocardial perfusion. For similar reasons, excessive chamber dilatation secondary to intravascular volume loading may actually diminish RV perfusion and performance. It is more difficult to understand why performance of the LV should also deteriorate during the evolution of ARDS. Nonetheless, pulmonary artery occlusion pressure (wedge, P_w), is often inappropriately elevated, especially in fatal cases. Reduced LV compliance may account for at least a part of this pressure change—an attractive way to link RV afterloading to apparent LV dysfunction is through the phenomenon of *ventricular interdependence* (see p. 79).

Other factors act to limit CO in the setting of ARDS. Preload may be reduced by PEEP, capillary leakage, and myocardial stiffening secondary to ischemia or catecholamine stimulation. Contractility may be impaired by hypotension, ischemia, electrolyte abnormalities, or cardiodepressant factors released from injured tissue.

Assessing Perfusion Adequacy

The assessment of perfusion adequacy in ARDS is addressed in detail elsewhere (see Respiratory Failure, Chapter 20). However, a few points deserve emphasis. Individual organs vary widely with regard to requirements for O_2, completeness of O_2 extraction, and adaptability to ischemia or hypoxia. Cerebral and cardiac tissues are especially vulnerable to anoxia. In these organs, the O_2 requirement per gram of tissue is high, and O_2 extraction is relatively complete, even under normal circumstances. Subtle changes in mental status may be the first indication of hypoxemia, but the multiplicity of potential causes renders such signs difficult to interpret. Because cutaneous arteries normally constrict when vital organ perfusion is jeopardized, cool skin often provides a valuable clue to inadequate perfusion. Unfortunately, vasopressor use and disorders of vasoregulation common to the critically ill reduce the utility of this finding. The normal kidney provides a window on the adequacy of vital organ perfusion through variation of its urine output. Although adequate urine volume suggests sufficient renal blood flow, reductions in urine volume may reflect glomerular or tubular dysfunction, rather than inadequate perfusion.

Sustained hypoperfusion precipitates metabolic acidosis. As anaerobic metabolic pathways are activated, arterial blood pH and bicarbonate concentrations decline and lactic acid levels rise. A widening anion gap provides a major clue to hypoperfusion-related acidosis. A pulmonary artery catheter may also provide valuable information. Indices derived from the O_2 contents of arterial and mixed venous blood are valuable when addressing questions of tissue O_2 supply and utilization (see p. 23). Unfortunately, adequacy of CO cannot be determined by any single calculated index. Perhaps it is judged best from a battery of indicators, including the clinical examination of perfusion-sensitive organ systems, the cardiac index, the presence or absence of anion gap acidosis, and the mixed venous oxygen saturation ($S\bar{v}O_2$).

Apart from efforts to maximize CO, tissue oxygenation and perfusion may be improved by reducing metabolic need and optimizing hemoglobin concentration and function. For example, *metabolic needs* (and perfusion requirements) may be reduced strikingly by control of sepsis and fever, elimination of agitation, and institution of mechanical assistance to reduce the work of breathing. In the setting of ARDS, therapy directed at improving CO should be guided by assessing its primary determinants—HR, preload, afterload, and contractility—in each ventricle independently. Although the general principles of CO adjustment have already been described, ARDS requires special consideration in that minor elevations of pulmonary venous pressure may flood the lung, necessitating higher levels of PEEP and supplemental O_2. Because perfusion failure may relate as much to RV dysfunction as to LV dysfunction, every attempt should be made to reduce RV afterload by correcting hypoxemia and acidosis, and by using the minimal PEEP required to fully saturate arterial blood.

Cor Pulmonale

Cor pulmonale is hypertrophy, dilatation, or failure of the RV in response to extreme afterload. By definition, this term excludes changes in RV function resulting from pulmonary venous hypertension or LV failure. Three important factors reinforce each other as causes of resting pulmonary hypertension: a *restricted capillary bed*, *alveolar hypoxia*, and *acidosis*. Although extensive obliteration of the capillary bed is the fundamental cause of pulmonary hypertension, superimposed hypoxemia or acidosis may elevate pulmonary arterial pressure (P_{PA}) dramatically. Conversely, relief of these "reversible" factors can be lifesaving.

The normal RV cannot sustain its forward output at mean pulmonary arterial pressures > 35–40 mmHg. However, when given time to hypertrophy, an RV can thicken sufficiently to generate pressures that rival those in the systemic circuit without failing. Hypertrophy of the arterial smooth muscle also occurs over time, enabling an exaggerated response to alveolar hypoxemia and other vasoconstrictors. Most acute diffuse pulmonary insults increase PVR; however, massive pulmonary embolism is the most common cause of *acute cor pulmonale* in a previously healthy patient. Conversely, *chronic cor pulmonale* can result from severe lung disease of virtually any etiology (especially those that produce chronic hypoxemia and pulmonary capillary obliteration). Acute decompensation of chronic cor pulmonale occurs frequently in patients with chronic obstructive pulmonary disease (COPD). In such patients, P_{PA} can fall dramatically with correction of bronchospasm, hypoxemia, and acidosis.

Since $\approx 1/2$ of the normal pulmonary capillary bed can be obstructed without raising resting mean P_{PA} ($\overline{P_{PA}}$) outside the normal range, pulmonary hypertension in a normoxemic person at rest signifies an important reduction in the number of patent pulmonary capillaries. P_{PA} varies markedly with CO when the capillary reserve has been exhausted. Thus, an elevation of P_{PA} does not necessarily indicate worsening of lung pathology—an elevation in P_{PA} may simply reflect increasing CO, whereas a reduction in P_{PA} may indicate a falling CO. The measurement of P_w and the computation of PVR are essential measurements in separating right from left heart disease.

The *physical findings* of acute cor pulmonale are those of pulmonary hypertension: hypoperfusion, RV gallop, a loud P2, pulsatile hepatomegaly, and systemic venous congestion. Right heart abnormalities are accentuated by inspiration as blood flow returning to the thorax increases stress on the RV. Pulmonic and tricuspid regurgitation, hepatomegaly, a palpable P_2, and a right parasternal lift usually indicate severe longstanding pulmonary hypertension. Unfortunately, many of these signs are difficult to elicit in patients with hyperinflated, or noisy lungs. Clinical suspicion can be confirmed by documenting elevations in P_{RA}, P_{PA}, PVR, and by measurement of normal or depressed CO, P_w, and $S\bar{v}O_2$.

Chest x-ray signs of pulmonary arterial hypertension include: dilated central pulmonary arteries with rapid tapering and peripheral vascular pruning. Although precise measurements are difficult, a right lower lobar artery > 18 mm diameter (on PA film) or main pulmonary arteries > 25 mm in diameter (judged on lateral) probably reflect pulmonary hypertension. Overall heart size may appear normal until disease is advanced; however, encroachment of the RV on the retrosternal airspace is an early sign.

Electrocardiographic (ECG) criteria for RV hypertrophy are insensitive and/or nonspecific. In acute cor pulmonale the changes of hypertrophy are lacking. P-pulmonale and a progressive decrease in the R/S ratio across the precordium are sensitive but non-specific signs. Conversely, the "S1, Q3, T3"

pattern, right axis deviation >110 degrees, R/S ratio in V5 or V6 <1.0, and a QR pattern in V1, are relatively specific but insensitive signs.

A radionuclide ventriculogram or 2-D ECHO may help document LV function non-invasively. In patients with true cor pulmonale, LV systolic function should be unaffected. At the present time, RV ejection fractions determined by echocardiography, radionuclide ventriculography, or thermodilution techniques are of questionable accuracy.

Management of Acute Cor Pulmonale

The key features in management are to reverse hypoxemia and acidosis and to treat the underlying illness. The majority of patients with decompensated COPD and cor pulmonale have a reversible *hypoxemic* component. Although oxygen must be administered cautiously, patients with CO_2 retention should not be denied O_2 therapy. *Acidosis* markedly accentuates the effect of hypoxemia on PVR, whereas hypercarbia has a less notable effect. *Bronchospasm*, *infection*, and *retained secretions* should be treated. If severe polycythemia exists, careful *lowering of the hematocrit to $< 55\%$* may significantly reduce RV afterload and improve myocardial perfusion.

The roles of *digitalis* and *diuretics* in acute cor pulmonale are highly questionable. Digitalis has only a small inotropic effect on RV performance unless there is unequivocal hypertrophy; however, it may be valuable for controlling atrial arrhythmias. Gentle diuresis helps to relieve symptomatic passive congestion of the lower extremities, gut, and portal circulation. Diuresis may also decrease CO, thereby lowering P_{PA}. It must be recognized, however, that the beneficial effects of diuresis are linked primarily to improved RV performance. In patients requiring very high RV preload to sustain adequate SV, vigorous diuresis or phlebotomy may have disastrous consequences.

The role of cardiotonic agents in the treatment of acute cor pulmonale is likewise uncertain. However, such inotropes as dopamine can exert important effects on LV function, boosting the perfusion pressure of the RV myocardium. Furthermore, because the ventricles share the septum and circumferential muscle fibers, it is likely that improved LV contraction benefits the RV through systolic ventricular interdependence.

Pericardial Constriction and Tamponade

The pericardium (PC), normally supports the heart and shields it from damage or infection. PC prevents acute cardiac dilatation and enhances diastolic ventricular coupling. In the ICU, three types of pericardial disease are noteworthy: *acute pericarditis*, *pericardial tamponade*, and *constrictive pericarditis*.

Acute Pericarditis

Acute pericardial inflammation can result from diverse causes (Table 1.2).

The primary complaint is chest pain eased by sitting and leaning forward and aggrevated by supine positioning, coughing, deep inspiration, or swallowing. Dyspnea and a sense of chest or abdominal pressure are frequent. On physical examination, pericarditis without effusion can be detected by a one-, two-, or three-component friction rub. The rub is often evanescent, best heard with the patient leaning forward and is easily confused with the "mediastinal crunch" of pneumomediastinum, a pleural rub, coarse ronchi, or artifact of the stethoscope moving against the skin. Early ECG changes include ST segment elevation which, unlike the pattern in acute myocardial infarction, is concave upward and usually present in all leads except V1. Initially, the T waves are upright in leads with ST segment elevation—another distinction from acute infarction. PR segment depression is also a common early occurrence in acute pericarditis. Over several days the ST segments return to baseline, and the T waves flatten. (ST segments usually normalize before T wave inversion, unlike those accompanying acute myocardial infarction.) Eventually T wave changes revert to normal, a process that may require weeks or months.

Management of uncomplicated pericarditis (without tamponade) includes careful monitoring, treatment of the underlying cause, and in selected cases judicious use of non-steroidal anti-inflammatory agents. Occasionally, pericarditis is complicated by cardiac compression (tamponade) or the development of a constrictive pericardial sac.

Table 1.2
Causes of Pericarditis

Infections	Dissecting	Malignancy
Viral	aneurysm	Trauma
TB	Dressler's	Uremia
Bacterial	syndrome	Radiation
Fungal	Anticoagulation	Drugs
Rheumatologic	Myocardial	
diseases	infarction	

Pericardial Tamponade

Although the accumulation of pericardial fluid reduces the sensation of pain and dyspnea by buffering friction between the heart and pericardium, rapid development of pericardial fluid may compress the heart, resulting in tamponade. On the chest roentgenogram, at least 250 ml of fluid must accumulate before an enlargement of the heart shadow is noted: a normal or unchanged chest film does *not* exclude the presence of a hemodynamically important effusion. On ECG, non-specific findings—reduced QRS voltage and T wave flattening—occur as fluid accumulates. In this setting *electrical alternans* suggests the presence of massive effusion and tamponade. Although echocardiographic quantification of effusion size is imprecise, it is the most rapid and widely used technique (see p. 26). In the supine patient small effusions pool posteriorly. Large pericardial effusions (> 350 ml) give rise to anterior echo-free spaces and exaggerated cardiac swinging motion. Diastolic collapse of right heart chambers suggests a critical degree of fluid accumulation.

Physiology of Pericardial Tamponade

Pericardial tamponade (PT) is a hemodynamic crisis characterized by increased intracardiac pressures, limitation of ventricular diastolic filling, and reduction of SV. Normally, intrapericardial pressure is very close to intrapleural pressure and less than both RV and LV diastolic pressures. Accumulation of sufficient fluid to exceed RA and LA pressures equalizes intrapericardial and ventricular filling pressures, reducing the diastolic volume and SV of both ventricles. Initially, reflex increases in adrenergic tone produce tachycardia and increased ejection fraction to maintain CO. Any process which causes bradycardia (e.g., hypoxemia, beta blockade) can be lethal. Tamponade alters the dynamics of systemic venous return and cardiac filling. As cardiac volume transiently decreases during ejection, pericardial pressure falls, resulting in a prominent "X descent" on the venous pressure tracing.

The usual surge of ventricular filling that occurs in early diastole is attenuated, and its representation on the venous pressure tracing, the "Y descent", is abolished. Simultaneously, pulsus paradoxus (PP) may develop. PP results from an exaggeration of normal physiology. Inspiration is normally accompanied by an increase in diastolic dimensions of the RV, and a small decrease in LV volume. These changes lower LV ejection volume during early inspiration, reducing systolic pressure. PT accentuates this normal fluctuation (< 10 mmHg) to produce PP. *Paradoxical pulse* is best detected by lowering the cuff pressure of a sphygmomanometer slowly from a point 20 mmHg above systolic pressure until the Korotkoff sounds are heard equally well in inspiration and expiration. The paradox is the difference between the pressure at which systolic sound is first heard and the point at which the systolic sound is heard uniformly throughout the respiratory cycle. Pulsus paradoxus and other manifestations of PT are critically dependent on inspiratory augmentation of systemic venous return on RV swelling and on curtailment of LV size. Paradox may be absent in PT if underlying heart disease causes marked elevation in LV diastolic pressure, so that the two ventricles are unequally compressed, or if the left ventricle fills by a mechanism independent of respiratory variation (e.g., aortic regurgitation).

Clinical Manifestations of Pericardial Tamponade

In PT, *reduced* systemic arterial pressure and *pulse volume*, *systemic venous congestion* and a *small, quiet heart* comprise a classic presentation. However, other disorders, including obstructive pulmonary disease, restrictive cardiomyopathy, RV infarction, massive pulmonary embolism, and constrictive pericarditis may present with systemic venous distention, pulsus paradoxus, and clear lungs. Hyperactivity of the adrenergic nervous system is evidenced by tachycardia and *cold, clammy extremities*. The most common physical findings are jugular venous distention and pulsus paradoxus. However, jugular venous pressure may be difficult to assess because of tachypnea.

Laboratory Evaluation

There are no features that are diagnostic of PT on chest x-ray. Similarly, the development of electrical *(QRS) alternans* on the ECG in a patient with a known pericardial effusion is highly suggestive, but not diagnostic. (Electrical alternans may also occur in constrictive pericarditis, tension pneumothorax, severe myocardial dysfunction, and after myocardial infarction.) Adjunctive studies are needed to confirm tamponade physiology. Apart from demonstrating pericardial fluid, the *echocardiogram* can provide additional clues to PT. These include reduction of the E:F slope, sudden posterior motion of the intraventricular septum during inspiration, RV *diastolic collapse*, and an exaggerated inspiratory increase and expiratory decrease in RV size. However suggestive they may

be, the findings of a single ECHO study cannot predict the presence or severity of PT.

Cardiac catheterization confirms the diagnosis, quantifies the magnitude of hemodynamic compromise, and permits detection of co-existing hemodynamic problems. Typically, catheterization demonstrates elevation of P_{RA} with characteristically prominent, systolic X descent and diminutive or absent Y descent. There is elevation and diastolic equilibration of intrapericardial, RV and LV pressures. RV diastolic pressures lack the dip and plateau configuration characteristic of a constrictive pericarditis. Because the pressure volume curve of the pericardium is steep, aspirating 50–100 ml of fluid usually leads to a striking reduction in intrapericardial pressure and dramatic improvements in systemic arterial pressure and CO. Pericardiocentesis lowers the diastolic pressures in the pericardium, RA, RV, and LV and re-establishes their normal gradients.

Management

In PT, it is essential to *maintain adequate filling pressure and heart rate*. Volume depletion (e.g., excessive diuresis), hypoxemia, beta blockade (and other causes of bradycardia), can be life-threatening. Pericardial *fluid* can be *evacuated* by one of three methods: needle pericardiocentesis, pericardiotomy via a subxyphoid window (often under local anesthesia), or pericardiectomy. During pericardiocentesis the probability of success and the safety of the procedure are directly related to the size of the pericardial effusion. Pericardiocentesis is unlikely to be helpful in the presence of a small pericardial effusion (< 200 ml in size), in the absence of a documented anterior effusion, or when clot and fibrin or loculations inhibit the free withdrawal of fluid. Pericardiocentesis is not a housestaff procedure; it should be performed whenever possible under fluoroscopic and needle-ECG guidance in the cardiac catheterization suite by an experienced cardiologist. Complications include coronary laceration, myocardial injury, and life-threatening arrhythmias.

Subxyphoid pericardiotomy (SXP) can be performed safely under local anesthesia in critically ill patients. SXP allows continuous drainage of the pericardium as well as pericardial biopsy. Regardless of drainage method, successful relief of tamponade is documented by the fall of intrapericardial pressure to normal, the reduction of elevated P_{RA}, separation between right and left heart filling pressures, augmentation of CO, and disappearance of pulsus paradoxus. After drainage the majority of patients should be observed for at least 24 hours in the intensive care unit (ICU) for evidence of recurrent tamponade. Continued elevation and equilibration of RV and LV diastolic pressures after pericardiocentesis or SXP suggest a component of pericardial constriction. Pericardiectomy may be required in patients with a component of constriction and in those with recurrent tamponade despite repeated needle drainage or SXP.

Constrictive Pericarditis

Constrictive pericarditis (CP) results from a restrictive pericardial shell that prevents adequate chamber filling. Although both CP and tamponade are characterized by elevation and equilibration of RV and LV diastolic pressures, they can be differentiated by several key hemodynamic features (see Table 1.3). Although CP does demonstrate the atrial pressure changes of PT, the *RV pressure contour* shows a prominent *dip and plateau* configuration.

CP can be mimicked by restrictive or ischemic cardiomyopathy: in both conditions RV and LV diastolic pressures are elevated, SV and CO are depressed, LV end-diastolic volume is normal or decreased, and end-diastolic filling is impaired. However, restrictive cardiomyopathy is more likely when marked RV systolic hypertension is present

and LV diastolic pressure exceeds RV diastolic pressure by > 5 mmHg. Differentiation between these two entities, however, may require an exploratory thoracotomy for confirmation.

CP should be suspected in patients with right-sided congestive symptoms. Supportive (but non-diagnostic) clinical features of CP include a history of prior cardiothoracic trauma, acute pericarditis, or mediastinal radiation. Physical examination may reveal an early diastolic sound ("knock") and mild cardiac enlargement. Whereas pulsus paradoxus is usually absent, *Kussmaul's sign* (inspiratory augmentation of the venous pulse wave) is usually present. The RV pulse tracing shows a prominent "dip and plateau" waveform whereas the venous or RA waveform shows a prominent Y descent. Common ECG findings include: low QRS voltage, generalized T wave flattening or inversion, and an atrial abnormality suggestive of P-mitrale. Because CP is a progressive disease, *surgical intervention is required*. Hemodynamic and symptomatic improvement is evident in some patients immediately after operation; however, in others improvement may be delayed for weeks or months.

SUGGESTED READINGS

1. Braunwald E (ed): *Heart Disease. A textbook of Cardiovascular Medicine*. Philadelphia, WB Saunders, pp. 409–466, 1984.
2. Braunwald E: Regulation of the circulation (parts 1 and 2). *N Engl J Med* 290:1124–1129, 1420–1425, 1974.
3. Guyton AC: Regulation of cardiac output. *N Engl J Med* 277:805–812, 1967.
4. Guyton AC, Jones CE, Coleman TG: *Circulatory physiology. Cardiac Output and Its Regulation*. Philadelphia, WB Saunders, 1973.
5. Harizi RC, Bianco JA, Alpert JS: Diastolic function of the heart in clinical cardiology. *Arch Int Med* 148:99–109, 1988.
6. Marini JJ: Hemodynamic assessment and management of patients with respiratory failure. Chapter 9. In Fallat RJ, Luce JM, (eds): *Cardiopulmonary critical care management*. New York, Churchill Livingston, 1988.
7. Ross J: Afterload mismatch and preload reserve: a conceptual framework for the analysis of ventricular function. *Prog Cardiovasc Dis* 18:255–264, 1976.
8. Wiedemann HP, Matthay RA: Acute right heart failure. *Crit Care Clinics* 1:631–662, 1985.

Table 1.3
Tamponade versus Constriction

Feature	Pericardial Tamponade	Constrictive Pericarditis
Heart Size	↑ or ↑↑	↔ to ↑↑
Kussmaul's Sign	Usually absent	Usually present
Pulsus paradoxus	Very prominent	May be absent
RV tracing	Prominent X descent	Dip and plateau
RA tracing	Negligible Y descent	Prominent Y descent
Pericardial fluid	Always present	May be present
ECG	Alternans	Low QRS T wave depression

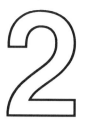

Hemodynamic Monitoring

BALLOON FLOTATION (SWAN-GANZ) CATHETER

The balloon flotation catheter allows acquisition of three types of primary data: *pulmonary artery and wedge pressure measurements*, *cardiac output* (CO) determination, and sampling of *mixed-venous blood*. This information can be used in its primary form or manipulated to provide useful indices of fluid volume status, ventricular performance, or tissue perfusion (Table 2.1).

Measurement of Pulmonary Vascular Pressures

Used in conjunction with the CO, the pulmonary arterial and balloon-occluded (''wedge'') pressures yield important diagnostic information regarding intravascular filling, the tendency for pulmonary edema formation, the status of the pulmonary vasculature, and the vigor of left ventricular contraction.

System Requirements for Accurate Pressure Measurement

Accurate recording of intravascular pressure requires error-free measurement of static pressure

Table 2.1
Hemodynamic Data Provided by the Pulmonary Artery Catheter

Direct	Derived[a]
Cardiac output	Vascular resistance
Mixed-venous oxygen	Pulmonary
saturation	Systemic
Vascular pressures	
Right atrium	Stroke-work index
Right ventricle	
Pulmonary artery	Arteriovenous O_2 content
Balloon occlusion	difference
(wedge)	

[a]Partial listing

and faithful tracking of an undulating (dynamic) waveform. Close attention must be paid to the technical details of data acquisition to avoid error.

A continuous fluid column must exist from the left atrium (LA) through the catheter to the flexible diaphragm of an electromechanical transducer. The transducer membrane deforms in response to pressure exerted by the fluid column and generates proportional electrical signals for amplification and display. Because this segment of the system is fluid filled, the vertical distance separating the LA from the top of the transducer dome exerts a hydrostatic pressure against the membrane that adds to or subtracts from the actual (left atrial) pressure (Fig. 2.1).

To eliminate the bias induced by transducer position, two approaches can be taken that are variants of the same technique. In one, the top of the transducer dome is placed at the LA level. The display is then adjusted to read zero pressure, with the dome closed to the patient and open to atmosphere. In the second approach, the transducer can be placed at any convenient level. (However, the tubing length necessary to connect the transducer and catheter may impair dynamic response characteristics, setting practical limitations on transducer placement.) The fluid line is opened to atmosphere via a stopcock held at the LA level, as before. By adjusting the display to register zero pressure under those circumstances, any difference developed between the transducer dome and the open stopcock is offset electronically, compensating for the hydrostatic pressure bias with an electrical one. With either method, the transducer level relative to the LA and the zero offset adjustment must not be changed without ''re-zeroing''.

Once the transducer is balanced (''zeroed'') at the LA level, a known pressure is applied to the transducer membrane to complete the calibration. This is easily accomplished by creating an open

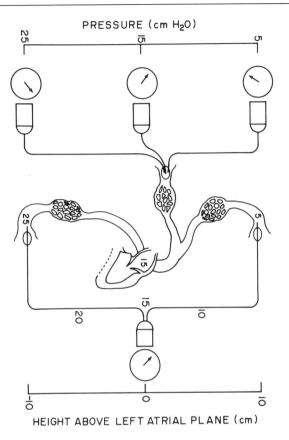

Figure 2.1 The transducer must not be moved from its original position after the display has been adjusted to record "zero" pressure, with the liquid-filled system exposed to atmospheric pressure at the left atrial level. After zeroing, a hydrostatic column develops that influences the recorded value when the transducer is lifted or lowered from its original position (left). Conversely, when the transducer remains at the "zeroed" position (right), movement of the catheter tip makes no difference, provided that a continuous column of fluid extends from the left atrium, through the catheter, to the transducer dome.

water column from the connecting tubing which links the transducer and catheter. A stopcock is closed to the patient, opened to atmosphere at the LA level, and lifted a known vertical distance. The electronics are then adjusted to display the applied pressure. Calibration can easily be accomplished before insertion by raising the distal tip of the fluid-filled catheter (on line to the zeroed transducer) a known distance above the left atrial level. Because the electronic display expresses pressure in mmHg, whereas the calibrating pressure is applied in cmH$_2$O, an appropriate conversion must be made:

$$1 \text{ mmHg} = 1.34 \text{ cmH}_2\text{O} \text{ or}$$
$$0.7 \text{ mmHg} = 1 \text{ cmH}_2\text{O}$$

Whatever the components and linkages, this newly calibrated system measures *static pressure* accurately. However, to track *dynamic pressures*

faithfully, the liquid-filled portions of the system must have appropriate frequency-response characteristics. These properties are the natural *resonant frequency* (NRF) of the system and its degree of *damping*. Without an appropriate frequency response, the system may exaggerate or attenuate components of complex pressure waveforms. An improperly tuned system often generates erroneous systolic and diastolic pressure values, and may not allow differentiation between distorted pulmonary artery and wedge pressure tracings. Air bubbles, loose or damaged fittings, inefficient coupling of disposable transducer domes to the sensing membrane, and excessively lengthy or compliant connecting tubing reduce the NRF, blunting the system's ability to respond. Damping is produced by air bubbles, multiple stopcocks, clot or protein debris within the catheter, impingement of the catheter tip against a vessel wall, and long, narrow, or kinked tubing. Partially occluded catheters connected to "continuous flush" devices can give rise to *falsely elevated* mean pressures as well. A simple check for adequate frequency response can be conducted using the rapid flush device of the catheter system (Fig. 2.2).

When this mechanism is actuated, a sustained pulse of high pressure is temporarily applied to the transducer membrane. Upon sudden closure of the flush stream, an abrupt change of pressure occurs. The tracing from a responsive system should overshoot and briefly oscillate before recovering a crisp, PA waveform. A poorly tuned system fails to overshoot or oscillate and recovers to a damped configuration after a noticeable delay.

Strip-chart records of pulmonary vascular pressure should be examined frequently, particularly when serious diagnostic or therapeutic questions arise. Influenced by fluctuations of intrathoracic pressure, electronically processed digital displays of "systolic, diastolic, and mean" pressures may be highly misleading, particularly during forceful or chaotic breathing. The strip-chart record allows the clinician to adjust for the influence of the respiratory cycle. The simultaneous recording of pulmonary wedge pressure (P_w), together with airway or (preferably) esophageal pressure, greatly facilitates interpretation.

Types of Pressure Measurement

Pulmonary Artery Pressure

The right ventricle (RV) develops the pulmonary arterial pressure (P_{PA}) in forcing the cardiac output through the pulmonary vascular network against resistance. Because the difference between mean arterial and venous pressures drives flow, P_{PA} can be made to rise by increasing either the downstream venous pressure (as in left ventricular (LV) failure) or flow resistance (as in primary lung diseases). With its large capillary reserve, the normal pulmonary vascular bed offers little resistance to runoff. Consequently, pulmonary artery diastolic pressure, (P_{PAD}) seldom exceeds LA pressure by more than a few mmHg, even when flow is increased. Obliteration of pulmonary vascular channels, however, increases resistance, obligating a larger gradient of pressure. Under these conditions P_{PAD} may greatly exceed the pressure within pulmonary veins and LA. Just as important, the lack of recruitable vasculature removes the reserve which normally buffers P_{PA} against fluctuations in CO. Thus, major variations in P_{PA} often attend changes in output or vascular tone, making P_{PAD} an unreliable index of LV filling pressure in serious lung disorders.

The pulmonary vascular network is designed to accept large (5–10 fold) variations in CO without building sufficient pressure across the delicate endothelial membrane to cause interstitial fluid accumulation and alveolar flooding. The RV normally develops only enough power to pump against modest impedance. As a rule, the normal RV cannot sustain acute loading to mean systolic pressures > 35 mmHg without decompensating. Over long periods, however, as during a protracted course of adult respiratory distress syndrome (ARDS), the RV strengthens and P_{PA} builds. Given adequate time to adapt to increased afterload, systemic levels of arterial pressure can be sustained.

Once the pulmonary vascular reserve is exhausted, additional obliteration or narrowing by embolism, hypoxia, acidosis, or infusion of va-

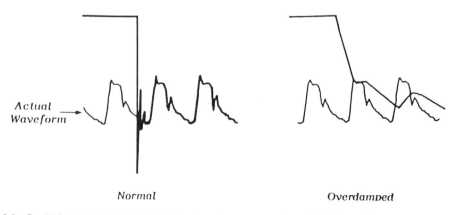

Actual Waveform →

Normal   *Overdamped*

Figure 2.2   Rapid flush test for determining the dynamic response of a catheter-transducer system.

soactive drugs may evoke a marked pressor response. Such elevations of hydrostatic pressure may
cause fluid leakage, even across precapillary vessels. It is certainly possible, therefore, that hydrostatic pulmonary edema can form even when LA
and pulmonary venous pressures (P_v) remain within
the normal range, especially if serum oncotic pressure is low.

Wedge Pressure

Balloon inflation encourages migration of the
catheter tip from a main pulmonary artery into a
smaller-caliber vessel where it impacts and wedges.
With the distal catheter orifice isolated from P_{PA},
fluid motion stops along the microvascular channels served by the occluded artery (Fig. 2.3).

Because no resistive pressure drop occurs along
this newly created static column, the pressure at
the catheter tip equilibrates with that existing at
the downstream junction of flowing and nonflow-
ing venous blood (the "j" point). It is believed
that this junction normally occurs in a vessel of
similar size to that of the occluded artery—that is,
in a large vein. P_w therefore provides a *low- range*
estimate of the mean hydrostatic pressure within
the more proximal fluid-exchanging vessels. (When
resistance in the small veins is high, P_w may not
accurately reflect the true tendency for edema formation.)

It should be noted that the validity of the P_w
measurement rests on the assumption that the oc-

clusion of a major vessel by the balloon does not
interfere with blood flow through the lungs. It has
been convincingly shown, however, that this is not
always a good assumption when the pulmonary
vascular reserve is limited—as after pneumonectomy. In these circumstances balloon inflation can
detrimentally afterload the right ventricle, reducing pulmonary blood flow and P_w during its measurement.

Because *large* pulmonary veins are inherently
low-resistance vessels, P_w normally varies little
from P_{LA}. Mean P_{LA}, in turn, closely approximates
left ventricular end-diastolic pressure (P_{LVED}) in
the absence of mitral valvular obstruction or incompetence, or markedly reduced ventricular compliance. Since P_{LVED} is the intravascular force
component determining preload, P_w not only provides a low-range estimate of the hydrostatic pressure in the pulmonary venous circuit, but also gives
an indication of presystolic LV fiber stretch. Unfortunately, a number of technical and physiologic
factors encourage errors of data acquisition as well
as misinterpretation of the recorded value.

Obtaining a Valid Wedge Pressure. The validity of P_w as a measure of pulmonary venous
pressure depends on the existence of open vascular
channels connecting the LA with the transducer.
However, flaccid capillaries exposed to alveolar
pressure separate the catheter tip from the downstream j point. Because of the collapsible nature
of the these vessels, the inter-relation between alveolar gas and fluid pressures governs the patency
of vascular pathways.

Conceptually, the upright lung can be divided
into three zones, viewing the pulmonary vascular
network as a variable (Starling) resistor vulnerable
to external compression by alveolar gas pressure
(Fig. 2.4). These zones extend vertically, because
regional vascular pressures are modulated by gravity, unlike the uniform gas pressure shared among
the alveoli. In zone 1, near the apex of the upright
lung, alveolar pressure exceeds both P_{PA} and P_v,
flattens alveolar capillaries, and stops flow. In zone
2 alveolar pressure is intermediate between P_{PA}
and P_V, so that flow in this region is limited by
the arterial-alveolar pressure gradient. In zone 3,
near the lung base, alveolar pressure is less than
either vein or artery pressures and does not influence flow.

Inflation of the catheter balloon isolates downstream alveoli from P_{PA}. To sense pressure at the
j point, the catheter tip must communicate with
the pulmonary veins via a channel whose vascular
pressure exceeds alveolar pressure. Intuitively, it

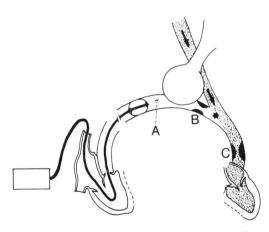

Figure 2.3 Definition of the wedge pressure (P_w). The
P_w, measured at point A, is nearly identical to the pressure at the junction of static and flowing venous blood
(*). P_w will not be influenced by partial occlusions of
the static column (B). However, obstructions (C) downstream of the junction point dissipate pressure, causing
P_w to significantly exceed the mean P_{LA}.

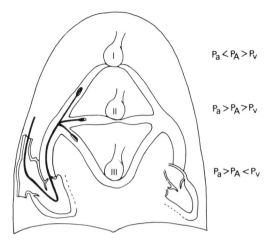

$P_a < P_A > P_v$

$P_a > P_A > P_v$

$P_a > P_A < P_v$

Figure 2.4   Ascending vertically in the lung, pulmonary arterial (P_a) and pulmonary venous (P_v) pressures decline relative to alveolar pressure (P_A), which remains uniform throughout. In both zones 1 and 2, P_A exceeds P_v during balloon occlusion, collapsing alveolar vessels. P_w is a valid measure of pulmonary venous pressure only when a continuous fluid column connects the catheter tip with the left atrium (e.g., zone 3).

would seem that only in zone 3, could patent vascular channels remain open to connect the catheter lumen and the LA. Outside zone 3, alveolar pressure would exceed P_v, collapsing the affected capillaries and forcing P_w to track alveolar, rather than P_{LA}. Although by and large true, it is now clear that this simple schema does not always apply, for several reasons. If a portion of the capillary bed in communication with the catheter tip extends below the LA reference level, the hydrostatic column extending down to those vessels will raise their intraluminal pressure (P_v) sufficiently to maintain a patent channel, even when the tip of the catheter lies in "Zone 2". Alveolar pressure will not collapse these lowermost vessels until it exceeds P_{LA} plus this hydrostatic pressure (often 5–10 cmH$_2$O). Thus "zoning" is not usually a problem with PEEP up to 10 cmH$_2$O, and it seldom occurs so long as the catheter tip lies at or below the level of the LA—its usual position. Furthermore, recent animal experiments indicate that densely infiltrated or flooded alveoli may protect the patency of vascular channels, despite an unfavorable relation between pulmonary venous pressure and the pressure within gas-filled alveoli. (When a problem with a zoning artifact does arise, lateral decubitus positioning may place the catheter tip in a dependent position and convert the wedged region from zone 2 to zone 3.)

During spontaneous breathing in the supine position, the great majority of lung vessels normally are in zone 3 throughout the respiratory cycle. The extent of zones 1 and 2 will increase when alveolar pressure rises relative to P_v, as during hypovolemia or mechanical ventilation. Because PEEP both augments alveolar pressure and reduces venous return, its application tends to diminish the zone 3 region. Catheter tip positioning in a vertical plane higher than the LA further increases the likelihood of zoning artifact. A catheter wedged outside zone 3 will show marked respiratory variation and an unnaturally smooth waveform. Although a marked rise in P_w during the respiratory cycle suggests zone 3 positioning, a valid P_w may still be restored at end exhalation. However, a *change in $P_w > \frac{1}{2}$ of an applied change in PEEP strongly suggests that end expiratory P_w reflects alveolar not LA pressure.*

Checklist for Verifying Position of Pulmonary Artery Catheter

	Zone 3	Zone 1 or 2
Respiratory variation of P_w	$< \frac{1}{2} \Delta P_{alv}$	$> \frac{1}{2} \Delta P_{alv}$
P_w contour	Cardiac ripple	Unnaturally smooth
Catheter tip location	LA level or below	Above LA level
PEEP trial	$\Delta P_w < \frac{1}{2} \Delta$ PEEP	$\Delta P_w > \frac{1}{2} \Delta$ PEEP
P_{PAD} versus P_w	$P_{PAD} > P_w$	$P_{PAD} < P_w$

Even when the catheter tip is positioned appropriately, asymmetrical balloon inflation or rotation of the catheter axis can artifactually elevate P_w ("over-wedging") by isolating the catheter tip from the vascular lumen. When this occurs, the blind pocket of fluid bounded by the balloon and vascular wall continues to receive inflow from the continuous flush system, forcing the recorded pressure baseline to rise. The overwedged P_w eventually exceeds $P_{\overline{PA}}$, an event without logical physiologic interpretation. (Such a pressure gradient situation would imply flow reversal.) Under these circumstances, the balloon should be deflated and the catheter gently flushed, and repositioned, if necessary.

Wedge Pressure as a Measure of Hydrostatic Filtration Pressure.   The pressure within the large pulmonary veins, the presumed j point, has long been regarded as a good reflection of the mean pressure within the fluid filtering vessels. Until recently, it was commonly believed that the small capillaries were the only vessels to conduct significant fluid exchange with the interstitium, and that very little pressure drop occurred beyond the capillary level. However, both assumptions now appear questionable; extra-alveolar vessels almost certainly participate actively in fluid exchange. Furthermore, as much as 40% of the pulmonary vascular resistance may reside within the capillaries and small veins. It is therefore *likely* that P_w may seriously underestimate the mean filtration pressure under certain conditions. Such discrepancies may help to account for hydrostatic edema occurring in the face of normal wedge pressure and presumably intact endothelium.

Furthermore, the j point may sometimes occur in a small vein (for example, when the underinflated catheter tip wedges within a small pulmonary artery). Under these circumstances, considerable resistance may be interposed between the j point and the LA, leading to a discrepancy between these two pressures. A $P_w - P_{LA}$ discrepancy may develop in the setting of endotoxemia or sepsis, and with conditions known to be associated with constriction of the small veins.

When P_w is used to estimate the hydrostatic contribution to edema formation, four additional factors should be considered: *chronicity of the pathologic process, extravascular pressure, plasma oncotic pressure*, and *endothelial permeability*. Over time, compensatory mechanisms for evacuation of interstitial fluid (e.g., improved lymphatic drainage) may allow high pulmonary venous pressures to exist without frank edema formation. Thus P_w can be chronically elevated in mitral valvular disease in the face of a clear chest x-ray.

Extramural pressure undoubtedly varies along the length of the filtering segment. For example, recruited capillaries are imbedded within the alveoli, whereas derecruited capillaries and larger filtering vessels may be surrounded by lower pressures closer to the pleural value. The hydrostatic gradient across the fluid exchanging vessels is the difference between intravascular pressure (estimated by P_w) and extravascular pressure. Therefore, pulmonary edema can form at a normal P_w if the interstitial pressure is sufficiently reduced by markedly negative pleural pressures (for example, during acute re-expansion edema, asthma or strangulation). Conversely, edema may not form with high interstitial pressures (PEEP, Auto-PEEP), despite marked elevation of P_w. Therefore, it is wise to interpret P_w in light of possible alterations of intrathoracic pressure. Although no precise correction can be made, one rational method is to approximate the change in interstitial pressure as

the change in pleural pressure, measured or estimated at the same point in the respiratory cycle.

Although an important role for *plasma oncotic pressure* is predicted by the Starling equation describing lung water dynamics, reduced plasma oncotic pressure alone rarely, if ever, is sufficient to cause edema. However, when the ratio of plasma/interstitial protein concentration falls, pulmonary edema may form at a lower transvascular pressure. Gross edema formation is unusual when the serum colloid osmotic pressure exceeds P_w by ≥ 4 mmHg, but is increasingly likely at lower values. Capillary oncotic pressure is reduced by the hypoproteinemia of cirrhosis, malnutrition, nephrosis, or excessive crystalloid administration.

Endothelial permeability is a major factor governing the influence of P_w on lung water accumulation. Unlike the curve relating P_w to edema formation when permeability is normal, the steep relationship between these variables exhibits no distinct point of inflection when permeability is increased. Thus, there does not appear to be a "safe range" of P_w values over which edema can be completely avoided; small changes in P_w greatly influence the tendency for alveolar flooding.

Wedge Pressure as a Measure of Left Ventricular Preload.   When afterload and contractility are held constant, end-diastolic muscle fiber length (preload) determines stroke volume. Over brief periods, fiber length parallels ventricular volume, and volume, in turn, is a function of myocardial distensibility (compliance) and the net pressure stretching the ventricle. The intracavitary pressure at end-diastole (P_{LVED}) pushes the ventricle from within, and is helped or hindered by the extramural pressure surrounding the heart ($\simeq$ pleural pressure). Mean left atrial pressure ($P_{\overline{LA}}$) closely approximates P_{LVED}, except at high filling pressures ($P_{LVED} > 20$ mmHg) or in the presence of mitral valve obstruction. In this upper range, atrial systole may boost P_{LVED} significantly above $P_{\overline{LA}}$. As a close estimate of $P_{\overline{LA}}$, P_w is used clinically to judge the intracavitary filling pressure of the LV and thereby to monitor preload.

Even when P_w accurately estimates P_{LVED}, intracavitary pressure is but one determinant of preload. Just as extravascular pressure must be considered when judging the hydrostatic tendency for fluid filtration, *transmural pressure* ($P_{LVED} - P_{pl}$) is the effective force distending the heart. Of equal importance, the fiber length achieved by any specific transmural pressure depends on *ventricular compliance*.

P_{pl} varies continuously throughout the respiratory cycle. Although P_{pl} is seldom measured directly, changes in P_{pl} can be measured easily and noninvasively with an esophageal balloon. (A catheter which combines the functions of a nasogastric tube and an esophageal balloon is now available.) Referencing P_w to esophageal pressure (P_{es}) provides a good approximation of LV transmural pressure under most conditions, independent of P_{pl} fluctuation. When used without a P_{es} reference, however, P_w must be interpreted cautiously, with attention directed toward the fluctuations in P_{pl} which influence its transmural value.

Compensation for Elevated Pleural Pressure

Positive End-Expiratory Pressure (PEEP)
Regardless of the mode of chest inflation, end-exhalation often provides a readily identified, convenient reference point for P_w interpretation because P_{pl} normally returns to a resting baseline. End-expiratory P_{pl} can exceed the normal value when the expiratory musculature actively contracts, tension pneumothorax is present, or when elevated airway pressure at end-exhalation increases lung volume (PEEP, auto-PEEP). If PEEP is intentionally applied and exhalation is passive, the relationship between the compliances of the lung (C_l) and chest wall (C_{cw}) determine the resulting elevation in pleural pressure:

$$\Delta P_{pl} = PEEP \times C_l/(C_l + C_{cw})$$

When the normal lung deflates passively, end-expiratory P_{pl} increases by $\simeq \frac{1}{2}$ of the applied PEEP because C_l and C_{cw} are similar over the tidal volume range. Under conditions of reduced lung compliance (e.g., ARDS), however, the "transmitted" fraction may be one quarter of the PEEP value or less. Thus, if a PEEP of 14 cmH$_2$0 (10 mmHg) is applied to the airways of a patient with ARDS, P_{pl} and P_w at end-exhalation should both increase by $\simeq$ 2.5 mmHg. These simple rules of thumb cannot be applied, however, during active expiratory efforts. Some clinicians seek to avoid confusion by transiently discontinuing PEEP and measuring P_w under conditions of ambient end-expiratory pressure. Because venous return usually increases when PEEP is interrupted, a low P_w measured *off* PEEP should indicate that intravascular filling pressures *on* PEEP are not excessive. Nonetheless, hemodynamic conditions often change rapidly and unpredictably after PEEP discontinuation, and a P_w in the middle or high range is of questionable value.

Auto-PEEP (Intrinsic PEEP). A ventilator discontinuation strategy cannot be applied when alveolar pressure remains unintentionally positive at end-exhalation. When a positive pressure ventilator powers inflation and insufficient time is allowed between ventilatory cycles for the chest to deflate to its relaxed volume, flow continues past critically narrowed airways throughout exhalation, resulting in an occult "auto-PEEP" (intrinsic PEEP) effect at the alveolar level. This phenomenon is most likely to occur in patients with airflow obstruction who require high minute volumes. Compliant lungs allow transmission of an unusually high percentage of alveolar pressure to the pleural space, producing large fractional increases in P_{pl} and P_w (often half or more of the auto-PEEP value). Unless accounted for, auto-PEEP encourages overestimation of intravascular volume and inappropriate therapy. Although unmeasured during normal ventilator operation, the auto-PEEP level is detectable by the simple bedside maneuver of expiratory port occlusion at the end of passive exhalation (Fig. 2.5).

Active Exhalation. Active exhalation and chaotic breathing present another difficult problem. Vigorous expiratory muscle contraction often elevates end-expiratory P_{pl} during acute respiratory distress. Large respiratory fluctuations of P_w (> 10 mmHg) should alert the clinician to this possibility. When the respiratory variation of P_w exceeds 10 mmHg, the end-expiratory P_w exceeds the post-paralysis value in direct (almost 1 for 1) proportion to the respiratory variation observed. The effect of vigorous breathing can be overcome by simultaneously recording P_{es} or by giving short-acting muscle relaxants during the measurement.

Even when transmural P_w can be computed with certainty, effective preload is difficult to estimate without knowledge of the myocardial pressure-volume relationship. Unfortunately, ventricular compliance is rarely known with precision and can change abruptly. The LV and RV are made interdependent by sharing muscle fibers, the septum, and the pericardial sac. Thus, the LV can functionally stiffen when the RV distends in response to changes in pulmonary vascular resistance or volume loading. Ischemia, inotropic drugs, and circulating catecholamines can also produce abrupt but reversible reductions in diastolic compliance. Shrinkage of RV chamber size, relief of ischemia, removal of adrenergic stimulation and administration of nitroglycerin or nitroprusside produce the opposite (relaxing) effects.

The Fluid Challenge. Uncertainty concerning LV compliance may be a major reason why absolute P_w values do not track LV volume or

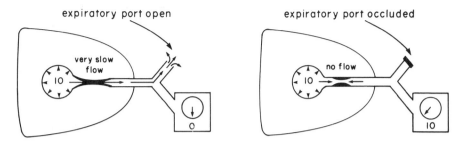

Figure 2.5 The auto-PEEP effect and its measurement. In the presence of severe airflow obstruction and high ventilation requirements, alveolar pressure at end-exhalation remains elevated as flow continues throughout expiration, driven by the recoil pressure of hyperexpanded lung (left). Transiently stopping flow *at end-exhalation* allows equilibration of pressure throughout the circuit. Occult alveolar pressure is then detectable on the ventilator manometer.

preload accurately in the setting of critical illness. Except when the calculated transmural P_w is very high or very low, decisions regarding fluid therapy of a patient in oxygenation or perfusion crisis are often best made by an empirical trial of rapid volume loading (a fluid challenge). P_w, systemic blood pressure, CO, heart rate, and the physical examination are monitored before and after a rapid infusion of fluid, preferably isotonic saline or colloid. A fluid bolus (50–200 ml) is administered over 5–20 minutes, depending on the suspected fragility of the patient. If hemodynamic variables improve with little change in the measured P_w, additional volume administration is prudent. Conversely, a marked increase in heart rate or P_w (> 5 to 7 mmHg), together with marginal improvement in blood pressure and CO, indicates that increasing the rate of volume infusion risks pulmonary edema with little benefit.

Cardiac Output Determination

Principle of the Measurement

The second primary function of the pulmonary artery (PA) catheter is to facilitate measurement of CO. Although all PA catheters can provide a sample of mixed venous blood for use in an oxygen-Fick determination, thermodilution capability allows more convenient and precise measurement. A sensitive, rapidly responding thermistor bonded to the catheter tip continuously senses temperature, altering resistance in response to thermal changes within PA blood. As a side benefit, the thermistor provides a highly reliable, continuous readout of core body temperature. When a bolus of cold fluid enters the right atrium (RA), it mixes with warm venous blood returning from the periphery. The churning action of the right

ventricle (RV) homogenizes the two fluids, and the thermistor records the dynamic thermal curve generated when the mixture washes past the proximal PA. The technique uses thermal deficit, or "cold", as a marker. The relation linking output to temperature is the Stewart-Hamilton formula:

$$\dot{Q} = V (T_B - T_I) K_1 K_2 / \int \Delta T_B (t) dt$$

where $\dot{Q}$ = cardiac output; V = injected volume; T_B = blood temperature; T_I = injectate temperature; $\Delta T_B(t)dt$ = change in blood temperature as a function of time; and K_1 and K_2 are computational constants. The components of the numerator are all known constants (V, K_1, K_2) or measured values (T_B, T_I). The denominator is the area beneath the time-temperature curve, derived by computer integration of the thermistor signal. When close attention is paid to the method of data acquisition, thermodilution CO values compare favorably with those obtained by the Fick method and by dye dilution.

Technical Considerations and Potential Errors

Thermistor Position—To generate a valid estimate of output, the thermistor should sample a well-mixed cold charge of known strength and must be positioned freely within the lumen of the central PA. Impaction against a vessel wall tends to insulate the thermistor from the cool stream, falsely elevating the reported values. A P_{PA} waveform that appears damped or wedged may indicate malpositioning and potential problems. It is good clinical practice to inspect the temperature-time profile periodically, especially when a question of temperature accuracy exists. A valid curve shows a rapid early descent to a trough value, smoothly returning to baseline within 10 to 15 seconds of injection.

Distorted curves should alert the clinician to inadequate blending of injectate with blood, thermistor contact with the wall of the vessel, abnormal respiratory patterns, and arrhythmias or abrupt changes in heart rate. Information from irregular curves should be discarded.

Injectate Volume and Temperature—Icing the injectate accentuates the thermal difference between marker and vehicle fluids, increasing signal strength. Although icing theoretically enhances output accuracy and reproducibility, the extreme sensitivity of the thermistor/computer systems currently available allows the use of room temperature injectates without appreciable loss of accuracy. Room temperature injectates do not require the 45-minute equilibration period necessary for cooling, maintenance of proper injectate temperature is facilitated, and errors induced by rewarming during handling are minimized. Furthermore, bradycardia and atrial arrhythmias during injection occur less commonly. Although 10-ml injectate volumes are normally used, 5-ml volumes (with computer adjustment) can be used with acceptable results when frequent measurements introduce a significant danger of volume overload. Seriously hypothermic patients, however, require the larger volume for an acceptable signal-to-background ratio. Whatever volume is chosen for injection, syringes should be filled carefully; variation in injected volume contributes significantly to measurement error. The composition of the fluid chosen for injection—saline or dextrose—does not materially influence the output calculation. When completed within 4 seconds, the speed of injection has little influence on outcome; automated, gas-powered injectors offer no convincing advantage over manual technique.

Respiratory Variation—The temperature of PA blood tends to vary throughout the respiratory cycle, particularly during mechanical ventilation. The cause of this variation is uncertain, but one likely possibility is that the composition of mixed venous blood returning from individual organs varies with respiration. Although it has been suggested that injection be timed to begin consistently at a single point in the ventilatory cycle, the need for this practice is controversial. Perhaps the best compromise is to obtain at least three injections spaced equally along the respiratory cycle, averaging the results.

Catheter-Computer Mismatch—Inadvertent mismatching of the computational coefficient to the catheter is an important and surprisingly frequent error, particularly when catheters of varied manufacture are used with the same computer. Coefficients vary widely with the volume and temperature of the injectate and the type of catheter used. Mismatching should be suspected when measured CO does not fit well with the clinical picture.

Anatomical Variation—Thermodilution values for CO are usually accurate when computational constants are correctly entered, the catheter is well positioned, and appropriate injection technique is utilized. However, such non-operator-dependent variables as intracardiac shunting, incompetence of the tricuspid valve, or thermistor malfunction due to thermal shielding by wall contact or clot may compromise validity. Errors can also result from inadvertent augmentation of the cold charge by concomitant administration of intravenous fluids at a contiguous site.

Clinical Interpretation

By combining measures of CO and ventricular filling pressure, important diagnostic information can often be obtained regarding the functional status of the heart and the vasculature. The fluid challenge is particularly helpful for this purpose. However, CO must be interpreted in relation to the mass and the metabolism of the patient. A CO of 3 l/min may suffice for the needs of a hypothermic, cachectic 40-kg patient, but the same CO may be associated with a circulatory crisis in a previously healthy 100-kg burn victim. The cardiac index (CI, cardiac output/surface area) attempts to adjust for variations in tissue mass. Body surface area (BSA) can be determined from standard nomograms or can be approximated by this regression equation:

$$BSA = 0.202 \times Wt^{0.425} \times Ht^{0.725}$$

where BSA is expressed in square meters, weight (wt) in kilograms, and height (ht) in meters. Used alone, however, even the CI is of limited help in assessing perfusion adequacy. Over a broad range, any given value for CI may be associated with luxuriant, barely adequate, or suboptimal tissue O_2 transport, depending on hemoglobin concentration, metabolic requirements, and blood flow distribution. Measures of urine output and metabolic acid production together with indices of tissue O_2 utilization provide better guides of perfusion adequacy.

Indices of Vascular Resistance

The CO measurement can be used in conjunction with pulmonary and systemic pressure measurements to compute the parameters of vascular resistance needed to gauge ventricular afterload. These indices of vascular resistance, not mean blood pressure *per se*, should guide vasodilator and vasopressor therapy (see p. 34). Pulmonary vascular resistance (PVR) and systemic vascular resistance (SVR) are crude indices, calculated as if blood flow fulfilled the assumptions of Poiseuille's law for laminar flow:

$$PVR = (P_{\overline{PA}} - P_w)/CO \text{ and}$$
$$SVR = (P_{\overline{a}} - P_{RA})/CO$$

where CO = cardiac output, $P\overline{a}$ = mean systemic arterial pressure, and P_{RA} = mean right atrial pressure. Although PVR and SVR are commonly computed in the clinical setting, vascular resistance calculations should preferably be made using cardiac index. The resulting values, the systemic (SVRI) and pulmonary (PVRI) indices, avoid the misleading variations of the raw parameters with body size. Significant elevations of PVRI virtually always indicate underlying lung pathology, reflecting the interplay of constrictive and occlusive forces on a compromised pulmonary capillary bed. Unfortunately, however, the complex relation between PVR and CO often confounds physiologic interpretation. Changes in the PVRI should be evaluated with full awareness that the PVRI is output dependent. SVRI, on the other hand, may rise homeostatically to high values in support of a failing output. However, excessive elevations in SVRI can be detrimental to the performance of the weakened ventricle. The SVRI generally serves well in following compensatory and pharmacologic responses of the stressed, critically ill patient.

CO data find one of their most useful applications in the management of disordered gas exchange. Because tissues attempt to extract normal amounts of oxygen, the mixed-venous tension falls when O_2 delivery (the product of CO and blood O_2 content) becomes insufficient for tissue needs. If the fraction of venous blood admixed through the lung remains unchanged, *arterial* O_2 tension may fall precipitously. Thus, depressed CO values may contribute to hypoxemia, and variation in output may sometimes explain otherwise puzzling changes in arterial O_2 tension (see p. 24).

As a primary determinant of O_2 delivery, CO measurements often prove helpful during selection of the appropriate PEEP level for the patient with life-threatening hypoxemia. Depression of venous return coincident with PEEP application may nullify any beneficial effect of improved pulmonary gas exchange on tissue O_2 delivery.

Sampling Of Mixed-Venous Blood

Oxygen Supply and Demand

Analysis of mixed-venous blood provides valuable information in evaluating the oxygen supply—demand axis. Blood flow to individual organs is not precisely matched to metabolic rate, so that venous O_2 content varies widely among sites. Normally, blood from the inferior vena cava is more fully saturated than is blood from the superior vena cava. During shock states, however, the obverse occurs. Samples drawn from either of these central vessels or from the incompletely blended pool within the RA are not entirely representative of the true mixed-venous value. Blood withdrawn from the proximal pulmonary artery, however, has been blended in the right ventricle, and is therefore appropriate for analysis. Care should be taken to withdraw blood slowly, with the balloon deflated and the catheter tip positioned in a major vessel. Otherwise, contamination from the post-capillary region may artifactually increase the oxygen content.

The value of mixed-venous blood analysis can only be understood in the framework of *tissue O_2 demand-supply dynamics*. Briefly, the product of CO and arterial oxygen content defines the overall rate of O_2 delivery. Each organ receives a variable fraction of the total amount, a flow that may be luxuriant, just adequate, or insufficient to satisfy its aerobic metabolic demand. The O_2 tension ($P\overline{v}O_2$) and saturation ($S\overline{v}O_2$) of the venous effluent reflect the balance between supply and need. When flow does not rise to meet increased tissue demands for O_2, each milliliter of blood yields more of its O_2 content, and $P\overline{v}O_2$ and $S\overline{v}O_2$ fall. Conversely, when the O_2 transport/demand ratio increases, the arteriovenous oxygen difference narrows and $P\overline{v}O_2$ and $S\overline{v}O_2$ rise. However, $P\overline{v}O_2$ and $S\overline{v}O_2$ may not reflect serious perfusion deficits if arterial blood is anatomically or functionally shunted past metabolizing tissue. For example, in cirrhosis, cyanide poisoning or the early phases of septic shock, nonnutritive flow may cause $S\overline{v}O_2$ to remain misleadingly high, despite serious tissue hypoxia. Because of these distribution and utilization pitfalls, it is always wise to monitor metabolic (lactic) acid production simultaneously.

Low venous O_2 tensions, however, more reliably signal an impending perfusion crisis. Reduced flow and diminished arterial O_2 concentration (due to reductions in SaO_2 or hemoglobin) depress effective O_2 transport, encouraging lower values for $P\overline{v}O_2$ and $S\overline{v}O_2$. $S\overline{v}O_2$ has been shown to correlate with survival in acute myocardial infarction, acute respiratory failure, and shock.

As O_2 delivery is reduced from the normal level without changing tissue O_2 demand, tissues initially compensate by maintaining oxygen consumption ($\dot{V}O_2$) at the expense of a falling $S\bar{v}O_2$ (Fig. 2.6). However, beyond a certain critical value of O_2 delivery, the O_2 extraction mechanism reaches the limits of compensation, $S\bar{v}O_2$ stabilizes, and $\dot{V}O_2$ becomes delivery dependent. Once this critical value is reached, $S\bar{v}O_2$ becomes an insensitive monitor of changes in perfusion. Such delivery dependence has been demonstrated for acute lung injury both in experimental animal models and in the clinical setting. Below this critical value of O_2 delivery, anaerobic metabolism must supplement the aerobic mechanism if energy production is to be maintained. The $S\bar{v}O_2$ at which this limit occurs varies, depending on whether delivery was reduced by anemia, arterial hypoxemia, or falling CO.

Despite the importance of $P\bar{v}O_2$ as a global indicator of end-capillary tissue O_2 tension, $P\bar{v}O_2$ can vary with alterations in the affinity of hemoglobin for O_2, even when O_2 content remains stable. Therefore, direct assessment of $S\bar{v}O_2$ is the preferred index for clinical assessment of the oxygen-perfusion axis; estimation of $S\bar{v}O_2$ from $P\bar{v}O_2$, pH, and temperature is frought with error due to the steepness of the O_2 tension-saturation relation.

Traditionally, $S\bar{v}O_2$ has been determined on individual blood samples analyzed by laboratory instruments that measure SaO_2 by transmission oximetry (co-oximeter) or O_2 content by fuel cell determination. The recent application of fiberoptic reflectance oximetry to the flotation catheter has enabled continuous bedside monitoring of $S\bar{v}O_2$. Although currently available instruments appear accurate, reliable, and convenient, the range of clinical applications of the fiberoptic catheter is just now being explored. For example, O_2 saturation rises when blood is withdrawn past the wedged fiberoptic tip, facilitating the distinction between wedged and damped P_{PA} tracings. (This feature may also help to avoid tissue infarction consequent to inadvertent distal migration of the catheter.) Continuous measurement of $S\bar{v}O_2$ should also speed the process of determining the optimal PEEP level, because alterations in net tissue O_2 flux are made quickly apparent.

Changes in $S\bar{v}O_2$ have no unique interpretation and must be viewed in light of the variables which determine O_2 transport and demand—the volume and distribution of CO, hemoglobin concentration and function, arterial O_2 tension, and metabolic rate.

Although a change in $S\bar{v}O_2$ does not indicate which of the multiple factors comprising the Fick equation is responsible, integration of $S\bar{v}O_2$ with clinical observations, blood gas information, and cardiac output data often establishes an early, if presumptive, diagnosis (Fig. 2.7). For example, declining $S\bar{v}O_2$ and CO, together with unchanging PaO_2, implies hemodynamic deterioration, whereas a rising CO with a falling $S\bar{v}O_2$ is consistent with

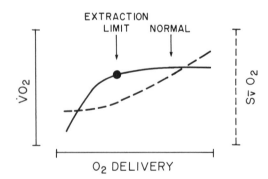

Figure 2.6 Relation of oxygen delivery to oxygen consumption ($\dot{V}O_2$) and to the saturation of mixed venous blood ($S\bar{v}O_2$). As oxygen delivery is reduced from the normal value (for example, by reducing cardiac output) while the metabolic demand remains unchanged, increased extraction can initially maintain oxygen consumption, at the cost of a falling $S\bar{v}O_2$. At some critical level of oxygen delivery the limits of extraction are reached, forcing $\dot{V}O_2$ to become delivery-dependent.

DETERMINANTS OF $S\bar{v}O_2$

$$\dot{V}O_2 = \dot{Q}(C_aO_2 - C\bar{v}O_2)$$

$$\dot{V}O_2 \propto \dot{Q}\,Hgb\,(SaO_2 - S\bar{v}O_2)$$

$$S\bar{v}O_2 \propto SaO_2 - \dot{V}O_2/\dot{Q}\,Hgb$$

Figure 2.7 Oxygen consumption ($\dot{V}O_2$) is the product of cardiac output ($\dot{Q}$) and the oxygen content difference between arterial and mixed venous blood (CaO_2-$C\bar{v}O_2$). Hemoglobin concentration (Hgb) and saturation (SaO_2, $S\bar{v}O_2$) determine blood oxygen content. Therefore, the saturation of mixed-venous blood ($S\bar{v}O_2$) is determined by four interacting variables: A decrease in $S\bar{v}O_2$ can be caused by reductions in SaO_2, $\dot{Q}$, or Hgb or by an increase in $\dot{V}O_2$. Changes in any one of these determinants can be nullified by an offsetting change in another. For example, if metabolism changes, $\dot{V}O_2$ and $\dot{Q}$ can fall or rise in proportion to one another, leaving $S\bar{v}O_2$ unchanged.

increased metabolic demand or acute blood loss. Initial experience with the fiberoptic catheter as an on-line monitor has underscored the rapidity with which $S\bar{v}O_2$ responds to transient changes in metabolism or altered O_2 delivery. Sensitivity to such changes is undoubtedly enhanced when the heart is unable to augment its output in response to stress. Then, $S\bar{v}O_2$ must reflect altered arterial oxygenation or increased O_2 demand, undampened by the buffering effect of cardiac compensation. Such wide fluctuations may help to explain why SaO_2 often varies markedly in the absence of convincing clinical improvement or deterioration. From initial clinical experience, it appears that $S\bar{v}O_2$ often falls in advance of dectectable changes in the primary hemodynamic variables, and a downward trend may serve to alert the clinician to intervene. A decline in $S\bar{v}O_2$ may be the first indication of occult bleeding, incipient pump failure, or impending cardiac arrest. Conversely, an increasing $S\bar{v}O_2$ may signal the onset of sepsis.

A growing amount of literature documents rapid and convincing changes in $S\bar{v}O_2$ accompanying drug therapy (vasopressors, vasodilators, sedatives), intravascular volume manipulation (diuresis, fluid infusion, transfusion), and ventilatory changes. Although fiberoptic oximetry appears to be an exciting adjunct to pulmonary artery catheterization, the clinical value of these instruments cannot be considered proven. Yet monitoring $S\bar{v}O_2$ has a distinct physiologic rationale and may well find a recognized place as an on-line indicator of perfusion adequacy.

Echocardiography and Radionuclide Ventriculography

Neither echocardiography (ECHO) nor radionuclide ventriculography provides continuous information and therefore cannot properly be considered true monitoring techniques. Yet, each has an important place in characterizing the *nature* of cardiac pathology in the intensive care unit (ICU). These methods allow the physician to answer specific diagnostic questions and to categorize the overall structure and performance of the heart. In a sense, they can be considered adjuncts to Swan-Ganz and arterial monitoring.

Echocardiography

Definition And Principles

ECHO provides a valuable bedside method for the non-invasive assessment of cardiac function. The ECHO probe both emits a high frequency (1–10 MHz) rapidly pulsed ultrasonic signal and re-

ceives its acoustic reflection. These data are then integrated to form an interpretable image. Three different ECHO techniques are currently in use: *M-mode*, which provides a 1– dimensional view of the heart, *real time or sector scanning* in which a 2– dimensional, dynamic view is produced, and *Doppler echocardiography*, a technique to quantify blood flow velocity and estimate intravascular pressures.

ECHO is non-invasive, inexpensive, rapidly performed, and diagnostic in a wide variety of valvular, myocardial, and pericardial disorders. Ambiguity and limited resolution are its most important limitations. Because the ultrasound signal is attenuated by fat and reflected by air-tissue boundaries, ECHO is of limited value in patients with obesity or obstructive lung disease. Chest wall deformities, dressings, and occlusive coverings prevent optimal transducer positioning. Skilled technical support and an experienced interpreter are essential for optimal results.

M-Mode Echocardiography

M-mode echocardiography provides a 1–dimensional "ice pick" view through the heart, forming images from sound reflected along the narrow axis of the beam. M-mode examines the movements of a tissue core over time. Broad structures lying perpendicular to the ECHO axis reflect the acoustic beam efficiently and are well delineated. The anterior and posterior ventricular walls, intraventricular septum, aortic root, and valve leaflets (particularly the anterior mitral valve) are seen clearly. Conversely, the pulmonic and tricuspid valves are more difficult to visualize; thickening, vegetations, or abnormal motions of the aortic and mitral valve are frequently detected, while those of the pulmonic or tricuspid valves are often missed. M-mode is perhaps the best ECHO method for determining changes in chamber dimension during various phases of the cardiac cycle. Because only a single axis or view can be obtained at any particular instant, M-mode is distinctly inferior to real time (2-D) ECHO for detecting valve or wall motion abnormalities. M-mode usually allows accurate measurements of chamber dimension, but its narrow sampling area may not be representative of the entire atrium or ventricle. Similarly, loculated pericardial effusions, pleural fluid collections contiguous to the pericardial surface, and small intraventricular defects may be missed entirely.

Two-dimensional Echocardiography

Two-dimensional (real time or 2-D) ECHO is the best technique for examining wall and valve motion. Because 2-D ECHO provides a wider field of view than M-mode, any process localized to a segment of the pericardium or myocardium is better seen (e.g., loculated pericardial fluid, small ventricular septal defects, and small left ventricular aneurysms). Superior resolution and the ability to delineate valve motion make 2-D ECHO superior to M-mode for examining right-sided cardiac valves and for detecting mitral prolapse and vegetations. 2-D ECHO is also the preferred technique for calculation of valve areas.

Doppler Echocardiography

Doppler echocardiography deduces velocity of moving blood by interpreting changes in the frequency of reflected sound waves. Either M-mode or 2-D ECHO can be used in conjunction with Doppler technology to estimate cardiac output or flow through a valvular orifice. Once valve area is determined and blood velocity is known, flow may be calculated. Thus, Doppler potentially provides a means for estimating cardiac output noninvasively. Pressures in various cardiac chambers may also be inferred from Doppler flow estimates. Finally, Doppler helps to detect the regurgitant jets of blood characteristic of valvular insufficiency.

Specific Diagnostic Problems

Investigation of *pericardial effusion* and *tamponade* is one of the most frequent uses of ECHO in the ICU. Although optimal studies may detect effusions of 25–50 ml, delineation of such small pericardial effusions can be frought with difficulty, especially when pleural effusions coexist. Normally, the epicardium and pericardium are closely apposed, with only slight separation occasionally seen in systole. Accumulated pericardial fluid separates these two structures throughout both phases of the cardiac cyle. Small amounts of fluid in the pericardial sac pool posteriorly in supine patients. Because M-mode ECHO occasionally fails to distinguish pleural from pericardial effusions, 2-D ECHO is superior for detecting small amounts of pericardial fluid. In such cases visualizing the left atrium may be revealing. (Pericardial fluid rarely accumulates behind the left atrium because of the anatomic arrangement of the pericardium.) When larger effusions accumulate, diagnosis becomes much easier, as fluid may also be seen anteriorly as well as posteriorly in the pericardial space. When pericardial effusions become very large, the heart may swing to and fro within the sac, producing artifactual wall motion and apparent abnormalities of mitral and tricuspid valve function. Apparent

mitral prolapse is perhaps the most common abnormality mimicked by pericardial effusion. The diagnosis of pericardial effusion is most commonly missed by ECHO when there is fibroadhesive pericardial disease, simultaneous pleural effusion, or massive left atrial enlargement.

The diagnosis of *tamponade* is a clinical one that cannot be made solely by ECHO criteria. Tamponade physiology may be suspected, however, when a large pericardial effusion is present, or when the right atrial or ventricular cavities show intermittent collapse. Evidence of decreased flow through the mitral valve during inspiration and relatively enlarged right ventricular dimensions are also suggestive.

ECHO may also be used in the ICU to detect intracardiac shunts in patients with refractory hypoxemia or suspected paradoxical embolism. In such cases, the contrast injected is either an echo dense dye or (more commonly) an intravenous fluid containing *micro* bubbles (e.g., agitated saline). In such testing the acoustic contrast agent is introduced by vein while the ECHO transducer probes the left heart chambers. If a right-to-left cardiac shunt is present, there is prompt appearance of acoustic noise in the left atrium or ventricle shortly after injection. (The legs are preferentially used for such injections because right atrial streaming patterns favor crossing of the contrast material into the left heart.) While this "bubble" technique has relatively high specificity for right to left shunt, it lacks the sensitivity of angiographic dye injections.

Nuclear Cardiology

Thallium and *technetium scanning* detects areas of reversible cardiac ischemia and acute myocardial infarction, respectively. (Both tests are discussed in Acute Myocardial Infarction, Chapter 17.) *Radionuclide ventriculography* (RVG) uses radio-labeled red blood cells to define the boundaries of the heart and track changes in its volume. Images may be obtained immediately after injection (single pass scanning) or, more frequently, after a period of equilibration (gated ventriculography). In gated ventriculography, multiple images are accumulated at various phases of the cardiac cycle by coupling the detector to an ECG trigger. Comparing ventricular volume (count density) during diastole and systole allows calculation of the change in ventricular volume—the ejection fraction. Ventricular size, contour, and segmental wall motion may also be assessed. Unfortunately, RVG does not visualize the atria or details of valvular anatomy. RVG proves useful in patients who demonstrate changes in ejection fraction or wall motion during ischemia; ischemic myocardium becomes dysfunctional and occasionally paradoxic in its motion. ECG-gated RVG studies require a relatively regular ventricular rhythm for computerized data collection. Therefore, patients with atrial fibrillation or frequent premature atrial or ventricular beats are poor candidates for this study. In most instances RVG must also be performed outside the ICU, necessitating patient transfer.

ARTERIAL BLOOD PRESSURE MONITORING

Normally, *mean* arterial pressure (MAP) is similar in all large arterial vessels of a supine subject; there is only a slight pressure gradient between aortic and radial vessels, for example. Posture-related hydrostatic increases of pressure are shared equally between arteries and veins, so that perfusion pressure is little affected. Although MAP is largely the same throughout the arterial tree, waveform contours differ with the caliber of the arterial vessel in question. Peak systolic pressure actually *rises* in the periphery, due to wave reflection. When a vessel is totally occluded by a monitoring catheter, wave reflection may amplify pressure fluctuations to produce sharp spikes of systolic arterial pressure (to over 300 mmHg in some cases).

Depending on the shape of the arterial pressure waveform, the peak systolic (P_S) and nadir diastolic (P_D) pressures contribute to varying degrees to MAP. At normal heart rates (60–100 beats/min)

$$MAP \simeq P_D + \frac{1}{3}(P_S - P_D).$$

(During tachycardia, P_S contributes relatively more, and during bradycardia, relatively less.) The diastolic pressure, therefore, is clearly the most important contributor to MAP. It is important to remember that flow does not equal pressure: Unlike pressure, flow is largely continuous, not pulsatile. More importantly, the ability of any specified difference between arterial and venous pressures to perfuse tissue depends directly on the resistance of the vascular bed. A MAP of 60 mmHg may produce luxuriant flow through a widely vasodilated vascular bed, whereas a MAP of 100 mmHg may be inadequate during a crisis of malignant hypertension.

Indications

The decision to initiate invasive arterial monitoring must be undertaken cautiously. Many critically ill patients can be adequately monitored by intermittent sphygmomanometry (manual or automated). Patients with *hemodynamic instability or shock*, *malignant hypertension*, or *oxygenation crises* are most likely to benefit from arterial cannulation. A well-adjusted catheter system provides accurate pressure information necessary for hemodynamic monitoring and facilitates blood sampling, often obviating the need for venapuncture.

Complications

Serious complications can arise due to local hemorrhage, infection and thrombosis. (For this reason the radial artery of the non-dominant arm should be used whenever possible.) Although common, regional thrombosis of the radial artery seldom results in tissue-damaging ischemia—digital embolization is the greater hazard. Large catheter size, low cardiac output, pre-existing arteriopathy, negative Allen test, and vasopressors increase the risk. (Artery caliber tends to parallel wrist size.) Although a positive Allen test is reassuring, it does *not* preclude the development of ischemic damage following arterial thrombosis. The Allen test is performed by raising the wrist well above the heart level and compressing the radial and ulnar arteries simultenously for 10 seconds, blanching the capillary bed. When the ulnar artery is then released, flushing should occur within seconds. A 20-gauge Teflon catheter is preferred for measurement and sampling, because it facilitates insertion, minimizes risk of thrombosis, and tends to exhibit the best dynamic frequency response characteristics. (Larger catheters occlude the vessel, creating standing waves. Smaller gauge catheters tend to kink or clot off.)

Rarely, the arterial catheter may erode the vessel wall to cause aneurysm, localized hematoma, compressive neuropathy, or arteriovenous fistula. Although local colonization is very common, frank tissue infections are rare during percutaneous cannulation when the puncture site is kept sterile, and precautions are taken during blood sampling to preserve sterility. Femoral catheters and "cutdowns" are most prone to infect.

The radial artery is not an appropriate site for injection of any drug. Intra-arterial injections of certain drugs, particularly calcium compounds and vasopressors, can cause ischemic necrosis of the hand, a functionally devastating injury. Prolonged, high pressure flushing can drive clot or gas bubbles retrograde to produce cerebral embolism.

Non-invasive Arterial Pressure Monitoring

Sphygmomanometer pressures are notoriously inaccurate when cuff width is $< \frac{2}{3}$ of arm circumference. Artifactual elevations of blood pressure (BP), occur during measurements made with an inappropriately narrow cuff and when arteriosclerosis prevents the brachial artery from collapsing under pressure. Conversely, because tight proximal occlusions can artifactually lower the blood pressure, BP should initially be checked in both arms. In many hypotensive patients with low cardiac output, the "muffle" and disappearance points of diastolic pressure cannot be detected with certainty. In shock, all Korotkoff sounds may be lost. In this setting Doppler ultrasonography may detect systolic pressures below the audible range.

Central Venous Pressure

Central venous catheters serve a wide variety of clinical purposes. Since the advent of the Swan Ganz catheter, many physicians have considered these lines primarily as secure and predictable routes for infusing drugs, nutrients and volume expanders. Yet, the central venous pressure (CVP) should not be ignored for the hemodynamic data it provides. When considered together with compliance and pleural pressure, mean CVP serves to index the preload of the right ventricle. Indeed, the CVP proves essential in diagnosing right ventricular infarction. Furthermore, the contour of the CVP tracing can indicate the tricuspid regurgitation of right ventricular overload, as well as suggest pericardial restriction and tamponade. In the absence of lung or heart disease, CVP serves well to indicate the degree of circulatory filling (e.g., during acute GI hemorrhage). CVP is an essential component of the systemic vascular resistance calculation. Fluctuations in CVP crudely reflect changes in intrapleural and pericardial pressures. In conjunction with the wedge pressure, CVP can therefore be used to estimate fluctuations in transmural filling pressure. Disproportionate elevations of CVP with respect to P_w accompany pulmonary embolism with clot or air, right ventricular infarction, or acute lung disorders (bronchospasm, aspiration, pneumothorax).

SUGGESTED READINGS

1. Cain SM: Peripheral oxygen uptake and delivery in health and disease. *Clin Chest Med* 4(2):139–148, 1983.
2. Culver BH: Hemodynamic monitoring: physiologic problems in interpretation. In Fallat RJ, Luce JM (eds): *Cardiopulmonary Critical Care Management.* New York, Churchill-Livingstone, 1988.
3. Gardner RM, Chapman RH: Trouble-shooting pressure monitoring systems: when do the numbers lie? In Fallat RJ, Luce JM (eds): *Cardiopulmonary Critical Care Management.* New York, Churchill-Livingstone, 1988.
4. Marini JJ: Hemodynamic monitoring with the pulmonary artery catheter. *Crit Care Clinics* 2(3):551–572, 1986.
5. O'Quin R, Marini JJ: Pulmonary artery occlusion pressure. Clinical physiology, measurement and interpretation. *Am Rev Respir Dis* 128:319–326, 1983.
6. Pepe PE, Marini JJ: Occult positive end-expiratory pressure in mechanically ventilated patients with airflow obstruction. The "auto-PEEP" effect. *Am Rev Respir Dis* 126:166–170, 1982.
7. Schuster DP, Seeman MD: Temporary muscle paralysis for accurate measurement of pulmonary artery occlusion pressure. *Chest* 84:593–597, 1983.
8. Sharpe M, Driedger AA, Sibbald WJ: Noninvasive clinical investigation of the cardiovascular system in the critically ill. *Crit Care Clin* 1(3):507–532, 1985.
9. Sprung Ch: *The Pulmonary Artery Catheter.* Baltimore, University Park Press, 1983.
10. Wiedemann HP, Matthay MA, Matthay RA: Cardiovascular-pulmonary monitoring in the Intensive Care Unit (Part l). *Chest* 85:537–549, 1984.

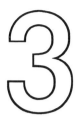

Support of the Circulation

PHYSIOLOGY OF THE FAILING CIRCULATION

Shock is a state of inadequate perfusion relative to tissue demand. Although certain physical and laboratory parameters may be suggestive, *shock is defined by dysfunction of vital organ systems*—not by such "supply side" parameters as blood pressure (BP) or cardiac output (CO), or by such "demand side" parameters as oxygen consumption ($\dot{V}O_2$). What might be considered a normal CO in a healthy patient at rest may inadequately perfuse the tissue beds of a critically ill patient. The objective of circulatory support, therefore, is to maintain vital organ perfusion, as reflected in mental status, urinary output, and systemic pH.

Organ perfusion is governed by *driving pressure* and vascular *resistance*. Ordinarily, adequate pressure is available, and vasomotor control regulates individual organ perfusion in proportion to metabolic demand. Under resting conditions, only a small percentage of all vascular channels are open. However, when pressure fails to maintain flow despite full vasodilation (e.g., during a cardiovascular crisis or hypovolemia) or when vasoregulation is defective (e.g., during sepsis), tissues are not adequately nourished and the shock syndrome begins. Once underway, *vasoactive mediators* and *myocardial depressants* are released into the circulation, perpetuating the circulatory crisis. Even with appropriate treatment, mortality exceeds 50% for septic shock and 85% for cardiogenic shock.

Normally, *stroke volume* (SV) and *heart rate* (HR) operate in unison to maintain output in proportion to metabolic need (see p. 4). Deficits in one parameter are largely compensated by adjustments in the other over a wide range. Circulatory function can, however, be compromised by abnormalities of either factor. Both extremes of HR can cause CO to fall to shock levels. During sinus rhythm the maximal sustainable physiologic HR can be estimated as ($HR_{max} = 220 -$ age). Heart rates exceeding this value are detrimental to CO and myocardial perfusion, even for normal people. When the heart is noncompliant or compromised by coronary insufficiency, CO may fall with much lower heart rates. Furthermore, the loss of atrial contraction that accompanies many tachyarrhythmias (i.e., atrial fibrillation) may cause the circulation to fail on this basis alone.

In the intensive care unit (ICU), *hypoxemia*, *enhanced vagal tone* and *advanced heart block* are three key mechanisms causing marked bradycardia. The normally compliant and contractile heart can adapt to physiologic or pathological depressions in HR via the Starling mechanism. (For example, young athletes often maintain resting heart rates $\simeq$ 40 beats/minute.) However, patients with impaired myocardial contractility or reduced effective compliance (e.g., ischemia, diastolic dysfunction, pericardial disease) may suffer marked depressions in CO and BP when heart rates fall into the low normal range ($\simeq$ 60 beats/min). This is especially true when the normally coordinated activation sequence is compromised or metabolic demands are high.

Determinants of Cardiac Output

Although attention usually focuses on the pump that energizes the circulation (the heart), the status of the vasculature is equally important (see p. 6). Thus, while the Frank-Starling relationship offers a restricted perspective on circulatory kinetics, CO can equally well be viewed as a function of the effective pressure driving blood centrally and the resistance to venous return (VR). The upstream force driving VR, the mean systemic pressure (MSP), is the equilibrium pressure that would exist throughout the vasculature if the heart abruptly stopped pumping. Because of the large capacitance of the venous bed relative to the arterial bed, MSP lies much closer in value to the central venous pressure (CVP) than to mean arterial pressure (normally $\approx$ 7–10 mmHg). MSP is influenced both by blood volume and by vascular tone. The downstream backpressure to VR is right atrial pressure (P_{RA}). If MSP fails to rise sufficiently to compensate for an increase in P_{RA}, CO falls. Indeed, the relationship between CO and P_{RA} is linear for any fixed value of MSP, and the slope of this relationship is influenced by the resistance to venous return. The tendency of the vena cava to collapse limits the extent to which effective driving pressure (MSP—P_{RA}) can be increased by reducing P_{RA} (Fig. 3.1).

The actual CO observed at any moment is defined by the intersection of Starling and VR curves. Thus, pump factors (HR, contractility) and vascular factors (intravascular volume, vessel tone) both have a major impact on circulatory performance.

Three basic mechanisms may cause or contribute to circulatory failure:

1. pump failure,
2. failure of vascular tone, and
3. hypovolemia.

Pump Failure

Cardiac output, the product of HR and SV, can be depressed by abnormalities of either factor (see Hemodynamics, Chapter 1). SV is determined by end-diastolic volume and ejection fraction. End-diastolic volume, in turn, is the product of transmural filling pressure and myocardial compliance.

Foremost among the primary depressants of contractility and ejection fraction during critical illness are: (1) *acute ischemia*; (2) *extensive myocardial necrosis*; (3) poorly characterized *humoral substances* (collectively known as ''myocardial depressant factors''); and (4) *drugs* that impair contractility (e.g., *beta-blockers*, *calcium channel blockers*, and *antiarrhythmics*, most notably type Ia drugs). Cardiogenic shock consequent to acute myocardial infarction implies a *tissue loss* exceeding 40% of myocardial mass. Its prognosis is grim, with mortality exceeding 85%.

Structural defects such as papillary muscle rupture or post-infarct ventriculoseptal defect (VSD), may compromise CO on a mechanical basis, even when there has been subcritical myocardial damage. The output of a failing heart may be greatly influenced by the impedance to ventricular ejection (afterload). Increased vascular tone may improve blood pressure at the expense of perfusion. Patients with ''tight'' aortic stenosis are especially sensitive to changes in preload and contractility.

To scale for metabolic need, the CO must be referenced to body surface area. The resulting quotient, the *cardiac index* (CI), attempts to take the mass of metabolizing tissue into account (normal

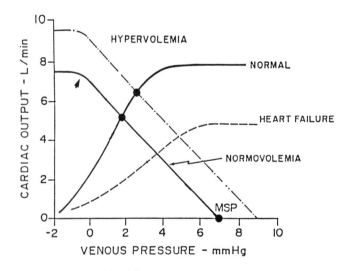

Figure 3.1 Control of cardiac output (CO). CO is determined by the intersection of Starling and venous return curves. Venous return, driven by the difference between mean systemic pressure and central venous pressure (CVP), tends to improve as CVP falls, until the point of vessel collapse (broad arrow). For the same VR curve, the failing heart reduces its output despite a higher filling pressure. CO can be restored toward normal by raising intravascular volume and MSP (hypervolemia).

> 2.5 l/min/m^2). CO adequacy can only be judged with respect to metabolic demands. Under some circumstances even a normal CI may be insufficient for vital organ support. Such "high ouput" cardiac failure can be precipitated by fever, anemia, thiamine deficiency, thyrotoxicosis, and arteriovenous shunting. Patients with extensive burns, septic shock, and cirrhosis may have vastly different CO requirements than the average resting patient.

Failure of Vascular Tone

Because organ perfusion depends on perfusion pressure and resistance to flow through the tissue bed, failure of vasomotor tone and/or distributive control may produce the shock syndrome even when the CI is maintained in the normal range. In its earliest phase, sepsis provides the prime example of maldistributive shock, characterized by reduced afterload, and normal or elevated CO and $\dot{V}O_2$, despite underperfusion of vital tissue beds. (General and spinal anesthesia, autonomic failure resulting from acute spinal cord injury, and certain drugs may also produce generalized, nonselective vasodilation that leads to underperfusion of critical organs.) Recently, endogenous peptides (endorphins) have also been demonstrated to cause vasodilatory hypotension during acute illness. In certain patients, endorphin antagonists (e.g., naloxone) may transiently increase systemic BP.

Hypovolemia

Although marked inadequacy of plasma volume is itself a primary cause of circulatory failure, *relative* deficiency is often a *contributing* cause in the setting of impaired pump function or reduced vascular tone. Primary hypovolemic shock develops during hemorrhage or when extensive extracellular volume losses result from burns, pancreatitis, vomiting, diarrhea, or long bone fractures. Right ventricular infarction and pericardial disease mimic hypovolemia because inadequate fluid is delivered to prime the left ventricle, despite systemic venous congestion.

Systemic *acidosis* aggravates the shock state by causing myocardial depression, catecholamine resistance, and potentially irreversible precapillary arteriolar dilation. *Selective* arteriolar dilation produces direct cellular injury, and massive transudation of fluid into the extracellular space. *Adrenal insufficiency* and *myxedema* are two frequently ignored endocrine problems that may contribute to circulatory failure.

Effect of Shock on Organ Systems

The closely autoregulated *central nervous system* can tolerate marked reductions in mean arterial pressure (to 50–60 mmHg) without irreversible tissue damage. However, cortical *functions* are among the first to be impaired as shock develops.

As a general rule, reductions of mean arterial pressure (MAP) are poorly tolerated by the *gastrointestinal (GI) tract*. Early in shock, the gut suffers marked reductions in flow, impairing bowel wall integrity—occasionally to the point of frank ischemic necrosis. Hepatic ischemia may elevate liver function tests, alter the metabolism of drugs, and impair removal of toxins and coagulation products. Hypotension and shock may convert uncomplicated pancreatitis into the hemorrhagic variant.

Shock often impairs the *clotting system* sufficiently to cause disseminated intravascular coagulation (DIC). The mechanism is multifactorial: vascular endothelial injury, cell death, and reduced hepatic clearance of fibrin degradation products.

In response to hypotension, the *kidneys* secrete renin to increase sodium and water retention. Intense vasoconstriction of the afferent arterioles shunts blood from the cortex to the medulla, reducing glomerular filtration to a greater degree than total renal blood flow or cardiac ouput. If profound or prolonged, underperfusion may culminate in acute tubular necrosis.

During the hyperpnea that accompanies shock, *respiratory muscles* may consume large amounts of oxygen, outstripping the heart's ability to deliver adequate flow. Ventilatory failure may result. However, even when the ventilatory mechanism remains compensated, intubation and mechanical ventilation may decrease respiratory muscle O_2 consumption, allowing for improved O_2 transport to other critical organs, including the heart, brain, and kidneys. Thus, mechanical ventilation reduces circulatory demands.

THERAPY OF THE FAILING CIRCULATION

Indications for Monitoring

Repeated examinations of mental status, urine output, and skin perfusion provide essential information to help guide the adequacy of therapy. *Although a specific blood pressure should not be the sole end-point of circulatory support, a minimal MAP of ≈ 70 mmHg is normally required to perfuse the heart and brain.* For additional information see Chapter 2, Hemodynamic Monitoring.

When hypotension produces *signs of vital organ*

dysfunction that are not rapidly reversible, arterial and ventricular filling pressures should be continuously monitored. In young patients without underlying heart or lung disease, a central venous pressure (CVP) catheter may suffice to monitor filling pressures or may be helpful until a pulmonary artery (PA) catheter is placed. However, when data are carefully obtained and analyzed, the PA catheter provides the most accurate assessment of LV filling pressures and CO (see Chapter 2). PA catheters can be helpful in both diagnosing the etiology of shock and guiding therapy. Most hypotensive patients receiving *vasopressors* other than low-dose dopamine or dobutamine should be invasively monitored. *Severe peripheral vasoconstriction* and the reduction in pulse pressure in shock states make determination of BP by standard cuff methods difficult. Consequently, blood pressure should usually be invasively monitored. Arterial catheterization allows frequent determinations of blood gases, other laboratory parameters, and *continuous* on-line assessment of BP. Because pressures within the glomerular vessels closely parallel systemic BP, urinary output is a sensitive indicator of renal perfusion. Therefore, a Foley catheter should also be placed in patients with hypotension to monitor urine output as an index of renal perfusion.

Fluid Therapy

Water comprises $\simeq 60\%$ of body weight. Of this total $\simeq\frac{2}{3}$ is intracellular and $\frac{1}{3}$ extracellular. Of the extracellular fluid $\frac{1}{4}$ is intravascular and $\frac{3}{4}$ interstitial (Fig. 3.2). *Isotonic solutions* (e.g., normal saline and Ringer's lactate) initially distribute only into the *extracellular space* while the distributive space of hypotonic or potentially hypotonic fluids approximates that of total body water. Therefore, hypotonic fluids (e.g., $\frac{1}{4}$ NS) or those subject to rapid metabolism of their osmotic components (e.g., D5W) have only transient effects on intravascular volume (i.e., $\simeq\frac{1}{12}$ of the volume of D5W remains intravascular following dextrose metabolism). Because the majority of *isotonic* crystalloid ultimately migrates to the interstitial space, edema should be expected following crystalloid resuscitation. As a result of the normal pattern of fluid partitioning, replacing a particular volume of lost plasma requires at least 4 times as much isotonic crystalloid and even larger volumes of hypotonic fluids.

When large volumes of fluid are administered, dilution of the packed cell volume (PCV) and serum protein occurs. As fluid redistributes out of the vascular space these values tend to return toward baseline. The time required for this equilibration or *"circulation dwell time"* is brief for crystalloid. Redistribution begins within minutes and is complete within hours.

Use of the Fluid Challenge

Fluid challenge is useful to assess the need for volume replacement in hypotensive patients (see p. 20). The keys to use of the fluid challenge are to: (1) use *crystalloid* as the replacement fluid; (2) use a relatively *large volume* ($\simeq 500$ ml) to maximize chances of detecting hemodynamic effect; (3) *infuse the fluid rapidly*, (< 10 minutes); and (4) *closely monitor the patient's response*. Because the majority of an isotonic fluid load diffuses into the interstitial space within hours, crystalloid infusions are a relatively "reversible" method to expand volume. *Large volumes* (at least 500 ml) of fluid are infused rapidly to minimize dissipation of their hemodynamic impact. Fluid challenge should not be performed in absentia. To safely obtain meaningful information it is critical that the physical examination, CVP, wedge pressure, CO and arterial pressure be closely monitored. A rapid or sustained increase in filling pressure following fluid infusion signals that the heart is operating on the flat portion of the Starling curve, particularly if CO or MAP fail to rise. In such patients, further fluid administration may overload the circulation causing pulmonary edema. Conversely, if the fluid infusion causes small, transient increases in filling pressure, accompanied by substantial increases in CO and MAP, further preload augmentation is likely to be beneficial.

Selection of Fluids

There is continuing controversy over the merits of colloid versus crystalloid for fluid resuscitation. The major difference between these fluids resides in the marked superiority of colloid for remaining in the vascular space. One hour after infusion, only $\simeq\frac{1}{5}$ of the volume of administered isotonic crystalloid remains intravascular. Therefore, it requires 5 times more crystalloid than colloid to replace acute blood loss, making crystalloid an inferior fluid choice for patients with *hemorrhagic* shock. Conversely, the vast majority of infused colloid remains intravascular for many hours. However, colloid is expensive, frequently costing many times as much for similar volume expansion. Furthermore, crystalloid is free of allergic risk and is more easily transported and stored.

BODY FLUID DISTRIBUTION

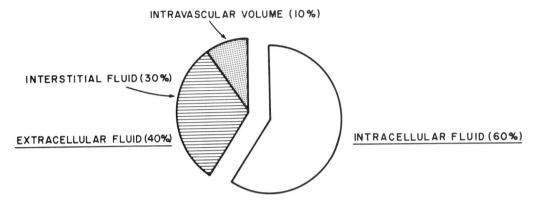

Figure 3.2 Distribution of total body fluid.

Crystalloid

Normal saline (NS) is the preferred crystalloid—except in patients with hyperchloremic acidosis, in which case NS may worsen the problem. Ringer's lactate (RL) has a slightly lower Na^+ than normal saline; therefore less volume remains intravascular. Additionally, RL contains 4 meq/l of K^+ that is undesirable in patients with renal failure, oliguria, or hyperkalemia. Although lactate in RL does *not* potentiate systemic lactic acidosis, its metabolism to bicarbonate occurs slowly in patients with shock or hepatic hypoperfusion. A 5:1 ratio of crystalloid to colloid is commonly used because it provides more effective volume resuscitation than crystalloid alone at less cost than using colloid exclusively. A crystalloid-containing regimen also helps to replete *intracellular* fluid losses. Blood is not essential for resuscitation unless there is acute *blood loss exceeding 2 units*, *marked anemia*, or *ongoing coagulopathy* (see Chapter 13).

Colloid Infusions

Albumin (the colloid to which all others are compared) is available as a 5% (isotonic) or a 25% (hypertonic) solution. Isotonic albumin contains up to 145 mEq/l of sodium. Therefore, the 25% solution may offer an advantage in edematous, volume depleted patients. The oncotic effect of 1 gram of albumin pulls $\simeq 18$ grams of H_2O into the vascular space. Contrary to popular teaching, albumin *does* leak out of the intravascular space with a circulating half life of about 16 hours. Albumin is *very expensive* and carries the risk of *allergic reaction*. Although unlikely, there is also concern that *infectious agents* may be transmitted. Albumin contains no viable coagulation factors. Albumin should not be used as a nutritional supplement in hypoalbuminemic patients (e.g., nephrotic syndrome or hepatic failure). Exogenous albumin is rapidly excreted in these conditions, negating its nutritional value and blunting its effect on volume expansion. However, albumin may be useful in such patients who develop acute bleeding and require volume resuscitation.

Fresh frozen plasma (FFP) provides another source of colloid protein. Because FFP carries significant risk of allergic reaction and hepatitis, it should not be used solely for volume expansion. However, when hypovolemia and coagulation disorders coexist, FFP may restore both functions.

Dextran is a heterogenous mixture of polysaccharides available as 40,000 or 70,000 molecular weight (MW) solutions. Clearance of small MW fractions occurs rapidly through renal filtration, whereas larger molecules are taken up and metabolized by the reticuloendothelial system. The effect of dextran on circulatory volume is relatively brief with only 20–30% remaining intravascular after 24 hours. Dextran has several potential advantages: It produces volume expansion greater than the volume infused, it promotes "microvascular" flow by coating vessel walls and decreasing red cell-vessel wall interaction, and it reduces serum viscosity.

Unfortunately, dextran has many adverse effects. Reductions in platelet adherence and degranulation may produce *bleeding* at doses > 1.5 g/kg/day. *Renal failure* may occur secondary to tubular obstruction, an effect probably preventable if low tubular flow rates are avoided. Minor *allergic reactions* are seen in ≃ 5% of patients. (Patients with previous streptococcal or salmonella infections are particularly predisposed.) Fatal *anaphylactic reactions* occur rarely. The *osmotic diuresis* following initial dextran resuscitation necessitates continued fluid replacement. Finally, dextran *interferes with several common laboratory tests*, occasionally producing false elevations in the serum glucose, bilirubin, and serum protein concentrations. Dextran also mimics antibody-induced red cell agglutination, making crossmatching of blood difficult.

Hydroxyethyl starch (HES) is a polysaccharide structurally similar to glycogen, supplied as a mixture of MW fractions from 10,000 to 1,000,000. HES expands plasma volume in direct relationship to the amount infused.

Small MW fractions of HES are cleared predominantly by the kidney while reticuloendothelial cells metabolize larger MW fractions. HES is also degraded by serum alpha amylase. Trace amounts of HES have been detected as long as 17 weeks following administration. Prolonged or massive infusions may accumulate in phagocytes, with unknown effects on immune function.

HES *prolongs the partial thromboplastin time (PTT)* modestly in most patients, but the mechanism is uncertain. HES also causes a transient *decrease in platelet count* and clot tensile strength. Very recently, intracerebral hemorrhage has been reported in patients receiving HES. Its causative role, however, remains uncertain. Clotting abnormalities may be reversed with transfusions of FFP and platelets. Of patients receiving HES, *allergic reactions* occur in < 1% of patients, and anaphylactic reactions are *extremely* rare. HES may artifactually *increase the sedimentation rate* and often *doubles serum amylase* determinations. In a minority of patients, *indirect bilirubin* may be spuriously elevated by up to 1 mg/dl. HES costs about 1/4 of what 5% albumin does but is more expensive than dextran.

Vasopressors

The goal of vasopressor therapy is to assure vital organ perfusion—not to achieve any particular blood pressure. Because vasoactive drugs are less effective in acidotic or volume-depleted patients, an adequate circulating volume and pH > 7.1 are needed for maximal pressor effect. Making an optimal choice of vasopressor requires an understanding of adrenergic receptor distribution and action. Simplistically, *alpha* effects are *vasoconstrictive* in the peripheral circulation. *Beta 1* receptor activation provides *chronotropic* and *ionotropic* stimuli. *Beta 2* effects induce *vasodilation* and *bronchodilation* (Table 3.1).

Epinephrine

Epinephrine has *balanced alpha and beta-agonist* properties and serves as the standard to which all other vasopressors are compared. Epinephrine "coarsens" ventricular fibrillation and augments arterial tone during cardiac arrest. Mean arterial pressure (MAP), systemic vascular resistance (SVR), and CO are boosted in patients with an organized rhythm. Potential side effects include palpitations, arrhythmias, and angina, due to increased myocardial oxygen consumption. In patients with hypotension due to ischemia-induced pump dysfunction, epinephrine may increase myocardial oxygen delivery to a greater degree than it increases myocardial oxygen consumption. Patients chronically taking beta-blocking drugs may paradoxically experience unopposed *alpha effects* when given a balanced alpha and beta-agonist such as epinephrine.

Norepinephrine

Norepinephrine (NE) is primarily an *alpha agonist with mild beta-1 activity*. The primary effect of NE is to vasoconstrict. Despite increases in SVR, CO usually remains stable because of mild increases in HR and contractility. However, excessive increases in afterload induced by NE may reduce CO. Perhaps NE is most useful in the early phases of septic shock in which CO is normal but SVR is reduced. Side effects include hypertension and increased myocardial oxygen consumption.

Isoproterenol

Isoproterenol (ISO) has primarily beta-1 (chronotropic and inotropic) actions but also possesses beta-2 effects of vasodilation and bronchodilation. It is most commonly used to increase HR and hence CO in the setting of marked bradycardia [e.g., 3° atrioventricular (AV) block]. Increases in CO are boosted predominately by increases in HR. MAP may actually *fall* in spite of rising CO as a result of peripheral vasodilation. ISO is also useful to increase HR and shorten the QT interval in patients

Table 3.1
Inotropic Drugs[a]

	Adrenergic Recepeptor Activation	Relative Effects in Midrange of Dosage		
		Inotropic	Chronotropic	Vasoconstrictor
Amrinone	0	+ + +	0	−
Dobutamine	$\beta_1\beta_2\alpha$	+ + +	+	− to +[b]
Dopamine	$\beta_1\Delta\alpha$	+ + +	+ +	− to + + +[b]
Epinephrine	$\beta_1\alpha\beta_2$	+ + +	+ + +	+ +
Isoproterenol	$\beta_1\beta_2$	+ + + +	+ + + +	− −
Methoxamine	α	0	0	+ + + +
Norepinephrine	$\beta_1\alpha$	+ + +	+ + +	+ + + +
Phenylephrine	$\alpha\beta_1$	+	0	+ + + +

[a]Reprinted with permission from Marini JJ: Hemodynamic assessment and management of patients with respiratory failure. In Fallat RJ, Luce JM (eds): *Cardiopulmonary Critical Care Management.* New York, Churchill-Livingstone, pp 179–214, 1988.
[b]Effect dependent on dosage range.

with arrhythmias resulting from QT prolongation (i.e., Torsades de Pointes).

Neosynephrine

Neosynephrine (NEO) is a pure alpha agonist that lacks cardiac stimulant properties. In high doses, increases in afterload may decrease CO, but such effects are less marked than with NE. NEO is useful to increase blood pressure in the treatment of supraventricular tachycardias and has become popular in combination with intravenous nitroglycerine to provide *decreased preload* and *coronary vasodilation* while *maintaining arterial blood pressure* in patients with acute cardiac ischemia.

Dopamine

Dopamine (DA) is a naturally occurring precursor of norepinephrine whose *effects vary with the dose administered.* At doses of 2–5 µg/kg/min DA has primarily beta-1 effects with mild beta-2 effects. At such doses DA independently stimulates renal dopamine receptors increasing renal blood flow, glomerular filtration rate (GFR), and promoting Na^+ excretion. At 5–10 µg/kg/min alpha effects become more prominent, and with doses > 10 µg/kg/min alpha effects predominate. In high doses, DA possesses a pharmacologic profile much like NE. *Even when using potent alpha agonists such as NE, low doses of DA help to promote diuresis.*

DA increases the potential for arrhythmias in patients receiving halogenated hydrocarbon anesthetics or monoamine oxidase (MAO) inhibitors. DA causes intense vasoconstriction and if extravasated may induce tissue necrosis, an effect antagonized by local infiltration of phentolamine.

Dobutamine

Dobutamine (DB) is an ISO analog that has *primarily beta-1 actions* but also possesses mild beta-2 activity. DB causes much less alpha stimulation than DA and less beta-2 activity than ISO. Unlike ISO, DB boosts CO primarily by increasing stroke volume, not heart rate. Because DB has only modest beta-2 activity, it is best suited to the treatment of low cardiac output states in patients with a near-normal BP. At commonly used doses, DB is less likely than ISO to produce tachycardia, but increases in heart rate of up to 15 beats per minute are common. In some patients with a very high baseline SVR, DB may induce hypotension by causing peripheral vasodilation. Rarely, DB increases AV conduction in patients with atrial fibrillation or flutter, leading to rapid heart rates.

Amrinone

Although the mechanism of action is unclear, amrinone has ionotropic properties distinct from the catecholamines or digitalis glycosides. (Its effect may be due to increased cAMP activity.) Amrinone is a positive ionotrope and vasodilator that raises CO by increasing stroke volume—not by increasing HR. Although renal excretion provides the primary route of clearance, hepatic metabolism is significant. Therefore, patients with either hepatic or renal failure may accumulate the drug. Increases in ionotropic activity may aggrevate outflow obstruction in hypertrophic cardiomyopathy. Increased ventricular rates in atrial fibrillation or flutter have been reported. Thrombocytopenia occurs in a small minority of patients. High doses of amrinone for long periods of time may elevate liver function tests and cause frank hepatic necrosis.

Mechanical Devices

Fluid and vasopressors have traditionally been the only options for support of the failing circulation, but recently several mechanical devices have been used. *Artificial hearts* and *implanted left ventricular (LV) assist devices* now provide temporary support options for patients with myocardial failure. Problems of infection, immobility, embolism and cost have limited use of implantable devices. Much more experience has accumulated with the *intra-aortic balloon pump* (IABP). This device is inserted in a retrograde fashion through the femoral artery into the descending aorta. Diastolic inflation of the large tubular aortic balloon augments diastolic pressure, hence coronary perfusion. Balloon deflation during systole lowers LV afterload, improving systemic perfusion. Peripheral arterial ischemia, stroke, coagulopathy, hemolysis, and aortic dissection constitute major hazards. IABP has proven most useful in temporary preoperative support of patients with acute valvular disorders, ventricular-septal defects, or angina refractory to medical therapy. IABP may be life-sustaining in patients awaiting cardiac transplant. In patients without correctable mechanical defects, IABP is of unproven benefit and potential risk.

SUGGESTED READINGS

1. Bregman D, Kaskel P: Advances in percutaneous intra-aortic balloon pumping. *Crit Care Clinics* 2(2):221–236, 1986.
2. Campbell S: Pharmacologic principles of cardiovascular drug administration to the critically ill. *Crit Care Clinics* 1(3):471–490, 1985.
3. Colucci WS, Wright RF, Braunwald E: New positive inotropic agents in the treatment of congestive heart failure. *N Engl J Med* 314:290–299, 349–358, 1986.
4. Forrester JS, Diamond G, Chatterjee K, Swan HJC: Medical therapy of acute myocardial infarction by application of hemodynamic subsets. Parts I and II. *N Engl J Med* 295:1356–1362, 1976.
5. Gunnan RM, Lambrew CT, Abrams W, Adolph RJ, et al: Task force IV: pharmacologic interventions. *Am J Cardiol* 50:393–408, 1982.
6. Herling IM: Intravenous nitroglycerin: clinical pharmacology and therapeutic considerations. *Am Heart J* 108:141–149, 1984.
7. Marini JJ: Hemodynamic assessment and management of patients with respiratory failure. In Fallat RJ, Luce JM (eds): *Cardiopulmonary Critical Care Management*. New York, Churchill-Livingstone, pp 179–214, 1988.
8. Scholz H: Inotropic drugs and their mechanisms of action. *J Am Coll Cardiol* 4:389–397, 1984.
9. Sibbald WJ (ed): Cardiovascular crises in the critically ill (symposium). *Crit Care Clin* 1(3):433–731, 1985.
10. Sobel BE: Cardiac and noncardiac forms of acute circulatory failure (shock). In Braunwald E (ed): *Heart Disease. A Textbook of Cardiovascular Medicine*. Philadelphia, WB Saunders, pp. 578–604, 1984.
11. Teich S, Chernow B: Specific cardiovascular drugs used in the critically ill. *Crit Care Clin* 1(3):491–505, 1985.
12. Virgilio RW, Rice CL: Crystalloid versus colloid resuscitation: is one better? A randomized clinical study. *Surgery* 85:129–139, 1979.

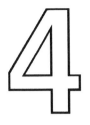

Arrhythmias and Cardioversion

COMPONENTS OF THE ECG

The first step in evaluation of the electrocardiogram (ECG) is to *identify atrial activity (P waves)*. P waves are best seen in the inferior leads (II, III, and aVF). P wave shape and pattern should be specifically examined for evidence of atrial flutter or atrial fibrillation. P wave inversion in limb lead II signifies retrograde depolarization. The atrial rate should be examined for regularity.

Once the atrial rhythm has been characterized, *ventricular activity (QRS complex)* should be examined. If the QRS is narrow, ventricular depolarization most likely occurs in response to normal sequential atrioventricular (AV) conduction. A wide QRS complex (> 0.12 sec) suggests (1) ectopic ventricular origin or (2) aberrant supraventricular conduction. The QRS should be examined for regularity and rate. The pattern of *grouped beats* may suggest a specific arrhythmia.

The *relationship between the P and QRS components* should be determined. If every P wave is not followed by a QRS complex, AV block, ventricular tachycardia, atrial flutter, or atrial fibrillation is possible. Because of the delays associated with AV nodal conduction, a QRS complex occurring <0.1 seconds after a P wave is unlikely to be related to it.

GENERAL APPROACH TO ARRHYTHMIAS

Cardiac arrhythmias are detrimental when they reduce tissue perfusion or increase myocardial oxygen demand. In making decisions regarding management, the *state of perfusion*, the *risks of treatment* versus simple observation, and a variety of *patient factors* must be considered. Tachyarrhythmias evoking hypotension or angina should be terminated immediately with cardioversion or drugs. Symptomatic bradycardia should be corrected with medications or pacing. The drug necessary for control and its potential side effects should be carefully considered. For example, young patients with frequent, isolated premature ventricular contractions (PVCs) lacking evidence of heart failure or myocardial ischemia have an excellent prognosis. In such patients drug suppression of the arrhythmia is unlikely to alter outcome but may produce untoward side effects. A past history of well-tolerated arrhythmia of a similar type suggests that acute treatment is not necessary. Conversely, patients with acute myocardial ischemia and those with a history of malignant or degenerative arrhythmias should be treated aggressively.

Arrhythmias are often provoked by drugs, electrolyte disturbances, and cardiac ischemia. Thus, hypokalemia, hypomagnesemia, acidosis, alkalosis, anemia, and hypoxemia exacerbate an arrhythmic tendency. Intracardiac catheter irritation, pacemaker dysfunction, digitalis, and theophylline provoke a wide variety of arrhythmias that reverse with their removal. Electrical stability can also be disturbed by ischemia. For example, hypotension reduces myocardial perfusion, whereas excesses of intravascular volume or ventricular afterload can increase wall tension and oxygen demand.

What to Do when Uncertain

Specific diagnosis is often difficult, especially in the setting of wide complex tachycardia (WCT). When patients are hemodynamically compromised, it is generally best to treat arrhythmias as if they were life threatening and ventricular in origin, once AV block has been ruled out. (Infranodal escape rhythms must not be terminated before treating the underlying block.) Hemodynamic status is *not* a guide to diagnosis. Patients with coronary disease and WCT should be assumed to have ventricular tachycardia. Patients with WCT in distress should receive procainamide or cardioversion, depending upon urgency. Verapamil is not a good choice for empirical therapy of WCT of uncertain origin.

Electrical *artifacts* may occur as a result of poor surface electrode contact or electromechanical devices such as aortic balloon pumps or infusion pumps. Muscle tremors, seizure activity, and Parkinson's disease may also lead to ECG artifacts that may be confused with serious arrhythmias.

Specialized electrocardiographic techniques may be of particular value in selected patients. These include esophageal, Lewis, and intracavitary recordings to detect occult atrial activity or right sided chest leads to detect right ventricular (RV) infarction.

TACHYARRHYTHMIAS

Sinus Tachycardia

Sinus tachycardia (ST) is the primary means by which cardiac output rises in response to metabolic demands; thus, ST is physiologic in the setting of *exercise, fever,* or *hyperthyroidism.* ST may also be an appropriate physiologic attempt to compensate for *hypovolemia, limited stroke volume,* or *reduced myocardial compliance.* Anxiety, pain, circulatory reflexes, and circulating drugs may also be responsible. Unless ST precipitates myocardial ischemia, it is important primarily as a clue to the underlying disorder. In the intensive care unit (ICU), ST usually signifies an important problem that requires treatment. Inappropriate ST reduces diastolic perfusion time and increases myocardial oxygen consumption. In patients with symptomatic ischemia beta blockade may prove helpful. However, beta-blockers should be used with extreme caution in the settings of hypotension, acute infarction or underlying myocardial dysfunction, because ST often reflects incipient heart failure in this setting.

Non-sinus Supraventricular Tachycardias

Re-entrant Tachycardias

Diagnosis—The nomenclature surrounding supraventricular tachycardia (SVT) is confusing. SVT usually results from a *re-entry* mechanism and less commonly from the rapid discharge of an ectopic atrial focus. The most common form is *AV nodal re-entrant tachycardia* (NRT) in which an atrial re-entry circuit involves the AV node. Less common forms of SVT include *AV re-entrant tachycardia,* in which the conducting circuit uses a bypass tract circumventing the AV node (e.g., Wolf-Parkinson-White syndrome). Rarely, intra-SA node

re-entry may occur. Although sometimes confused with atrial flutter with 2:1 conduction, NRT can usually be distinguished as a slightly irregular, narrow QRS tachycardia occurring at a rate < 200 beats/min. The inter-QRS baseline is isoelectric. Unlike atrial flutter or fibrillation which slow in response to vagal stimulation, NRT either remains unaffected or terminates abruptly. QRS complexes frequently exhibit a rate related right bundle branch block pattern that may simulate ventricular tachycardia. (P waves are often buried in the QRS complex or T wave.) When visible, P waves are frequently inverted in the inferior leads because atrial depolarization characteristically begins from a focus low in the right atrium and spreads cephalad. The diagnosis of SVT may be confirmed using esophageal or intracavitary electrodes demonstrating atrial activity. Non-sustained SVT is generally well tolerated and requires no treatment.

Treatment—Because NRT is a *re-entrant arrhythmia* that usually involves the AV node and a refractory atrial pathway, therapy is directed at disrupting the most accessible portion of the reverberating circuit, the AV node. Thus, NRT is most commonly terminated by maneuvers or drugs that increase acetylcholine concentration in the AV node, slowing conduction through this region. Conversely, AV re-entrant tachycardia is interrupted by slowing conduction through the bypass tract. *Massage of the non-dominant carotid artery* for 10–15 seconds, used alone or in conjunction with the Valsalva maneuver, often interrupts the arrhythmia. To avoid cerebral ischemia both carotid arteries should not be compressed simultaneously and vessels with bruits should not be massaged. Other vagal maneuvers (e.g., ocular compression) are potentially dangerous.

Verapamil is the drug of choice for NRT when vagal maneuvers fail. It should not be used when the chamber of origin is in doubt or in patients with systolic pressures < 100 mmHg; its vasodilating effects may cause hypotension unless rhythm conversion occurs. Doses of 2.5 to 5 mg intravenously are usually adequate. *Propranolol* in doses of 0.5 to 1.0 mg every 5 minutes (up to a 4-mg total dose) may also be effective. *Digoxin* has long been used in the treatment of NRT but often requires hours for effect, making it most useful in hemodynamically stable patients and in those requiring prophylaxis.

In boosting systemic blood pressure, *vasoconstrictive drugs* may reflexly decrease AV nodal conduction. However, vasopressors may precipitate cardiac or cerebrovascular complications in the elderly. *Type Ia antiarrhythmics* (quinidine, procainamide, and diisopyramide) exert vagolytic effects and *may worsen* arrhythmias by accelerating AV conduction. Lidocaine has no effect on SVT. In refractory SVT temporary *overdrive atrial pacing* may restore sinus rhythm. Overdrive pacing is particularly convenient when an atrial pacer or pacing Swan-Ganz catheter is already in place, as after cardiac surgery. Hemodynamically unstable SVT should be treated with low-energy synchronized cardioversion (see p. 45).

Ectopic Supraventricular Tachycardias

Multifocal Atrial Tachycardia

Diagnosis—Multifocal atrial tachycardia (MAT) most often occurs in association with obstructive lung disease or metabolic crisis, but it also complicates left ventricular failure, coronary artery disease, sepsis, and toxicity with digitalis and theophylline. MAT usually portends a poor prognosis. Because MAT (unlike SVT) is an *ectopic* tachycardia, measures to increase AV nodal refractoriness are ineffective. MAT is recognized by irregularly irregular supraventricular QRS complexes, varying PR intervals, and the presence of at least 3 morphologically distinct P waveforms. Comparable heart rates (100–180 beats/min) and beat-to-beat variation in PR and RR intervals often cause MAT to be confused with atrial fibrillation.

Treatment—Although verapamil may temporarily slow or convert MAT, the definitive treatment of MAT is to reverse hypoxemia, acidosis, and other underlying causes. Whereas theophylline and beta agonists may occasionally precipitate MAT, their cautious use after MAT onset may improve underlying bronchospasm sufficiently to reverse it. In patients who demonstrate MAT in response to theophylline or beta agonists, corticosteroids or inhaled anticholinergics represent attractive options for treating bronchospasm.

Atrial Fibrillation

Diagnosis—Atrial fibrillation (AF) is a chaotic atrial rhythm in which no single ectopic pacemaker captures the entire atrium. AF, a rhythm often seen in obstructive lung disease and hyperthyroidism, does not always signify heart disease. AF classically produces an irregularly irregular ventricular rhythm that may be confused with MAT, frequent premature atrial contractions, sinus tachycardia or atrial flutter with variable AV block. Because there is no organized atrial depolarization, there is no detectable P wave or effective atrial contraction. By preventing the normal atrial contraction that

facilitates left ventricular priming, cardiac output may fall by as much as 30% in patients with impaired ventricular distensibility.

Although the atria may depolarize 700 times per minute, the AV node usually fails to conduct impulses at rates > 180–200 beats/minute. Fever, sepsis, vagolytic drugs, and the presence of accessory conduction pathways may increase the ventricular response. On physical examination AF is suggested by a varying S1 (due to varying mitral valve position at the onset of ventricular systole) and a pulse deficit (due to occasional systoles with low ejection volumes).

Treatment is guided by ventricular response rate and hemodynamic status. Acute hemodynamic compromise mandates synchronized cardioversion (200–400 WS) to quickly terminate the arrhythmia. Ventricular rates > 200 beats/minute suggest accelerated conduction due to vagolytic drugs (e.g., type Ia antiarrhythmics) or an accelerated conduction pathway. If the *ventricular rate is < 60 beats/minute*, conduction system disease or digitalis toxicity should be suspected.

There should be no rush to correct chronic, hemodynamically stable AF. Before conversion is attempted, the *likelihood of attaining and maintaining sinus rhythm should be assessed.* When left atrial diameter exceeds 4 cm, conversion to stable sinus rhythm is unlikely. Although many clinicians advocate at least 1 attempt at restoring sinus rhythm, most patients do well if digoxin alone is used to maintain the resting ventricular response < 100 beats/minute.

The initial therapy of AF is to slow the resting ventricular rate to < 100 beats per minute with *digitalis.* (20% of patients with new onset AF treated with digoxin alone convert to normal sinus rhythm). In refractory cases, verapamil or beta blockers may be added. In chronic atrial fibrillation, *anticoagulation* should be undertaken for 2–6 weeks before attempts at rhythm conversion to minimize the risk of embolization. In patients with untreated AF and a slow ventricular response (< 80 beats/min) electrical *cardioversion,* digoxin, or verapamil may produce symptomatic bradycardia or asystole. The risk of bradycardia is sufficiently high that a temporary pacemaker should be inserted prior to attempting cardioversion in this group. *Quinidine* may chemically convert AF to sinus rhythm, but it should not be used alone because vagolysis may speed AV conduction and accelerate the ventricular rate to dangerous levels; digoxin pretreatment should first be given. This combination is effective in ≈ 40% of patients. (Procainamide is less effective.) Added to a stable dose of digoxin, quinidine may *increase serum digoxin levels by as much as 50%*. Electrocardioversion may change AF to sinus rhythm in patients failing the quinidine/digoxin regimen (see p. 46.) AF recurs following cardioversion in most patients unless digoxin and quinidine are continued; therefore, it makes little sense to cardiovert patients intolerant of these medications.

Atrial Flutter

Atrial flutter (FL), a rhythm that usually implies organic heart disease, arises in a localized region of re-entry outside the AV node or less commonly in a rapidly firing *ectopic focus*. FL frequently complicates the postoperative course of thoracic surgery but seldom occurs following myocardial infarction. FL is *intrinsically unstable*, often converting to AF spontaneously or in response to digitalis. Because the FL pathway does not involve the AV node, *atrial rates in FL are usually rapid* (260–340 beats/minute) *and the rhythm cannot be terminated by vagal maneuvers*. Depolarizations usually originate from a focus low in the right atrium, producing inverted P waves in the inferior leads and upright P deflections in lead V1. The frequency of ventricular response depends on the underlying atrial rate and the extent of AV block. Most commonly a 2:1 AV block leads to a regular ventricular rate of $\simeq$ 150 beats/minute and uncovers the "saw tooth" baseline pattern of atrial depolarization. Ventricular rate may be slowed further by conduction system disease or drugs (digitalis, beta blockers). Patients receiving digoxin sometimes show irregular AV conduction or higher degrees of block (3:1 or 4:1). *Vagal maneuvers* facilitate the identification of FL by transiently increasing AV block in stepwise fashion, *allowing flutter waves to emerge*. With a success rate > 95%, direct current (DC) cardioversion is the most effective method of restoring sinus rhythm, even when low doses of electrical energy are used. Overdrive atrial pacing also effectively terminates this rhythm. Because a high percentage of patients revert to flutter after conversion, prophylaxis with digoxin and quinidine is indicated.

Ventricular Extrasystoles

Ventricular extrasystoles are commonly associated with *organic heart disease, ischemia*, and *digitalis toxicity*. These autonomous discharges usually occur before the next expected sinus depolarization and are therefore termed *premature ventricular contractions* (PVCs). A PVC is rec-

ognized by an abnormally wide QRS complex accompanied by an ST segment and a T wave whose axes are directed opposite to that of the QRS. "Electrically insulated" from the ventricles, the sino-atrial (SA) node continues to discharge autonomously during the PVC but usually fails to influence the ventricle. Occasionally, when the timing is conducive, a combined supraventricular/ventricular electrical impulse may form a *"fusion beat"*. Because the SA node is not reset by the PVC, the first conducted sinus beat following the PVC appears only after a *fully compensatory pause*. (A PVC may be interpolated between two sinus beats without a compensatory pause in patients with bradycardia.) It is often difficult to distinguish PVCs from aberrantly conducted supraventricular beats. Factors favoring PVCs are listed in Table 4.1.

Aberrantly conducted supraventricular beats (usually in a right bundle branch block configuration) often appear when a short R-R interval follows a long R-R interval in patients with AF or MAT. This *Ashman phenomenon* results from variable, rate-related recovery of the conduction system after depolarization.

Occasionally, ventricular extrasystoles are not premature but delayed. These *escape beats*, usually occurring at a rate of 30–40 beats/minute, function as a safety mechanism to produce ventricular contraction when normal sinus conduction fails. Ventricular extrasystoles that occur in succession at rates < 40 beats/minute are referred to as "idioventricular". A rate of 40–100 beats/minute defines an "accelerated" idioventricular rhythm. For obvious reasons, ventricular *escape beats should not be suppressed*. The primary treatment of idioventricular rhythm is to increase the SA nodal rate with atropine, isoproterenol, or pacing.

The prognosis and treatment of PVCs depends upon their cause and frequency. *Not all PVCs require treatment*. Although some patterns are clearly

---

Table 4.1

Factors Favoring PVCs versus Supraventricular Aberrancy

1. Monophasic or diaphasic complex in lead V1
2. Notched QRS complex with R > R'
3. QS in V6 or an R/S ratio in V6 < 1.0
4. Absent P waves or PR interval < .10 seconds
5. QRS duration > 0.14 seconds
6. Fully compensatory pause
7. Fusion beat

more dangerous than others, ventricular tachycardia or ventricular fibrillation may develop without a "warning rhythm". Except in the setting of heart failure or acute myocardial ischemia, there is little evidence that pharmacologic suppression of PVCs improves outcome. Generally accepted indications for treatment of PVCs in the critically ill include: (1) *new PVCs* in the setting of cardiac ischemia; (2) *couplets or ventricular tachycardia* (three or more closely linked PVCs); (3) *multifocal PVCs*; (4) > 5 *PVCs/minute*; or (5) *an "R on T" configuration* (PVC interrupts ascending portion of preceding T wave). Common underlying causes of PVCs include *ischemia, acidosis, hypoxemia, electrolyte disorders, drugs,* and *toxins.*

Treatment

Intravenous lidocaine is the drug of choice for ventricular extrasystoles requiring treatment. Procainamide is an alternative drug that may be administered parenterally. Quinidine should not be used in the acute setting because it is frequently ineffective, has a delayed onset of action, and is available only as an oral preparation. Bretylium and a host of other new antiarrhythmics (flecainide, encainide, mexiletine, etc.) may prove useful in refractory cases.

Ventricular Tachycardia

Diagnosis

Ventricular tachycardia (VT) is defined as 3 or more consecutive ventricular beats occurring at a rate > 100/minute (commonly 140–220/minute). Some clinicians prefer the more stringent definition of 10 or more consecutive ventricular beats. The beats of VT are recognized by *wide QRS complexes with T waves of opposite polarity.* The ECG hallmark of VT is *AV dissociation* (a phenomenon resulting from the independent firing of the SA node and the ventricular focus). Mild beat-to-beat variation in R-R interval is usually present. VT is usually symptomatic and generally occurs in patients with underlying heart disease. The mechanism is the rapid firing of an ectopic ventricular pacemaker or electrical re-entry at the level of the His-Purkinje network. Antecedent isolated PVCs are not consistently present. VT is usually initiated by a PVC with delayed linkage to the preceding QRS. Occasionally, retrograde atrial depolarization may occur.

Differentiating SVT from VT may be difficult, particularly when supraventricular beats are aberrantly conducted or a bundle branch block is present. A varying S1 or Cannon A waves in the jugular venous pulse suggest VT, as do capture or fusion beats observed on the ECG. The arrhythmia is usually supraventricular if regular, upright P waves occur at an appropriate time *before* each QRS complex. However, if an inverted P wave follows each QRS, VT or junctional tachycardia is more likely. In contrast to NRT, VT fails to respond to vagal stimulation. Esophageal or special precordial leads may help to demonstrate atrial activity. The ECG characteristics proposed to distinguish SVT from VT by Wellens are helpful but not infallible (Table 4.1 and Ref. 6).

Treatment

In the hemodynamically compromised patient, VT should be treated by *synchronized* cardioversion, beginning with 100 WS of energy. Precordial thump is worth trying in *witnessed* VT but is rarely successful. Following cardioversion of VT to a stable rhythm, lidocaine or procainamide is indicated to prevent recurrence. If hemodynamically stable, lidocaine, procainamide, or bretylium may be used as primary therapy to interrupt VT.

Torsades de pointes ("the twisting of points") is a specific subset of VT recognized by its bizarre *polymorphism, constantly changing QRS axis,* and *propensity to begin after the peak of the preceding T wave* (see p. 150).

Symptomatic torsades require immediate treatment. Lidocaine or cardioversion are temporarily effective, but definitive therapy requires intervention to shorten the QT interval. Withdrawal of type Ia antiarrhythmics and cardio-acceleration with atropine, isoproterenol, or ventricular pacing are commonly used.

BRADYARRHYTHMIAS

Except when caused by intrinsic disease of the sinus mechanism or conduction system, bradycardia tends to reflect a non-cardiogenic etiology. Such stimuli include vagal reflexes, hypoxemia, hypothyroidism, and drug effects (particularly beta blockers, calcium channel blockers, or digoxin). Bradycardia is usually of little import in patients with normally compliant hearts, adequate preload reserves, and the ability to peripherally vasoconstrict. However, if stroke volume cannot be increased (e.g., dehydration, pericardial disease, noncompliant myocardium, or depressed contractility), bradycardia may precipitously lower cardiac output and blood pressure.

Sinus Bradycardia

Bradycardia may be physiologic when metabolic demands are reduced (hypothermia, hypothyroidism, starvation). Sinus bradycardia (SB) is characterized by normal P wave morphology and 1:1 AV conduction at a rate < 60 beats/minute. The association of SB with inferior and posterior myocardial infarctions may be related to ischemia of nodal tissue and increased vagal tone. The vagotonic actions of morphine and beta blockers aggrevate bradycardia in such patients.

SB does not require treatment unless it causes hypotension or angina or precipitates *ventricular escape beats*. However SB may be a marker of other pathologic processes important to reverse (e.g., hypoxemia, visceral distention, pain). SB may be treated with atropine or isoproterenol, but both drugs have the potential to increase myocardial O_2 consumption when used in the setting of myocardial ischemia.

Atrioventricular Block

First Degree Atrioventricular Block

In itself, first degree AV block (1° AVB) is physiologically unimportant. However, 1° AVB may signal drug toxicity or progressive disease of the conduction system. In 1° AVB, AV nodal or infranodal conduction is slowed, prolonging the PR interval (> 0.2 sec). In the ICU, 1° AVB is usually a temporary phenomenon caused by increased *vagal tone* or *digitalis*. Isolated 1° AVB does not require therapy. However, pacing is indicated if 1° AVB accompanies right bundle branch block and left anterior fasicular block in the setting of an acute myocardial infarction (MI). Complete heart block often follows in such patients.

Second Degree AV Block

There are two forms of second degree (2° AVB), an arrhythmia in which some atrial impulses are conducted while others are blocked.

Mobitz I (Wenkebach) conduction is characterized by sequential and progressive prolongation of the PR interval, culminating in periodic failure to transmit the atrial impulse. (While the PR intervals of successive beats progressively lengthen, the RR intervals shorten.) After QRS depolarization is blocked, the sequence is repeated, resulting in a recurring rhythm. The blockage site almost always resides *within the AV node* and is most frequently the result of digitalis toxicity or intrinsic heart disease, (e.g., infarction, myocarditis or cardiac surgery). Because the right coronary supplies the AV node in most patients, Mobitz 1 block often accompanies inferior MI. In this setting, Mobitz I block is usually benign and self limited. Conversely, Mobitz 1 block complicating *anterior* in-

farction, suggests extensive myocardial damage and a guarded prognosis.

Although atropine or isoproterenol may be used to improve conduction, no treatment is usually required. Pacemakers are effective but rarely necessary.

Mobitz II AV block originates *below* the level of the AV node (in the His-Purkinje system). In contrast to Mobitz 1 block, the PR interval remains constant. Some atrial depolarizations fail to conduct, usually on an unpredictable basis. The QRS complex may be prolonged if the HIS bundle is the site of blockade. Mobitz II block is usually *not* transient and, because it often progresses to symptomatic AV block of higher degree, almost always requires treatment. Mobitz II block with 2:1 conduction is difficult or impossible to separate from Mobitz I block in which every other P wave is non-conducted. (One helpful clue may be that QRS prolongation is more common in Mobitz II block.) Atropine fails to influence the infranodal site of blockade, making transvenous pacing necessary in most cases.

Third Degree AV Block

During complete (3°) AVB, the atria and ventricles fire independently, usually at different but regular rates. 3° AVB may result from degenerative myocardial disease or inflammation, myocardial infarction, or infiltration of the conducting system (e.g., sarcoidosis, amyloidosis). Toxic concentrations of digitalis and other drugs may also produce 3° AVB.

On physical examination, AV dissociation produces a *varying first heart sound* and *Cannon a waves* in the jugular venous pulse, the result of occasional simultaneous atrial and ventricular contraction.

Blockage of the AV node itself produces a "narrow complex" junctional rhythm at a rate of 40–60 beats/minute and usually results from myocardial infarction. In most cases, it is transient and asymptomatic. On the other hand, *infranodal AV block*, a pattern associated with a wide QRS (> 0.10 sec), is almost always symptomatic because it tends to produce slower heart rates (30–45 beats/min). The inherent instability of pacemakers originating distal to the AV node renders infranodal 3° AVB worthy of treatment, regardless of rate. Immediate insertion of a transvenous pacemaker is indicated.

ANTIARRHYTHMIC DRUGS

Antiarrhythmic therapy is far from ideal. Antiarrhythmics often fail to suppress the rhythm disorder and prevention may not improve outcome. Furthermore, all antiarrhythmic drugs have adverse side effects, including the tendency to exacerbate the underlying problem *("proarrhythmic" effects)*. Preoccupation with the drug management of physiologically insignificant arrhythmias may distract the physician from addressing the primary disorder (e.g., ischemia, electrolyte disturbance, heart failure, thyrotoxicosis, or drug intoxication). Normalizing arterial oxygenation, pH, potassium, and magnesium often improves or abolishes the arrhythmic tendency. In hypotensive or pulseless patients with tachyarrhythmias, electrical cardioversion (not drugs) is the treatment of choice. *Synchronized cardioversion* is the preferred method, except in ventricular fibrillation (see p. 45). Drugs used in the treatment of symptomatic arrhythmias are reviewed in Table 4.2.

Specific Antiarrhythmic Drugs

Lidocaine

Lidocaine, a type II antiarrhythmic, effectively suppresses ventricular irritability but has little effect on atrial disorders. Although a survival benefit has not been demonstrated, prophylactic therapy in myocardial infarction decreases the risk of VF and VT.

Because lidocaine distributes into multiple compartments, it requires one or more loading doses to maintain effective serum concentration. Without loading, constant infusion may require hours to achieve therapeutic serum levels. Loading is usually accomplished by giving three decremental doses (e.g., 100, 75, and 50 mg) spaced 7–10 minutes apart. For similar reasons, a modified drug bolus should accompany increased infusion rates in the correction of an inadequate serum concentration. Lidocaine doses should be reduced in the elderly and in patients with heart failure, shock, or liver disease (see Chapter 14).

Although no adjustment is needed for renal dysfunction, patients should be closely monitored after institution or withdrawal of drugs interfering with the hepatic metabolism of lidocaine (e.g., cimetidine, propranolol). Neurologic toxicity, confusion, lethargy, and seizures emerge when lidocaine levels exceed 5 μg/ml. Lidocaine may also exacerbate the neuromuscular blocking effects of paralytic drugs. The hemodynamic effects of lidocaine are usually inconsequential but include mild depression of blood pressure and cardiac contractility.

In the setting of infarction, the infusion is usually continued through the high risk period ($\simeq$ 36 hr). After this time, the need for continued medication must be reassessed. In most patients, lidocaine is discontinued as the patient is monitored for return of ventricular ectopy. Because of its multi-compartment distribution, lidocaine washes out slowly (over 6 hours) after abrupt discontinuation. Therefore, although tapering of the drug is not required, ECG monitoring is indicated for 6–12 hours after discontinuation.

Bretylium

Bretylium is a "second line" drug indicated for the treatment of *ventricular arrhythmias* refractory to lidocaine. Bretylium suppresses PVCs, prevents VT, increases fibrillation threshold, and may "chemically cardiovert" some patients with VF. Loading doses of 5–10 mg/kg may be given before initiating a constant infusion of 1–2 mg/min. Bretylium can produce hypotension if given rapidly. Bradycardia, nausea, vomiting, and orthostatic blood pressure changes are common.

Procainamide

Procainamide (PA) is a type Ia antiarrhythmic, useful for both *supraventricular* and *ventricular* arrhythmias. It effectively controls PVCs and VT and may convert supraventricular to sinus rhythm. Like other type Ia drugs (quinidine and disopyramide), PA may accelerate the ventricular rate in AF or FL unless AV conduction is slowed with digitalis or beta blockers.

In an average-sized patient, a total loading dose of 1 gram is given by injecting sequential boluses of 100 mg every 5 minutes. When continuous intravenous therapy is required, loading may be followed by constant infusion (2–6 mg/min).

PA acts as a vasodilator and negative ionotrope, thereby decreasing blood pressure and contractility. Both the QRS and QT intervals of the ECG often increase modestly. Like quinidine, PA may precipitate "torsades des pointes". PA is less likely than quinidine to cause gastrointestinal (GI) distress but over long periods induces a lupus-like syndrome in as many as 1 in 5 patients. A positive antinuclear antibody (ANA) develops in $\simeq$ 50% of all patients using the drug chronically. Rare cases of hemolysis or agranulocytosis have been reported.

Quinidine

Quinidine is a type Ia antiarrhythmic, most effective in restoring sinus rhythm in patients with AF or FL. Although not useful for emergent in-

Table 4.2
Treatment of Symptomatic Arrhythmias

Arrhythmia	Primary Treatment[a]	Alternative or Supplemental Measures	Comment
Atrial fibrillation/flutter	Cardioversion	Rate Control Digoxin Propranolol Verapamil	Supression of recurrent arrythmia may be achieved with quinidine, procainamide, disopyrimide.
Nodal re-entrant tachycardia	Vagal stimulation	Verapamil Edrophonium Propranolol Digoxin Alpha-adrenergic stimulant	Cardioversion useful when drug therapy fails or reversal urgent.
Multifocal atrial tachycardia	Correction of underlying metabolic or cardio-pulmonary disorder	Verapamil	Verapamil usually slows rate and occasionally re-establishes sinus mechanism. Digoxin or propranolol may slow rate but may prove toxic.
Bradycardia Supranodal	Atropine/oxygen	Isoproterenol	Hypoxemia and vagal reflexes are common precipitants.
Infranodal	Isoproterenol	Pacing	
Ventricular premature contractions	Lidocaine	Procainamide Quinidine Disopyrimide	A host of newer agents are available or in the process of development but cannot yet be therapy.
Ventricular tachycardia	Cardioversion	Lidocaine Procainamide Bretylium	
Ventricular fibrillation	Cardioversion	Lidocaine Bretylium	Successful cardioversion correlates inversely with duration of fibrillation.
Digitoxic rhythms	Lidocaine KCl	Phenytoin Procainamide Propranolol	Bretylium contraindicated

[a]Correction of hypoxemia, hypotension, disturbances of pH and electrolytes (Ca^{2+}, Mg^{2+}, K^+) are key elements of therapy.

dications, quinidine may also suppress ventricular ectopy. There is little use for quinidine in the ICU because it has limited effectiveness, many side effects, and is available only as an oral preparation. Diarrhea is the most common side effect. Cardiac toxicity includes: (1) AV block; (2) aggrevation of ventricular arrhythmias; and (3) negative inotropy. Quinidine prolongs the QT interval and may precipitate torsades. When added to a stable regimen, quinidine may double serum levels of digoxin.

Digitalis

The major use of digitalis in arrhythmia management is to *slow AV conduction* in AF and FL.

In this role, digoxin is usually given in 0.125- to 0.25-mg doses IV every 4–6 hours until the ventricular response rate is ≤ 100/min. (If hemodynamically unstable, cardioversion is indicated.) When used as an antiarrhythmic, digoxin is usually titrated to the desired degree of AV block, with less regard for "standard therapeutic drug levels" than when used as an ionotropic medication. Nonetheless, levels above 3 ng/ml are poorly tolerated and usually not necessary. Heart block, increased myocardial irritability, gastrointestinal distress (nausea and vomiting), and central nervous system (CNS) disturbances (confusion, visual aberrations) are the most common toxic side effects.

Verapamil

Verapamil, a calcium channel blocker, routinely converts NRT and slows the ventricular response of AF and FL. Verapamil often slows or abolishes MAT but rarely converts AF or FL to sinus rhythm. In hemodynamically compromised patients, cardioversion (not verapamil) is the treatment of choice. Intravenous doses of 2.5–5 mg at 5 to 10 minute intervals are usually promptly effective. Verapamil must be used with extreme caution; even with commonly used doses, high grade AV block (occasionally asystole) may result. (This effect is more common in VT than in SVT.) Because of its vasodilating effects, hypotension is common in the volume-depleted and elderly. Some recent evidence suggests that the vasodilating action of verapamil can be avoided by pretreatment with intravenous calcium.

Phenytoin

Phenytoin is a group II antiarrhythmic most useful in treating digitalis-induced ventricular tachyarrhythmias. Phenytoin shortens the QT and PR intervals and increases AV block. Phenytoin is usually administered IV in loading doses of $\simeq$ 1 gram but must be given slowly ($<$ 50 mg/min) as the cardiac rhythm is monitored. The drug and its solvent, propylene glycol, may provoke serious arrhythmias or hypotension during rapid administration. Phenytoin lowers blood pressure by decreasing cardiac output and systemic vascular resistance. Cerebellar ataxia is the major toxicity of phenytoin levels $>$ 20 mg/dl. Phenytoin potentiates the effects of other drugs that are highly protein bound (e.g., warfarin, phenylbutazone).

Beta-Adrenergic Blockers

A wide range of beta-adrenergic blocking drugs is currently available. These differ with respect to speed of onset, receptor selectivity, duration of action, and side effects. The prototype is propranolol, whose primary actions are shared among most members of the class. Propranolol, a nonspecific beta-blocker, is a negative ionotrope and chronotrope. Propranolol decreases the rate of SA node depolarization and conduction velocity. Although useful in states of catecholamine excess, beta-blockade may produce disastrous results in patients who depend on catecholamine stimulation to remain compensated. Such problems are likely to arise in patients with asthma, impaired cardiac contractility, or stroke volume limited by constriction.

Propranolol helps slow the rate in supraventricular tachyarrhythmias such as SVT, AF, FL, and Wolf-Parkinson-White syndrome. The drug is a poor choice for treating most ventricular arrhythmias, except when these are exacerbated by tachycardia or ischemia. In emergency situations propranolol may be administered in intravenous doses of 0.5 to 1.0 mg every ten minutes. Contraindications include severe bradycardia or high-grade AV block, heart failure, asthma, or digitalis toxicity. Beta-blocking drugs may aggrevate coronary spasm in variant (Prinzmetal's) angina. When selecting a beta-blocker, the desired duration of action should be a key consideration. The antiarrhythmic and antihypertensive effects of altenolol may last for 24 hours. Conversely, the ultra-short action of esmolol may help in the acute management of supraventricular tachyarrhythmias (AF, FL, SVT) without depressing myocardial function for protracted periods.

ELECTRICAL CARDIOVERSION

Electrical shock terminates re-entrant tachycardias and ventricular fibrillation by simultaneously depolarizing the entire heart. In pulseless tachyarrhythmias or VF, *unsynchronized shock* interrupts the arrhythmia, allowing a more stable pacemaker to emerge (see Chapter 16, Cardiopulmonary Arrest). A stable supraventricular pacemaker is less likely to predominate after cardioversion in patients with slow AF or evidence of infranodal disease. *Synchronized cardioversion* (SC) is preferred whenever an organized rhythm is present. Synchronization times the electrical discharge to occur slightly after the R wave (a ''non-vulnerable'' point in the cardiac cycle, where shock is unlikely to induce VF). To trigger the discharge SC requires monitoring of an ECG lead that demonstrates a tall R wave (usually lead I or II). Rarely, tall, steeply sloping T waves may trigger discharge at inappropriate times.

If possible, patients undergoing elective SC should take *nothing by mouth (NPO)* for 8 hours before the procedure to minimize the risk of aspiration. An *anesthesiologist* should be present to monitor airway patency, ventilation, oxygenation, and level of sedation. Midazolam, ultrashort acting barbituates, or diazepam can produce sufficient *sedation* and amnesia for patient comfort. *Digitalis* preparations should be withheld for 24–48 hours before the procedure to minimize the risk of postcardioversion arrhythmias. Hypokalemia, digitalis toxicity, and hyperthyroidism contraindicate elective SC. Hypoxemia and other *electrolyte disorders* should also be corrected before the procedure.

It should be emphasized that the appropriate dose of electricity depends upon the underlying rhythm. Unsuccessful attempts should be followed by another shock with *double* electrical energy. Being relatively unstable, FL may convert with as little as 5 joules (watt-seconds, WS). AF may convert with a 50 WS shock. Patients with re-entrant SVT frequently require > 100 WS. Ventricular tachycardia often needs 200 WS for conversion. In patients with re-entrant SVT, electrical "fatigue" of the SA or AV nodes may delay recovery of normal conduction and automaticity. For this reason, the physician should be prepared to immediately insert a temporary transvenous pacemaker.

Adverse effects of cardioversion include skin burns and disorders of conduction and repolarization. The myocardium may be dysfunctional for a variable period afterward. SGOT, CPK, and LDH may rise slightly. The most dreaded complication of cardioversion is systemic embolization, a problem most commonly seen in non-anticoagulated patients with mitral stenosis and chronic atrial fibrillation.

SUGGESTED READINGS

1. Levine JH, Michael JR, Guarnieri T: Treatment of multifocal atrial tachycardia with verapamil. *N Engl J Med* 312:21–25, 1985.
2. Reiser HJ, Sullivan ME: Antiarrhythmic drug therapy: new drugs and changing concepts. *Fed Proc* 45:2206–2212, 1986.
3. Shaw M, Niemann JT, Haskell RJ, et al: Esophageal electrocardiography in acute cardiac care: efficacy and diagnostic value of a new technique. *Am J Med* 82:689–696, 1987.
4. Stewart RB, Bardy GH, Greene HL: Wide-complex tachycardia: Misdiagnosis and outcome after emergent therapy. *Ann Intern Med* 104:766–771, 1986.
5. Waldo AL: Mechanisms of atrial fibrillation, atrial flutter, and ectopic atrial tachycardias—a brief review. *Circulation* 75:37–42, 1987.
6. Wellens HJJ: The wide QRS tachycardia. *Ann Intern Med* 104:879, 1986.

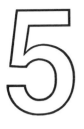

Respiratory Monitoring

Data relevant to the output, efficiency, and reserve of the respiratory system must be continually assessed to ensure appropriate management during cardiorespiratory failure. Techniques can be conveniently classified into those that characterize gas exchange, breathing workload, and ventilatory capability.

MONITORING GAS EXCHANGE

Monitoring Oxygenation

Arterial cannulation and blood gas analysis are discussed at length in other sections of this book (see Chapter 11, and *Respiratory Medicine for the House Officer*, Ref. 7). Perhaps the most popular innovation in gas exchange monitoring has been the application of oximetry to the on-line assessment of arterial (SaO_2) and mixed venous O_2 saturation ($S\bar{v}O_2$). Although intimately linked, O_2 saturation and tension provide complementary clinical data. PaO_2 reflects the maximal tension driving O_2 to the tissues, whereas saturation (interpreted in conjunction with hemoglobin concentration) reflects O_2 content. *Reflectance oximetry* is used when a pulmonary arterial (Swan-Ganz) catheter continuously samples $S\bar{v}O_2$ in the pulmonary arterial bloodstream. This technique and its interpretation are discussed elsewhere (see p. 24).

Transmission (Arterial Oximetry)

Transcutaneous *photometric (ear, pulse) oximetry* is most useful for patients with marginal or fluctuating oxygen exchange. In patients receiving mechanical ventilation, transcutaneous oximetry continuously measures SaO_2, enabling rapid adjustment of F_iO_2 and PEEP and warning of arterial desaturation during weaning, sleep, or changes of position.

Lightweight heated probes direct filtered light of selected wavelengths onto the surface of the earlobe or digit. The relative absorption of these beams as they pass through the tissue is continuously monitored and converted by spectrophotometric analysis to the appropriate saturation value. Pulse oximeter probes do not require tissue heating because phasic changes in blood volume and optical density cue the instrument to the arterial component of the blood contained in the nail bed of the finger or toe. Some units also display pulse rate and arterial waveform. Currently available instruments are highly accurate in their upper range (i.e., saturations $> 75\%$) but less reliable as the patient desaturates or perfusion falls. Although skin pigmentation and jaundice do not markedly affect the accuracy of pulse oximeters, carboxyhemoglobin and methemoglobin can produce falsely high saturation values.

Other gas measuring techniques (e.g., *transcutaneous and transconjuctival measurement of O_2 and CO_2*) are widely used in neonatology to monitor tissue gas tensions but are generally less successful in adults. Transcutaneous techniques require frequent calibration, skin and electrode preparation, and regular site changes to avoid burning the warmed patch of skin they monitor. More importantly, they are profoundly affected by perfusion crises and unreliably track arterial gas tensions in the critically ill. Transconjunctival probes are poorly tolerated by alert patients.

O_2 Consumption

Total body oxygen consumption ($\dot{V}O_2$) is surprisingly difficult to measure at the bedside of patients receiving mechanical ventilation. Two primary methods are in general use: direct analysis of inspired and expired gases, and the *Fick method:* computation of $\dot{V}O_2$ from the product of cardiac output (CO) and the difference in O_2 content between samples of arterial and mixed venous blood. Neither method is accurate when the patient's metabolic rate is changing at the time of data collection.

Expired Gas Analysis

Patients receiving mechanical ventilation are often administered high inspired fractions of oxygen (F_iO_2) and require large minute volumes to achieve effective alveolar ventilation. Such large amounts of O_2 flush through the lungs each minute that analyses of gas tensions and measurements of $\dot{V}E$ must be precise to distinguish the small oxygen deficits that correspond to $\dot{V}O_2$. Furthermore, the inspired gas mixture must be thoroughly blended to uniform composition. Precise measurement of inspired oxygen tension (P_iO_2) and $\dot{V}O_2$ in patients receiving high F_iO_2 remains a clinical challenge.

Fick Method

The Fick method analyzes arterial and mixed venous blood samples for O_2 content. The difference between them is then multiplied by CO to determine $\dot{V}O_2$. Unfortunately, this method is greatly influenced by small changes in either the activity of the patient or the CO over the period of the data collection. Furthermore, because of the unpredictable nature of the oxyhemoglobin desaturation curve, *O_2 content should be measured directly*—not calculated. Technical errors in blood analysis and CO determinations are multiplicative, further compromising the method.

Volumetric Analysis

Volumetric analysis is a method of estimating $\dot{V}O_2$ which uses a closed-circuit to absorb CO_2 while metering in sufficient O_2 to keep the total volume of the system constant. This technique avoids problems otherwise presented by elevated F_iO_2, but imposes significant airway resistance, as the necessary elements must be made part of the breathing circuit.

Applications of $\dot{V}O_2$

Although the $\dot{V}O_2$ is sometimes useful in determining nutritional requirements, its clinical utility is more questionable in other settings. In theory, assuming a stable tissue need for O_2, measurements of $\dot{V}O_2$ may be used to follow the hemodynamic response to therapeutic interventions. (An increasing $\dot{V}O_2$ suggests improvement, whereas failure of $\dot{V}O_2$ to change implies initial output adequacy or failure of the intervention.) Unfortunately, serial $\dot{V}O_2$ measurements are not highly reproducible and are subject to sudden changes in underlying metabolic status.

Efficiency of Oxygen Exchange

Computing Alveolar Oxygen Tension

To judge the efficiency of gas exchange, mean alveolar oxygen tension (PAO_2) must first be computed. The ideal PAO_2 is obtained from the modified alveolar gas equation:

$$PAO_2 = P_iO_2 - PaCO_2/R + (PaCO_2 \times F_iO_2 \times (1-R)/R)$$

where R is the respiratory exchange ratio and P_iO_2 is the inspired oxygen tension. [P_iO_2 = (barometric pressure $\times$ F_iO_2 − 47.] Under steady state conditions, R normally varies from $\simeq 0.7$ to 1.0, depending on the nature of the metabolic fuel. When the same patient is monitored over time, R is generally assumed to be 0.8 or neglected entirely. Under most clinical conditions the alveolar gas equation can be simplified to:

$$PAO_2 = P_iO_2 - 1.25 \times PaCO_2$$

For example, at sea level with the patient breathing room air:

$$PAO_2 = 150 - (1.25 \times PaCO_2)$$

Alveolar-Arterial Oxygen Tension Difference P(A-a)O₂

The difference between alveolar and arterial oxygen tensions, $P(A-a)O_2$, takes account of alveolar CO_2 tension and therefore eliminates hypoventilation and hypercapnia from consideration as the sole cause of hypoxemia. However, although useful, a single value of $P(A-a)O_2$ does not characterize the efficiency of gas exchange across all F_iO_2s, even in normal subjects. The $P(A-a)O_2$ normally ranges from $\simeq 10$ mmHg (on room air) to $\simeq 100$ mmHg (on an F_iO_2 of 1.0). Moreover, PAO_2 changes alinearly with respect to F_iO_2 as the extent of $\dot{V}/\dot{Q}$ mismatch increases. Thus, when the $\dot{V}/\dot{Q}$ abnormality is severe and inhomogeneously distributed among gas exchange units, the PAO_2 may vary little with F_iO_2 until high fractions of inspired oxygen are given (Fig. 5.1). Finally, the $P(A-a)O_2$ may be influenced by fluctuations in venous oxygen content.

Venous Admixture and Shunt

Under normal circumstances, fluctuations in $S\bar{v}O_2$ do not contribute significantly to hypoxemia. However, as ventilation/perfusion inequality or shunting develop, the O_2 content of mixed venous blood ($C\bar{v}O_2$) exerts an increasingly important effect on SaO_2. On-line measurements of $S\bar{v}O_2$ with a fiberoptic Swan-Ganz catheter enable venous ad-

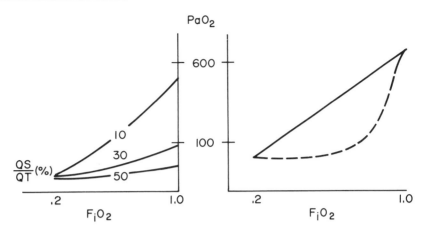

Figure 5.1 Effect of true shunt ($\dot{Q}s$ / $\dot{Q}t$) and $\dot{V}$ / $\dot{Q}$ mismatching (VQM) on the PaO_2/F_iO_2 relationship. Hypoxemia caused by shunt (left panel) is refractory to supplementary O_2, once $\dot{Q}s$ / $\dot{Q}t$ exceeds $\simeq$ 30%. Similar reductions in PaO_2 caused by VQM respond to O_2 (right panel); however, the F_iO_2 required depends on whether hypoxemia is caused by an extensive number of units with mildly abnormal VQM (solid line), or by a smaller number with very low $\dot{V}$ / $\dot{Q}$ ratios (dashed line).

mixture ($\dot{Q}s$ / $\dot{Q}t$) to be computed with relative ease. In the steady state, with hemoglobin expressed in grams/100 ml of blood:

$$\dot{Q}s / \dot{Q}t = (CAO_2 - CaO_2)/(CAO_2 - C\bar{v}O_2)$$

where oxygen content (CAO_2 or $C\bar{v}O_2$) in ml of O_2 per 100 ml of blood equals the product:

$$0.003 \times PO_2 + .0134 \times (\% SO_2 \times Hgb)$$

(In the latter equation PO_2 and SO_2 refer to the oxygen tension and saturation of blood at the respective sites.) Like $P(A-a)O_2$, $\dot{Q}s$ / $\dot{Q}t$ is also influenced by variations in $\dot{V}/\dot{Q}$ mismatching and by fluctuations in $S\bar{v}O_2$ and F_iO_2. If $\dot{Q}s$ / $\dot{Q}t$ is abnormally high but all alveoli are patent, calculated admixture will diminish toward the normal physiologic value ($\simeq$ 5%) as F_iO_2 increases. Conversely, if the $\dot{Q}s$ / $\dot{Q}t$ abnormality is due entirely to blood flowing through completely unventilated tissue, through intrapulmonary venoarterial communications, or through an intracardiac defect, there will be no change in $\dot{Q}s$ / $\dot{Q}t$ as F_iO_2 increases ("true" shunt).

Simplified Measures of Oxygen Exchange

Several pragmatic approaches have been taken to simplify bedside assessment of O_2 exchange efficiency. The first is to quantitate $P(A-a)O_2$ during the administration of pure O_2. After suitable wash-in time (5–15 minutes, depending on severity of disease) pure shunt accounts for the entire $P(A-a)O_2$. Furthermore, if hemoglobin is fully saturated with O_2, dividing the $P(A-a)O_2$ by 20 approximates shunt percentage (at F_iO_2 = 1). As pure O_2 replaces alveolar nitrogen, some patent but poorly ventilated units may collapse—the process of "absorption atelectasis". Whatever its shortcomings, determining shunt fraction is worthwhile because it can alert the clinician to consider nonparenchymal causes of hypoxemia (e.g., arteriovenous malformation, intracardiac shunting). Furthermore, because PaO_2 shows little response to variations in F_iO_2 at true shunt fractions > 25%, the clinician may be encouraged to reduce toxic and marginally effective concentrations of oxygen.

The *PAO_2/F_iO_2 (or "P/F") ratio* is a convenient and widely used bedside index of oxygen exchange that attempts to adjust for fluctuating F_iO_2. However, although simple to calculate, this ratio is sensitive to changes in $S\bar{v}O_2$ and does not remain equally sensitive across the entire range of F_iO_2—especially when shunt is the major cause for admixture. Another easily calculated index of oxygen exchange properties, *the PaO_2/PAO_2 (or "a/A") ratio*, offers similar advantages and disadvantages as F_iO_2 is varied. Like the P/F ratio, it is a useful bedside index that does not require blood sampling from the central circulation but loses reliability in proportion to the degree of shunting. Furthermore, in common with all measures that calculate an "ideal" PAO_2, even the a/A ratio can be misleading when fluctuations occur in the primary determinants of $P\bar{v}O_2$ (hemoglobin and the balance between oxygen consumption and delivery).

Monitoring Carbon Dioxide

CO$_2$ Production

Measurement of CO_2 excretion is valuable for metabolic studies, computations of deadspace ventilation, and the evaluation of hyperpnea. Measurements of CO_2 production are representative when the sample is carefully collected in the steady state over adequate time. The rate of CO_2 elimination is a product of $\dot{V}E$ and the expired fraction of CO_2 in the expelled gas. Provided that gas collection is timed accurately and the sample is adequately mixed and analyzed, an accurate value for excreted CO_2 can be obtained. However, whether this value represents metabolic CO_2 production will depend on the stability of the patient during the period of gas collection—not only with regard to $\dot{V}O_2$, but also in terms of acid-base fluctuations, perfusion constancy, and ventilation status with respect to metabolic needs. During acute hyperventilation or rapidly developing metabolic acidosis, for example, the rate of CO_2 excretion overestimates metabolic rate until surplus body stores of CO_2 are washed out or bicarbonate stores reach equilibrium. The opposite obtains during abrupt hypoventilation or transient reduction in cardiac output.

Efficiency of CO$_2$ Exchange

The CO_2 produced by the body tissues varies with metabolic rate (fever, pain, agitation, sepsis, etc.). The CO_2 load presented to the alveoli is eliminated by changes in minute ventilation, which are linked with varying efficiency to changes in alveolar ventilation. Alveolar and arterial CO_2 concentrations respond exponentially after step changes in ventilation, with a half-time of $\simeq 3$ minutes during hyperventilation, but a slower (16-min) half-time during CO_2 accumulation. These differing time courses should be taken into account when sampling blood gases after making ventilator adjustments. In the mechanically ventilated patient, many vagaries of CO_2 flux can be eliminated by controlling ventilation and quieting muscle activity with deep sedation with or without paralysis.

$PaCO_2$ must be interpreted in conjunction with the $\dot{V}E$. For example, the gas exchanging ability of the lung may be unimpaired even though $PaCO_2$ rises when reduced alveolar ventilation is the result of diminished respiratory drive or marked neuromuscular weakness.

Deadspace Fraction

The physiologic deadspace (V_D) quantifies the gas volume that fails to participate in CO_2 exchange. This fraction of wasted ventilation (V_D/V_T) can be estimated with analyzed specimens of arterial blood and mixed expired gas:

$$V_D/V_T = (PaCO_2 - PeCO_2)/PaCO_2$$

where $PeCO_2$ is the CO_2 concentration in a mixed expired gas sample. In collecting the expired gas sample during pressurized ventilator cycles, an adjustment should be made for the volume of gas stored in the compressible portions of the ventilator circuit (without gaining exposure to the patient, see p. 68). In healthy persons the normal V_D/V_T during spontaneous breathing varies from $\simeq 0.35$ to 0.15, depending on the vigor of respiration, the CO, and the tidal volume. (V_D/V_T tends to rise as tidal volume falls.) In the setting of critical illness, however, it is not uncommon for V_D/V_T to rise to values that exceed 0.7. Indeed, increased deadspace ventilation usually accounts for the majority of the increase in the $\dot{V}E$ requirement and CO_2 retention that occur in the terminal phase of acute hypoxemic respiratory failure.

In addition to pathologic processes that increase deadspace, *functional changes in V_D/V_T occur during periods of hypovolemia or overdistention by high airway pressures. This phenomenon is often apparent when progressive levels of positive end-expiratory pressure (PEEP) are applied to support oxygenation. Examination of the airway pressure tracing under conditions of controlled, squarewave ventilation may demonstrate concavity or a clear point of upward inflection, corresponding to a threshold pressure associated with overdistention, accelerated deadspace formation, and escalating risk of barotrauma. Small reductions in PEEP or tidal volume may then dramatically reduce peak cycling pressure and V_D/V_T.

CO$_2$ Monitoring of Exhaled Gas

Capnography analyzes the CO_2 concentration of the exhaled airstream. Once anatomic deadspace has been cleared, the CO_2 tension progressively rises to its maximal volume at end-exhalation, a number that tracks the mean alveolar value (P_ACO_2). Furthermore, when ventilation and perfusion are evenly distributed, end-tidal PCO_2 ($P_{ET}CO_2$) closely approximates $PaCO_2$. ($P_{ET}CO_2$ normally underestimates $PaCO_2$ by 1–3 mm Hg.) This difference widens when ventilation and perfusion are suboptimally matched.

As with other monitoring techniques, exhaled CO_2 values must be interpreted cautiously. The normal capnogram is composed of an ascending portion, a plateau, a descending portion, and a baseline (Fig. 5.2). $P_{ET}CO_2$ gives a low range estimate of $PaCO_2$ in virtually all clinical circumstances so that a high $P_{ET}CO_2$ strongly suggests hypoventilation. Abrupt changes in $P_{ET}CO_2$ may reflect such acute processes as aspiration or pulmonary embolism. Although breath-to-breath fluctuations in $P_{ET}CO_2$ can be extreme, the trend of $P_{ET}CO_2$ over time helps to identify underlying changes in CO_2 exchange. The capnogram also provides an excellent monitor of breathing rhythm. In evaluating the $P_{ET}CO_2$ it is essential to record and examine the entire capnographic tracing, not relying on digital readouts alone. Breathing pattern can be as influential as pathology, especially when gas flow is inhomogeneously distributed, as in airflow obstruction. Failure of the tracing to achieve a true plateau can occur because the sampling technique is inappropriate, exhalation is too brief, or ventilation is inhomogeneously distributed. Thus, the $P_{ET}CO_2$ may fluctuate for a variety of reasons, not all of which imply changes in lung disease.

The arterial to end-tidal CO_2 difference is minimized when perfused alveoli are maximally recruited. On this basis, the $(PaCO_2 - P_{ET}CO_2)$ difference has been suggested as helpful in identifying "best PEEP". This technique may have particular value in patients in whom a clear inflection point observed on the ascending limb of the airway pressure tracing suggests recruitable volume.

MONITORING LUNG AND CHEST WALL MECHANICS

In cooperative ambulatory patients, respiratory mechanics—those properties of the lung and chest wall that determine the ease of chest expansion—are best measured in the pulmonary function laboratory. However, because most patients with critical illness cannot cooperate and are often supported by a mechanical ventilator, the clinician must become his or her own pulmonary function analyst.

Pressure-Volume Relationships

A good understanding of static pressure-volume relationships is fundamental to the interpretation of chest mechanics. These elastic properties of the thorax are discussed at length in *Respiratory Medicine for the House Officer* (Ref. 7). Certain key concepts, however, deserve emphasis here. Gas flows to and from the alveoli driven by differences in pressure, however they may be generated. The difference between airway and atmospheric pressures dissipates in two primary ways: (1) in driving gas between the airway opening and the alveolus, and (2) in expanding the alveoli against the recoil forces of the lung and chest wall. The pressure required to expand the lung by a certain volume (ΔV) is the corresponding change in transpulmonary pressure: $\Delta P_l = \Delta (P_{alv} - P_{pl})$, where P_{alv} = alveolar pressure and P_{pl} = pleural pressure. The lung compliance

$$(C_L = \Delta V / \Delta P_l)$$

is the pressure required per unit volume to keep the lung expanded under no-flow (static) conditions. The distensibility of the relaxed chest wall is characterized by chest wall compliance $(C_w = \Delta V / \Delta P_{pl})$. The slope of the static pressure-volume relationship for the total respiratory system (C_{rs}) is $\Delta V / \Delta P_{alv}$. In ventilator-derived calculations of

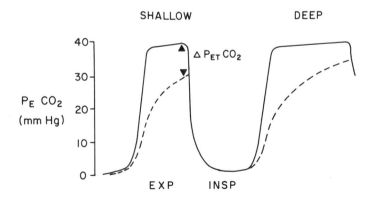

Figure 5.2 Capnographic tracing. Expired CO_2 tension (P_ECO_2) varies markedly during breathing cycle in 4 phases. Wide separation of end-expiratory values of end-tidal CO_2 ($\Delta P_{ET}CO_2$) for normal subject (solid line) and patient with increased anatomic deadspace (dashed line) narrows during more complete exhalation.

compliance, ΔV must be measured at the endotracheal tube, or expired volume must be adjusted for the volume stored during pressurized inflation in compressible circuit elements. As a useful rule of thumb, approximately 3 ml of volume are stored per cmH_2O of peak cycling pressure for an average adult circuit. The physician should be aware, however, that this figure may vary markedly, depending on the peak cycling pressure. The compression factor of the same circuit at 20 cmH_2O of peak cycling pressure may be much less than it is when 60 cmH_2O are required, and *delivered* tidal volume will fluctuate accordingly. Compliance measurements may have therapeutic and prognostic value in patients with arterial desaturation.

When PEEP is applied incrementally, C_L and C_{rs} tend to reach their highest values when lung units are maximally recruited. This point also tends to be that associated with minimal ventilatory deadspace and shunt fraction, and often coincides with the point of maximal oxygen delivery. Although this guideline does not always apply, it is a good general rule not to use values of end-expiratory pressure or tidal volume that depress thoracic compliance—unless objective evidence of improved oxygen delivery is available. Followed over time, serial changes in the respiratory pressure-volume curve and C_{rs} tend to reflect the nature and course of acute lung injury. Severe disease is implied when compliance falls to less than 25 ml/cmH_2O. Maximal depression of C_{rs} often requires 1–2 weeks to develop in the setting of acute lung injury.

Although C_{rs} provides useful information regarding the difficulty of chest inflation, C_{rs} *does not necessarily parallel underlying tissue elastance*—both the size of the alveolar compartment and the relative position on the pressure volume curve are important to consider. For example, identical pressures drive greatly different volumes into the chest of a patient before and after pneumonectomy. Ideally, compliance is referenced to a measure of absolute lung volume, such as FRC or TLC ("specific" compliance). Furthermore, C_{rs} may change greatly in the extremes of the vital capacity range, even in the same individual. Thus, most patients with hyperinflated lungs ventilated for acute exacerbations of asthma or chronic obstructive pulmonary disease exhibit depressed C_{rs}, despite normal or "super normal" tissue distensibility; C_{rs} would be better if measured in a lower volume range. Because compliances add in parallel, C_{rs} bears a complex relationship to the individual compliances of the lung and chest wall:

$C_{rs} = (C_l \times C_w)/(C_w + C_l)$. It should be kept in mind that the usual assumption that the pressure-volume characteristic of the chest wall is linear and unchanging throughout its range is often invalid in critically ill patients whose distensibility may be disturbed by abdominal distention, effusions, ascites, muscular tone, recent surgery, position, binders, braces, and so on. Such changes in C_w are important to consider, in that they influence the interpretation of hemodynamic data (e.g., pulmonary artery occlusion pressure, P_w), as well as calculations of chest mechanics. Specified values for peak airway pressure and C_{rs} have different prognostic significance, depending on whether the lung or chest wall accounts for the stiffness. Furthermore, the fraction of end-expiratory airway pressure (PEEP) transmitted to the pleural space depends on the relative compliances of the lungs and chest wall: $\Delta P_{pl} = PEEP \times (C_l/(C_l + C_w))$. Thus, apart from any effect on venous return, the relative stiffness of the lungs and chest wall determines the effect of PEEP on measured P_w (see p. 20).

Calculation of Compliance and Resistance During Mechanical Ventilation

Although not always elegantly presented or continuously displayed, all ventilators monitor external airway pressure (P_{aw}). When a mechanical ventilator expands the chest of a passive subject, inspiratory P_{aw} furnishes the entire force accomplishing ventilation, dissipating against frictional and elastic forces. Because the pressure volume relationships of the lung and chest wall are approximately linear over the tidal volume range, and because the increment in P_{aw} necessary to drive gas flow is nearly unchanging under constant flow conditions, the corresponding P_{aw} waveform resembles a trapezoid, a shape composed of a triangle of elastic pressure and a parallelogram of resistive pressure (Fig. 5.3).

Although the inspiratory resistance and compliance characteristics of the mechanically ventilated respiratory system can be gauged in several ways, in clinical practice, these data are usually estimated from P_{aw} alone. It should be emphasized, however, that calculations of C_{rs} and resistance from P_{aw} can only be made when inflation is passive. (During active effort, P_{aw} must be supplemented by esophageal pressure to make the relevant calculations.) When gas is prevented from exiting at the end of inspiration, P_{aw} falls quickly to a plateau value. If this end-inspiratory "stop flow", "plateau", or

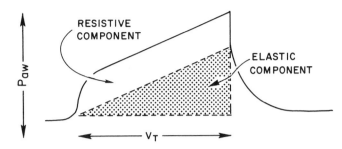

Figure 5.3 Airway pressure tracing during inflation of the passive respiratory system at a constant rate of inspiratory flow. Total inflation pressure is dissipated in expanding the lungs and chest wall (elastic work) and in driving gas from the airway opening to the alveolar level (resistive work). The slope of the elastic triangle is C_{rs}.

"peak static" (P_S) pressure is referenced to end-expiratory alveolar pressure (PEEP or Auto-PEEP), the difference determines the component of end-inspiratory pressure necessary to overcome the elastic forces of chest inflation. When tidal volume (adjusted for gas compression) is divided by (P_S − PEEP), effective compliance (C_{eff}) can be computed:

$$C_{eff} = (V_T − C_{cf} \times (P_S − PEEP))/$$
$$(P_S − PEEP)$$

where C_{cf} is the circuit compression factor, expressed in ml/cmH$_2$O.

The maximal pressure achieved just prior to the end of gas delivery (the peak dynamic pressure, P_D) is the total system pressure required to drive gas to the alveolar level at the selected flow rate and to expand the lungs and chest wall by the full V_T. The difference between P_D and P_S quantifies the gradient driving gas flow at end-inspiration, a difference that varies with the resistance of the patient and endotracheal tube as well as with the inspiratory gas flow setting. When corrected for the compression volume of the external circuit, the ratio of delivered volume to (P_D − PEEP) − the "dynamic characteristic"

$$DC = V_{Tcorr}/(P_D − PEEP)$$

reflects the overall difficulty of chest expansion, provided V_T and inspiratory flow settings do not change, and that inflation occurs passively. Because P_D is influenced both by the frictional and elastic properties of the thorax, it serves as a simple yet valuable indicator of bronchodilator response under passive conditions, again provided that flow rate and V_T remain unchanged.

During controlled inflation with squarewave inspiratory flow, and stable airway resistance (R_{aw}), the slope of the inspiratory pressure ramp should reflect C_{rs} (see Fig. 5.3). However, estimates of C_{rs} made by this technique (and those by the method previously described) are inappropriately low, unless auto-PEEP is taken into account. When there is occult positive end-expiratory pressure (Auto-PEEP) at the onset of inspiration, the relevant pressure for chest expansion is (P_S − Auto-PEEP), not P_S alone.

Whereas P_D and P_S can be measured rather precisely, the flow rate on which the bedside R_{aw} computation depends is not always reflected accurately by the peak flow setting of the machine. Indeed, flow rates at end-inflation are often lower than set, especially in patients with elevated chest impedance, because many ventilators do not maintain constant flow against increasing back pressure. Of course, a deliberately set decelerating flow profile is subject to the same misinterpretation.

Endotracheal Tube Resistance

The endotracheal tube often contributes greatly to R_{aw}. Depending on the nature, length, diameter, patency, and angulation of the endotracheal tube, computed values for R_{aw} may be dominated by the resistive properties of the external airway. Marked flow dependence of resistance may also be demonstrated in certain patients, a phenomenon usually attributed to turbulence developing in a narrow or partially occluded tube. If endogenous bronchial resistance must be monitored precisely, P_{aw} should be sensed beyond the carinal tip of the endotracheal tube. This can be done with an intraluminal catheter, or by using a tube specially designed for measuring pressures at this site during jet ventilation. Values for C_{rs} (computed under static conditions) remain valid, whatever the resistances of endotracheal tube or airway may be.

Auto-PEEP (Intrinsic PEEP) Effect

In the presence of increased airway resistance, the need for high levels of ventilation may cause hyperinflation when insufficient time elapses between inflation cycles to re-establish the equilibrium (resting) position of the respiratory system (Fig. 5.4). Consequently, when a mechanical ventilator powers inflation, alveolar pressure (P_{alv}) remains continuously positive through both phases of the respiratory cycle. Airflow is not stopped at end exhalation but continues very slowly as increased alveolar pressure decompresses through critically narrowed airways.

Although deliberate generation of lung distention by this mechanism can be useful as a ventilatory technique in patients with refractory hypoxemia (see p. 71), auto-PEEP is usually an inadvertent phenomenon with potentially adverse hemodynamic and mechanical consequences. *Barotrauma* is an obvious risk of hyperinflation. Unlike restrictive lung disease, obstructive lung disease allows normal transmission of alveolar pressure to the pleural space. Thus, the *hemodynamic consequences* of the auto-PEEP effect may be more severe than those incurred with intentionally applied PEEP of a similar level. Auto-PEEP also adds to the *work of breathing*, presenting an increased threshold load to inspiration and depressing the effective triggering sensitivity of the ventilator. In such cases, the addition of low levels of exogenous PEEP (less than the auto-PEEP level) to patients with quantifiable auto-PEEP may improve subject comfort and the work of breathing, without markedly increasing lung volume or peak cycling pressure. As already mentioned, auto-PEEP must be accounted for to accurately measure chest compliance. At the bedside, auto-PEEP can be quantified by occluding the expiratory port of the ventilator at the end of the period allowed for exhalation between mechanical breaths.

End-Expiratory Port Occlusion Method

For accuracy, occlusion must occur just prior to the subsequent ventilator-delivered breath—timing that is easiest to achieve during controlled ventilation. Alternative methods to quantify auto-PEEP require specialized sensing equipment and displays. For example, auto-PEEP can be detected without precise quantification simply by noting that *flow fails to cease during expiration*, remaining elevated above the zero flow line in the period immediately prior to machine activation.

Esophageal Pressure Monitoring

Knowledge of intrapleural pressure often facilitates clinical decision making. Fluctuations of global intrathoracic pressure can be estimated by a well-positioned esophageal balloon. Esophageal pressure (P_{es}) enables estimation of force generation during all patient-initiated breaths (spontaneous or machine-assisted) and allows partitioning of transthoracic pressure into its lung and chest wall components during passive inflation. Furthermore, P_{es} helps interpret pulmonary artery and wedge pressures under conditions of vigorous hyperpnea or elevated alveolar pressure (PEEP, Auto-PEEP). The knowledge of intrapleural pressure provided by the P_{es} tracing also permits calculation of lung compliance and airway resistance during spontaneous breathing.

The ΔP_{es} can be used to compute the work of breathing across the lung and external circuit or to calculate the product of developed pressure and the duration of inspiratory effort (the pressure-time product). It has been suggested that fluctuations in *central venous pressure can serve a similar purpose*, but the damped vascular pressure tracing

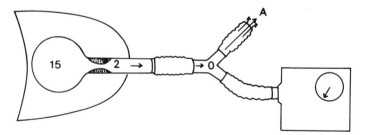

Figure 5.4 Dynamic hyperinflation and auto-PEEP. High levels of alveolar pressure go undetected as slow expiratory flow continues through an open expiratory port (*A*). An auto-PEEP effect may be seen in virtually any circumstance that causes high demand for ventilation—even in patients without severe airflow obstruction.

yields a low range estimate of effort. Such underestimation occurs because venous return tends to rise as intrathoracic pressure falls; conversely, venous return declines when intrathoracic pressure rises.

Transdiaphragmatic pressure (P_{Di}), the difference between P_{es} and gastric pressure, is generated by a single inspiratory muscle (the diaphragm) and can be used to quantify its effective contractile force. Clinically, the P_{Di} is occasionally used in conjunction with phrenic nerve stimulation or voluntary effort to investigate diaphragmatic paralysis.

Given its utility and ease of measurement, it is surprising that greater clinical use has not been made of the P_{es}. The thin esophageal catheter ($\simeq$ 2 mm diameter) is relatively comfortable to insert and poses little risk of esophageal perforation. Appropriate placement is achieved by first inflating the 10-cm long balloon with $\simeq$ 1 ml of air and passing it into the stomach. The catheter is carefully withdrawn until negative pressure deflections are observed during spontaneous inspiratory efforts. The balloon is then withdrawn another 10 cm, and its final position tested by occluding the airway and measuring the simultaneous deflections in P_{aw} and P_{es}. (With the airway occluded, these deflections should closely approximate one another.) As a general rule, P_{es} is best measured in an upright position. However, a lateral decubitus position may suffice if the patient must remain recumbent. (The supine position is suboptimal.) Although their absolute values differ, *fluctuations* in P_{es} more or less accurately reflect *fluctuations* in P_{pl} in all positions.

Value of Continuously Monitoring P_{aw}

A continuous tracing of P_{aw} provides useful information commonly neglected at the bedside (Fig. 5.5). Airway pressure can be continuously monitored using the transducer and display equipment normally used for measuring pressures in the pulmonary vasculature. A dedicated transducer must be used for this purpose, however, to avoid the risk of air embolism. Apart from enabling estimation of R_{aw} and C_{rs}, the waveform of inspiratory airway pressure traced during a controlled machine cycle provides graphic evidence of the inflation work performed by the ventilator at the particular combination of tidal volume and flow setting in use (and consequently the difficulty of chest inflation). When inflation occurs passively during constant flow, the area under the pressure-time curve is proportionate to the work performed by the machine to inflate the chest, and the pressure

measured halfway through the cycle ($\bar{P}$) is the work per liter of ventilation. When flow and tidal volume are matched to spontaneous values, $\bar{P}$ is a good estimate of the pressure needed to fully ventilate the patient during pressure support ventilation.

The shape of the airway pressure tracing should also be examined frequently. During constant flow, concavity of the airway pressure ramp indicates that C_{rs} is continuously deteriorating throughout inflation (as when the lung is hyperinflated), or more commonly that the patient expends effort during triggered cycles. An upward inflection of the terminal portion of the inspiratory airway pressure tracing (concavity) suggests that the combination of end-expiratory pressure and tidal volume chosen generate pressures that risk overdistention and barotrauma. Conversely, marked convexity of the P_{aw} tracing during constant flow indicates that inflation is becoming easier as the breath proceeds. Such a profile can be seen when volume is alternately recruited and derecruited during the breathing cycle, when auto-PEEP is present (requiring an initial counterbalancing pressure), or when resistance is highly volume dependent (Fig. 5.5). Cycle-to-cycle variations in the peak dynamic pressure of machine-aided breaths suggest that the durations of inspiratory effort and flow delivery are not well matched or synchronous (Fig. 5.6).

MONITORING BREATHING EFFORT

Oxygen Consumption of the Respiratory System

The oxygen consumed by the ventilatory pump ($\dot{V}O_{2R}$) estimates effort at its most basic level—cellular metabolism. In theory, $\dot{V}O_{2R}$ accounts for all factors that tax the respiratory muscles, i.e., the external workload ($\dot{W}$) and the efficiency (e) of the conversion mechanism

$$(\dot{V}O_{2R} = \dot{W}/e).$$

Two patients with different chest configurations, patterns of muscle activation, or degrees of coordination between the muscles of inspiration and expiration may perform identical external work ($\dot{W}$) but consume vastly different amounts of O_2 in the process. Because $\dot{V}O_{2R}$ cannot be measured directly, total body oxygen consumption ($\dot{V}O_2$) is tracked as ventilatory stresses are imposed or relieved, perturbing the respiratory system. Unfortunately, $\dot{V}O_2$ is difficult to measure in unstable intensive care unit (ICU) patients. Thus, other measures of respiratory muscle effort are usually sought.

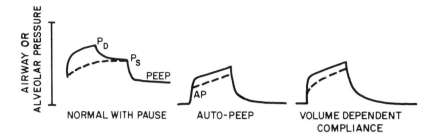

Figure 5.5 Continuous airway pressure tracings during controlled ventilation. Airway pressure (solid line) and alveolar pressure (dashed line) are represented. In a passive subject P_{aw} measured at end inflation and after a brief inspiratory pause provides the data needed to compute airway resistance: $(P_D - P_S)$/flow rate and C_{rs}: V_{Tcorr}/$(P_S - PEEP)$. Auto-PEEP (AP) and volume dependence of compliance cause the P_{aw} contour to "square-off".

Direct Measures of External Mechanical Output

External Work of Breathing

Mechanical work is accomplished when a pressure gradient (ΔP) moves the lung or relaxed chest wall (passive structures) through a volume change. At volumes (V) above relaxed functional residual capacity (FRC), pressure dissipates against frictional and elastic forces in the following way: $P = R_{aw} \times \dot{V} + V/C_{rs}$. Average developed pressure ($\bar{P}$) for the tidal inflation (V_T) can be expressed

$$\bar{P} = R_{aw} \times (V_T/t_i) + V_T/2C_{rs} + \text{Auto-PEEP}$$

and is numerically equivalent to the work per liter of ventilation. (Work per tidal breath (W_b) can be quantified from the product of $\bar{P}$ and V_T.) Thus, if R_{aw}, C_{rs}, t_i, and V_T are known for the spontaneously breathing subject, the external work rate for inspiration can be easily computed. (Exhalation normally proceeds passively, dissipating elastic energy stored during the inspiratory half cycle.) Such computations also serve to conveniently estimate the pressure support level needed to achieve most ventilatory needs. When the ventilator per-

forms the entire workload for a passive patient, total inflation pressure (P) is simply P_{aw}. (When inflation is achieved with a constant flow waveform, $\bar{P}$ is then approximated by the inflation pressure at mid-cycle.) However, no exertion must occur during inflation and to be relevant to spontaneous breathing, V_T and peak flow rate must approximate the appropriate values. With pressures and volumes expressed in the customary way, a convenient work unit is the joule (or watt-second) $\simeq 10$ cmH$_2$O $\times$ 1 liter (1 kg $\cdot$ m $\simeq 10$ joules.) Total inspiratory mechanical work per minute is the product of $\bar{P}$ and minute ventilation ($\dot{V}_e$) or of W_b and f, the breathing frequency.

Influence of Auto-PEEP on Work of Breathing

Auto-PEEP (AP) imposes a threshold load on inspiration in that the patient must supply a pressure sufficient to counterbalance AP before central airway pressure falls enough to trigger the ventilator. The threshold load imposed by AP effectively reduces the triggering sensitivity of the machine to a value equal to the sum of AP and the set trigger sensitivity value. In this setting,

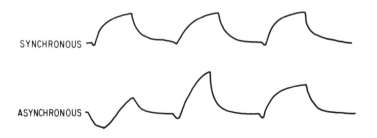

Figure 5.6 Airway pressure tracings during AMV. Variation in contour and peak cycling pressure characterize asynchrony between the respiratory rhythm of patient and ventilator.

judicious use of low levels of continuous positive airway pressure (CPAP) or PEEP ($\leq$ auto-PEEP level) can help restore trigger sensitivity and reduce the work of breathing. Additional PEEP should not be used if it causes the peak dynamic cycling pressure to rise.

Spontaneous Breathing Cycles

An esophageal balloon is required to directly measure work during spontaneous, machine-assisted, or pressure-supported breathing cycles. Fluctuations in P_{es} reflect patient efforts to overcome the impedance of the lung and external circuit. (Clues to the work done against the external apparatus can be gained by examining the P_{aw} tracing). Inspiratory inflections of the P_{aw} waveform quantify the pressure needed to suck gas through the inspiratory circuitry to the point of pressure measurement (Fig. 5.7). To include the resistance of the endotracheal tube, P_{aw} must be sampled between the tube tip and the carina, a site at which much deeper pressure fluctuations may be seen during inspiration. The resistance of standard endotracheal tubes often exceeds 10 cmH$_2$O/l/sec.

Machine-assisted Breathing Cycles

Volume-limited Machine Cycles. It is often assumed that patient work is negligible during patient initiated, machine-assisted breathing cycles. Indeed, the ventilator is fully capable of performing the entire work of breathing if the patient were

to cease effort immediately after triggering inspiration. However, relaxation does not occur abruptly once the machine cycle begins; instead, patient effort continues in direct proportion to the intensity of respiratory drive. When the ventilation requirement or sense of dyspnea is high (e.g., when the ventilator is poorly adjusted with respect to sensitivity, peak inspiratory flow rate, inspiratory duration, or tidal volume), exertion levels may approach those of unsupported breathing. Interestingly, resistance and compliance do not influence W_b during triggered cycles, provided that the machine fully satisfies the patient's peak flow demand ($\simeq 4 \times \dot{V}_e$, see p. 69). However, should the patient's flow demand exceed the delivery rate, the patient works against the resistance of the ventilator's circuitry as well as against the innate impedance characteristics of the chest. Clues to patient exertion during triggered machine cycles are provided by the airway pressure tracing, as already described. When a P_{aw} tracing is not used, the only clue to excessive patient effort during a triggered cycle may be the stuttering rise of the manometer needle to its peak value. P_D itself may not be much different from expected, inasmuch as inspiratory effort slackens near the end of inflation.

Pressure-Support Cycles. During pressure-support cycles, patient effort can only be gauged directly from the P_{es} tracing. Inspiratory airway pressure is maintained nearly constant by the machine at the preset level.

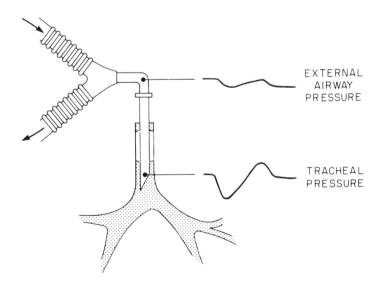

Figure 5.7 Airway and tracheal pressure tracings during spontaneous breathing. External recordings do not reflect exertion against the ET-tube.

Pressure Time Product and Pressure Time Index

Isometric components of muscle tension which consume oxygen without contributing to volume change fail to register as externally measured work, accounting in large part for the lack of agreement between $\dot{V}O_{2R}$ and W_b. A pressure time product (PTP = $\bar{P} \times t_i$) parallels effort and $\dot{V}O_{2R}$ more closely than W_b because it includes the isometric component of muscle pressure and is less influenced by the afterload to contraction. When $\bar{P}$ (as computed above) is referenced to the maximal isometric pressure that can be generated at FRC (P_{max}) and inspiratory time (t_i) is expressed as a fraction of total cycle length (t_{tot}), a useful effort index is derived: Pressure-time index (PTI) = $\bar{P}/P_{max} \times t_i/t_{tot}$. Values of PTI that exceed 0.15 identify highly stressful breathing workloads that may not be sustainable (see p. 88).

MONITORING VENTILATORY DRIVE AND BREATHING PATTERN

Importance of Assessing Ventilatory Drive

Remarkably little attention has previously been paid to drive measurement during critical illness. Heightened ventilatory drive increases work expenditure during triggered machine cycles and often signals pain, sepsis, and important perturbations of the cardiopulmonary system. During machine-assisted breathing cycles, ventilatory drive plays a more important role in determining the energy expenditure of the patient than any indicator of ventilatory mechanics—provided that the flow delivered by the machine exceeds the patient's flow demand. Derangements in ventilatory drive also furnish clues regarding the ability of the patient to wean from ventilator support. Recent clinical studies demonstrate that most patients who fail to wean from mechanical ventilation have elevated drives to breathe but may have blunted sensitivity to CO_2.

Ventilatory Drive Indices

Several methods can be used to index drive. When respiratory mechanics and strength reserves are normal, minute ventilation ($\dot{V}_e$) directly parallels the output of the ventilatory control center. Unfortunately, such conditions are seldom met in the clinical setting. $\dot{V}_e$ can be viewed as the product of mean inspiratory flow rate (the quotient of tidal volume and inspiratory time, V_T/t_i) and the inspiratory time fraction or duty cycle (t_i/t_{tot}): $\dot{V}E = V_T/t_i \times t_i/t_{tot}$). Both components yield useful

and largely ignored clinical information. Mean inspiratory flow (V_T/t_i), provides another potential index of drive but also depends upon the mechanical properties of the ventilatory system. The airway pressure generated against a surreptitiously occluded airway 100 msec after the onset of inspiratory effort (the $P_{0.1}$) is measured before the conscious recognition of occlusion, so that the corresponding outflow from the respiratory center is representative of the unimpeded cycles that preceeded it. As an isometric measurement, the $P_{0.1}$ is influenced by muscle strength and lung volume, but does *not* depend on respiratory mechanics. The delay imposed by the demand valve systems of certain ventilators in common use provide a quasi-occlusion period long enough to allow close estimation of $P_{0.1}$. However, the measurement of this index requires a sensitive pressure recording system and very rapid recording rates.

Breathing Pattern, Frequency, and Duty Cycle

The breathing pattern also offers valuable information. When muscular strength is limited, patients tend to meet $\dot{V}_E$ requirements by increasing frequency (f) without raising V_T. Although smaller breaths require less effort, the cost to the patient is increased deadspace ventilation and the need for a higher $\dot{V}_E$ to eliminate CO_2. Thus, although *work per breath* (W_b) is controlled by limiting tidal volume, *total work* (the product of f and W_b) per minute tends to increase when f exceeds some optimal value. A very high and continuously rising frequency (to rates > 30 breaths/min) is generally accepted as a sign of ventilatory muscle decompensation and impending fatigue. It should be noted, however, that some patients increase f to a stable value > 35 breaths per minute and remain compensated. As the ventilatory muscles fatigue, the duty cycle (t_i/t_{tot}), the fraction of each breathing cycle spent in inspiration, Also changes. When there is a breathing stress, t_i/t_{tot} normally increases from $\simeq$ 0.35 to a value of 0.40 to 0.50 during spontaneous breathing. ("Inspiratory time" may be fixed by chosen values of inspiratory flow rate and tidal volume during constant flow mechanical ventilation.) At the limits of compensation, the t_i/t_{tot} fails to increase with further stress and may actually decline.

At times of maximal effort, noteworthy alterations may be observed in the pattern of activation and coordination of the ventilatory muscle groups. Although normally passive, expiratory muscles may be called into play whenever the inspiratory muscles face a stressful burden in relation to their capability e.g., during expiratory airflow obstruction, when high levels of PEEP or CPAP are used, when the patient is anxious, when machine-controlled inspiratory duration is excessive, and at high levels of V_E. Visible use of the accessory muscles, especially the sternocleidomastoid group, may also signal the approach to the limits of ventilatory compensation.

Two indices once thought to always indicate diaphragmatic dysfunction or fatigue—*asynchrony* between the peak excursions of chest and abdominal compartments and *paradoxical inward movement of the abdomen* on inspiration—may sometimes reflect the normal response of a compensated system under extraordinary stress. Asynchrony between the excursions of rib cage and abdomen may be a stage in the development of full blown abdominal paradox. *Respiratory alternans*, another reported pattern of fatigue in which muscles of the chest cage and diaphragm alternate primary responsibility for achieving ventilation, is much less commonly observed than abdominal paradox.

Inductance (impedance) plethysmography yields a non-invasive means of monitoring f, V_T, t_i/t_{tot}, and respiratory muscle coordination. With this technique, loose elastic bands encircle the chest and abdomen. Changes in compartmental volume create proportional changes in the cross-sectional areas of electrical inductance loops. Fluctuations of compartmental motion can be summed to estimate overall tidal volume changes. The ratio of maximal compartmental amplitude to tidal volume (the MCA/V_T ratio) correlates with ventilatory distress and provides tangible evidence of mechanical inefficiency.

Impedance plethysmography can also be used as an apnea detector in non-intubated patients and may prove helpful in monitoring volume changes during pressure-cycled modes of ventilation (e.g., pressure support, pressure control, and intermittent positive pressure breathing (IPPB)).

MONITORING STRENGTH AND MUSCLE RESERVE (ENDURANCE)

The ability of a patient to sustain independent breathing must not be judged on the basis of any absolute value for workload, but rather on workload interpreted against the background of muscular strength and endurance.

Strength Measures

The two measures of respiratory muscle strength most commonly used in the clinical setting are the vital capacity (VC) and the maximal inspiratory pressure (MIP) generated against an occluded airway. Maximal activation of the respiratory musculature requires intense voluntary effort. Therefore, without full patient cooperation it is questionable that any measure of strength can reflect the full capability for pressure development.

Vital Capacity

In cooperative patients VC tends to be preserved relative to MIP for two primary reasons. First, the pressure volume relationship of the thorax is convex to the volume axis, so that small applied pressures achieve relatively large volume changes. Second, whereas many seriously ill patients can generate brief spikes of inspiratory pressure, few can sustain inspiratory effort long enough to achieve the plateau of their volume curve. Routine measurements of VC involve a single forceful effort from residual volume to total lung capacity (or the converse). However, many weak patients fail to sustain inspiratory effort long enough to achieve their potential maximum. Others simply refuse or cannot fully cooperate with the testing. Thus, in critically ill patients the VC has proven to be a disappointing measure of strength. Recently, a method has been described by which a one-way valve can be used to achieve a "stacked vital capacity", even when patients do not cooperate fully with testing.

Maximal Inspiratory Pressure

The maximal inspiratory pressure (MIP) is an isometric pressure measured in a totally occluded airway after 20 seconds or 10 breathing efforts. A one-way valve directed toward expiration can insure that inspiratory efforts begin from a lung volume low enough to achieve maximal mechanical advantage. The P_{aw} during the MIP maneuver should be measured continuously, either with a needle gauge or (preferably) by a pressure transducer linked to a recording apparatus. Ideally, the MIP is held for at least 1 second; a transient isometric pressure may bear little relation to true ventilatory muscle strength and endurance. The MIP is perhaps the only involuntary measure of muscle strength that is even moderately reliable. However, it should be kept in mind that the validity of MIP in uncooperative patients depends on the strength of ventilatory drive, and that the intensity of a voluntary effort in a fully cooperative patient is likely to exceed that elicited by simple airway occlusion.

Measures of Endurance

Mechanical Reserve

Simple indices of ventilatory power reserve, the ratio of $\dot{V}e$ requirement to maximal minute ventilation (MVV), and the V_T/VC have long been used to predict the outcome of machine withdrawal. On empirical grounds it has been suggested that ratios > 50% portend weaning failure. Interestingly, newer laboratory data confirm that only ≃ 50–60% of the MVV can be sustained > 15 minutes without ventilatory fatigue.

Electromyography

In the physiology laboratory an increasing ratio of the integrated diaphragmatic electromyographic (EMG) signal to $\bar{P}$ suggests a declining ability of the muscle pump to respond to neural stimulation (i.e., fatigue). Another EMG index of interest characterizes the spectrum of frequencies represented within the diaphragmatic EMG signal. The high frequency to low frequency ratio (H/L) is a good indicator of ventilatory stress and may be a sensitive and specific indicator of developing fatigue. Unfortunately, the diaphragmatic EMG (measured by surface or esophageal electrodes) is not commonly available, and advanced signal conditioning is required to compute the H/L ratio.

Pressure Time Index

Measured accurately, the MIP can be used in conjunction with $\bar{P}$ to judge endurance and the likelihood of weaning success. In the laboratory setting, a diaphragmatic $\bar{P}/P_{max}$ ratio > 40% (with $t_i/t_{tot} = 0.40$) or a pressure-time index (PTI = $\bar{P}/P_{max} \times t_i/t_{tot}$) > 0.15 predicts the inability to sustain a target workload. No confirmatory data are yet available for the specific clinical setting of the weaning trial.

Sequential Drive Indices

A practical indication of declining power reserve may also be provided by a comparison of sequential drive indices (such as the $P_{0.1}$) during the stress period. Recent work suggests that patients who fail to increase ventilatory drive in response to increasing $PaCO_2$ are prone to alveolar hypoventilation and weaning failure. In the future, monitoring the response of such indices as $P_{0.1}$ to imposed stress or CO_2 loading may provide valuable clinical indications of breathing reserve.

SUGGESTED READINGS

1. Bone RC: Respiratory Monitoring. Chapter 5. In Fallat RJ, Luce JM (eds): Cardiopulmonary Critical Care Management, Vol 14. In *Clinics in Critical Care Medicine*. New York, Churchill-Livingstone, pp 89–112, 1988.
2. Cohen C, Zagelbaum D, Gross D, et al: Clinical manifestations of inspiratory muscle fatigue. *Am J Med* 73:308–316, 1982.
3. Fallat RJ: Respiratory monitoring. In Bone RC (ed): *Critical Care: A Comprehensive Approach*. American College of Chest Physicians, Park Ridge, IL, pp 189–205, 1984.
4. Hess D, Maxwell C: Which is the best index of oxygenation: $P(A-a)O_2$, PaO_2/P_AO_2 or PaO_2/FIO_2? *Respir Care* 39:961–963, 1985.
5. Hubmayr RD, Gay PC, Tayyab M: Respiratory system mechanics in ventilated patients: techniques and indications. *Mayo Clin Proc* 62:358–368, 1987.
6. Marini JJ: Monitoring during mechanical ventilation. *Clin Chest Med* 9(1):73–100, 1988.
7. Marini JJ: *Respiratory Medicine for the House Officer*, ed 2. Baltimore, Williams & Wilkins, 1987.
8. Marini JJ, Rodriguez RM, Lamb VJ: The inspiratory workload of patient-initiated mechanical ventilation. *Am Rev Respir Dis* 134:902–909, 1986.
9. Milic-Emili J: Is weaning an art or a science? *Am Rev Respir Dis* 134:1107–1108, 1986.
10. Pepe PE, Marini JJ: Occult positive end-expiratory pressure in mechanically ventilated patients with airflow obstruction: the auto-PEEP effect. *Am Rev Respir Dis* 126:166–170, 1982.
11. Rossi A, Gottfried SB, Zocchi L, et al: Measurement of static compliance of the total respiratory system in patients with acute respiratory failure during mechanical ventilation. The effect of "intrinsic peep." *Am Rev Respir Dis* 131:672–677, 1985.
12. Smith TC, Marini JJ: Impact of PEEP on lung mechanics and work of breathing in severe airflow obstruction. *J Appl Physiol* 65:1488–1499, 1988.
13. Spence AA (ed): Respiratory monitoring in intensive care (Symposium). Vol 4. In *Clinics in Critical Care Medicine*. New York, Churchill-Livingstone, pp 1–162, 1982.
14. Tobin MJ, Perez W, Guenther SM, et al: The pattern of breathing during successful and unsuccessful trials of weaning from mechanical ventilation. *Am Rev Respir Dis* 134:1111–1118, 1986.
15. Truwit JD, Marini JJ: Evaluation of thoracic mechanics in the ventilated patient. Part I: Primary measurements. *J Crit Care* 3:133–150, 1988.
16. Truwit JD, Marini JJ: Evaluation of thoracic mechanics in the ventilated patient. Part II: Applied mechanics. *J Crit Care* 3:199– 213, 1988.
17. Tuxen DV, Lane S: The effects of ventilatory pattern on hyperinflation, airway pressures and circulation in mechanical ventilation of patients with severe airflow obstruction. *Am Rev Respir Dis* 136:872–879, 1987.

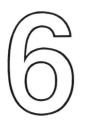

Endotracheal Intubation

INDICATIONS

Indications for endotracheal intubation include:

1. the need for assisted ventilation or high levels of inspired oxygen
2. airway protection against aspiration
3. clearance of secretions retained in central airways
4. relief of upper airway obstruction

ROUTES OF INTUBATION

Orotracheal (OT) *tubes* are generally easier to insert than nasotracheal (NT) tubes, making them the airway of choice in emergencies. The larger tube that may be passed by the oral route improves airway resistance and secretion management and allows passage of a fiberoptic bronchoscope (FOB) if the need arises. However, oral tubes are less stable, are less comfortable, and impair swallowing to a greater extent than do NT tubes. In addition, maintenance of oropharyngeal hygiene is difficult. Conventional OT intubation often cannot or should not be performed in patients with head injury, neck injury, or limited neck mobility (e.g., ankylosing spondylitis, rheumatoid arthritis). Fiberoptic intubating bronchoscopes and illuminated stylets make OT intubation feasible in such patients.

Nasotracheal tubes have relatively high resistance because they are long, kink easily, and tend to accumulate secretions. Furthermore, the nares do not admit tubes as large as those that the larynx will accept. NT tubes are more difficult to insert and, after several days,often cause purulent nasal discharge or sinusitis.

Tracheostomy improves comfort (potentially allowing the patient to eat, talk, and ambulate), affords excellent secretion management, minimizes airway resistance and anatomic deadspace, and eliminates the risk of laryngeal injury. However, tracheostomies have the highest associated risk of serious complications (bleeding, stenosis) and the highest incidence of post-extubation swallowing difficulty and aspiration. Unless carried out emergently for acute upper airway obstruction, tracheostomy should always be performed over an oral or nasal tube in an operating suite.

COMPLICATIONS

Endotracheal (ET) tubes bypass the mechanical defenses of the upper airway, contaminate the lower airways, and severely hamper effective coughing. Despite advances in materials and cuff design, all tubes have the potential of causing laryngeal and tracheal injury, and none completely protect against non-particulate aspiration.

Insertion Trauma

Inexpert placement of an ET tube may injure laryngeal, nasal, and pharyngeal tissues or cause dental or spinal trauma. Epistaxis occurs in a sizeable percentage of patients intubated via the NT route. Mandibular dislocation can result from forceful placement of an OT tube.

Hypoxemia/Ischemia

Patients who require supplemental O_2 are often exposed to room air during intubation, with consequent desaturation of arterial blood. Although this risk is reduced by "preoxygenation", O_2 stored in this way is quickly depleted by deep breathing. Therefore, intubation attempts should not be prolonged beyond 30 seconds before "re-oxygenating". Nasal prongs set to deliver 6–10 liters of oxygen can provide some supplemental O_2 during intubation.

Depletion of the pulmonary oxygen reservoir can be prevented by giving a rapidly acting hypnotic (e.g., thiopental 25–100 mg intravenously), followed by succinylcholine (1 mg/kg) to induce temporary paralysis. (If the patient is at risk for cardiac instability, vecuronium, although somewhat longer acting, is a safer choice.) This *apneic intubation* technique also facilitates cannulation of the larynx, shortens the time without ventilation, and lessens the hazards of laryngospasm and insertion trauma. Although apneic intubation is the preferred technique in difficult cases, the administration of sedatives and muscle relaxants is not without risk. Relaxation of the upper airway musculature may cause total obstruction if the intubation attempt is unsuccessful, and barbiturates may depress cardiac contractility. Rarely, succinylcholine can induce the syndrome of "malignant hyperthermia" (see p. 200).

Ischemia is less well tolerated than hypoxemia alone; therefore, intubation attempts should not interrupt cardiac compression for longer than 10–15 seconds during cardiopulmonary resuscitation, especially if the lungs can be effectively ventilated by mask.

In general, during emergent intubation the blind NT approach should not be attempted because of the uncertain length of time required to secure the airway. FOB often facilitates semi-emergent NT placement.

Gastric Aspiration

Stimulation of the oropharynx frequently causes vomiting, especially when the stomach is distended by food or air. Gentle cricothyroid pressure from the start of mask ventilation will help seal the esophagus against air entry. Evacuation of the stomach before intubation can also reduce the aspiration risk; however, such attempts should not delay emergent intubation.

Esophageal Intubation

Although usually of little consequence when rapidly corrected, esophageal intubation can be disastrous if unrecognized. The esophagus will not be intubated if the cords are visualized as the tube passes through. Use of a lighted stylet permits transcutaneous visualization of the tube tip as it passes the larynx, and minimizes the risk of this complication. Expansion of the upper chest, vesicular breath sounds, and rapid exhalation of air through the ET tube indicate proper placement. However, breath sounds may be remarkably normal even when the esophagus is intubated. Therefore, if tube position is uncertain, extubate, reoxygenate, and try again.

Laryngospasm

Reflex laryngospasm can prevent passage of the ET tube and may severely limit spontaneous ventilation. Rather than attempt forceful intubation (losing valuable time and causing laryngeal trauma), ventilate the patient with oxygen delivered by bag-mask insufflation. Spasm usually subsides promptly. However, if adequate ventilation cannot be achieved and the situation becomes urgent, intravenous succinylcholine (1 mg/kg) will release the spasm. Prior use of a topical anesthetic (lidocaine, 4%) minimizes the risk of laryngospasm.

Bronchospasm

Tube placement often triggers irritant receptors, producing cough and bronchospasm. Such receptors stop firing shortly after tube placement in most cases, unless the tip of the tube touches the carina. Coughing is often difficult to arrest, but an endotracheal lidocaine bolus (5 ml of 2%) may help. Infused aminophylline and nebulized atropine (2 mg) are good choices to relieve bronchospasm but do not reliably alleviate coughing.

Right Main Bronchus Intubation

There is a natural tendency to advance the ET tube beyond the carina, especially in emergent situations. The right main bronchus is less sharply angulated from the trachea than is the left and will be entered in 90% of low placements. The underventilated left lung may collapse rapidly, especially when previously ventilated with oxygen. The right upper lobe orifice may also be occluded. Although comparative auscultation is helpful, breath sounds are often surprisingly well transmitted to an underventilated lung.

ET tubes should be advanced a maximum of 2.5–5.0 cm beyond the point at which the tube cuff is seen to pass the cords. Use of a lighted stylet facilitates tip localization to the appropriate level. As a general rule, 22 cm at the 2nd molar will approximate the proper position in an average-size adult. A postprocedure chest film is necessary to check position. A generous distance between tube tip and main carina must be allowed for tube movement (see p. 97).

POINTS OF TECHNIQUE

Oral Intubation

Apart from being well prepared for emergent developments, perhaps the most important thing for the physician to do is to *relax and avoid panic*. After clearing the airway of secretions and debris, dislodge the base of the tongue from the retropharynx by lifting at the angles of the jaw. In obtunded or comatose patients, an oropharyngeal airway can be placed to maintain the passage, but such devices may stimulate vomiting in the conscious or agitated subject. The patient should be positioned with the head (not shoulders) resting on a thin pillow or a doubly folded towel. The optimal "sniffing" position is with the neck flexed and the head extended. Once this is done, the patient can generally be ventilated by mask without difficulty until the tube is inserted. Bag insufflations should be gentle and frequent, not forceful and slow.

If tube placement is not emergent, premedicate an alert patient with atropine (0.8 mg IM) and nebulized lidocaine (4%) as the patient pants to deposit the drug on the larynx and upper airway. As a general rule, agitated or seriously hypoxic patients should be quickly sedated and paralyzed (apneic intubation technique). However, this method must be used with special caution in patients who are massively obese and in those with upper airway pathology. The physician should be prepared to puncture the cricothyroid membrane with a 14-gauge needle in case the airway totally obstructs after paralysis and cannot be readily intubated. Oxygen insufflated through the needle at 2–4 l/min can maintain arterial oxygenation and a degree of ventilation until a secure airway is established.

A 9.0-mm (internal diameter) tube for an average-size male and an 8.0-mm tube for a female are good sizes to try first. Choose the largest tube that will easily pass the cords.

Curved laryngoscope blades are directed anterior to the epiglottis (Fig. 6.1). Straight-blade instruments are inserted immediately posterior to the epiglottis and allow a better view of the cords. Both instruments should lift the entire jaw upward to expose the larynx. Neither instrument should use the teeth as a fulcrum for leverage. During intubation, firm cricothyroid pressure helps to bring the cords into view and to seal the esophagus.

Flexible stylets can be used to direct the tip of the tube into a glottic opening that cannot be completely visualized. To avoid laryngeal trauma, care must be taken to ensure that the stylet does not project beyond the tip of the tube. After placement the cuff should be inflated with the minimum volume that seals without leakage under positive pressure. A standard ET tube is best anchored by a continuous single band of tape wrapped circumferentially around the neck and secured to the tube and bite block at both ends. The hands must be restrained if there is any possibility for self-extubation. In general, a nasogastric tube should decompress the stomach, especially when there is

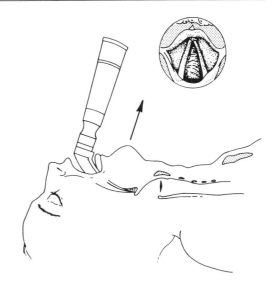

Figure 6.1 Orotracheal intubation. To align glottis, pharynx, and oral cavity, the neck is flexed and the head is extended. The laryngoscope lifts the tongue and lower jaw away from the posterior pharynx by a motion directed perpendicular to the oroglottic axis.

gut hypomotility or active air swallowing is evident in the orally intubated patient.

Flexible fiberoptic instruments (bronchoscope, laryngoscope) are advantageous when a difficult patient or one with limited neck mobility is being intubated. This is of particular importance in patients with ankylosing spondylitis or rheumatoid arthritis who have an increased risk of C1–2 subluxation with neck extension. Supplemental oxygen need not be interrupted if the fiberscope is inserted through a perforated T-piece adapter attached to the endotracheal tube. Modified NT intubation provides another safe option.

Nasotracheal Intubation

Blind NT intubation is not a technique to be performed by the inexperienced house officer. It should not be used in emergent situations and is especially inappropriate for securing the airway during apnea. Because it is usually performed in awake patients, topical anesthesia of the nose, pharynx, and larynx and sedation are mandatory. Selection of a small tube (e.g., size 7.0), generous nasal lubrication, and gentle insertion technique are necessary to prevent nasal, laryngeal, or tracheal injury. The NT tube should be initially inserted to a level just above the vocal cords. (This tube position can be detected by listening to the intensity of expired air flowing through the tube.) The tube is then rapidly but gently advanced in synchrony with the next inspiratory effort. Entrance to the larynx is usually signaled by a vigorous cough and subsequent inability to speak. Vigilance should be maintained against the development of sinusitis.

EXTUBATION

Extubation must not be performed casually. Inadvertent extubation can be lethal in acutely ill, agitated patients and must be avoided at all costs (see page 75). Extubation breaks the seal between the patient's upper and lower airway, potentially allowing secretions pooled above the cuff to enter the lung. Reflex stimulation may also provoke laryngospasm, bronchospasm, or cardiac arrhythmias.

Oxygen should be administered by nasal prongs, and the trachea and oropharynx should be cleared of secretions before the cuff is deflated. After a deep inspiration, the tube should be pulled quickly as the patient exhales forcefully from a high lung volume. Post-extubation stridor may occur due to laryngospasm or edema. This usually subsides within the first 6–24 hours, but such patients must be observed carefully to assess the need for urgent reintubation. Although not routinely necessary, racemic epinephrine and corticosteroids may be helpful in selected cases.

SUGGESTED READINGS

1. Ellis DG, Stewart RD, Kaplan RM, et al: Success rates of blind orotracheal intubation using a transillumination technique with a lighted stylet. *Ann Emerg Med* 15:138–142, 1986.
2. Heffner JE: Tracheal intubation in mechanically ventilated patients. *Clin Chest Med* 9(1):23–35, 1988.
3. Natanson C, Shelhammer JH, Parrillo JE: Intubation of the trachea in the critical care setting. *JAMA* 253:1160–1165, 1985.
4. O'Reilly MJ, Reddick EJ, Black W, et al: Sepsis from sinusitis in nasotracheally intubated patients. A diagnostic dilemma. *Am J Surg* 147:601–604, 1984.
5. Rashkin MC, Davis T: Acute complications of endotracheal intubation. Relationship to reintubation, route, urgency and duration. *Chest* 89:165–167, 1986.
6. Salem MR, Mathrabhutham M, Bennett EJ: Difficult intubation. *N Engl J Med* 295:879–881, 1976.
7. Selwyn AS: Endotracheal intubation. In Vander Salm TJ (ed): *Atlas of Bedside Procedures*. Boston, Little, Brown, pp. 159–168, 1979.
8. Stauffer JL, Silvestri RC: Complications of endotracheal intubation in tracheostomy and artificial airways. *Respir Care* 27:417–434, 1982.

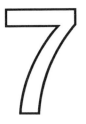

Mechanical Ventilation

INDICATIONS FOR MECHANICAL VENTILATION

The decision to institute mechanical support is independent of that to perform tracheal intubation or to use positive end-expiratory pressure (PEEP). Mechanical assistance may be necessary because ventilation is inadequate to control pH, because oxygenation cannot be achieved at a safe F_IO_2 without manipulating the pattern of ventilation, or because activity of the ventilatory muscles places excessive demands for blood flow on a compromised cardiovascular system.

Inadequate Alveolar Ventilation

Apnea is an absolute indication for instituting mechanical assistance. Likewise, patients with deteriorating ventilation despite other measures clearly need ventilatory support. In such cases, serial blood gas measurements show a falling pH and stable or rising $PaCO_2$. Although few physicians would withhold mechanical assistance when the pH trends steadily downward, there is less agreement regarding the absolute values of $PaCO_2$ and pH that warrant such intervention. In general, pH is a better indicator than $PaCO_2$ of ventilatory distress. High values of $PaCO_2$ themselves should not prompt intervention if pH remains acceptable and mental status is preserved.

Many patients require ventilatory assistance despite apparently adequate alveolar ventilation. For example, patients with metabolic acidosis and neuromuscular weakness or airflow obstruction may lower $PaCO_2$ to 40 mmHg or below, but not sufficiently to prevent acidemia.

If not reversed by simpler measures, a sustained pH > 7.65 or < 7.20 is sufficiently dangerous to require control by mechanical ventilation (and paralysis, if needed). Inside these extremes, the threshold for initiating support varies with the clinical setting. For example, a lethargic patient with asthma struggling to breathe can maintain a normal pH until shortly before suffering a respiratory arrest, whereas an alert cooperative patient with chronically blunted respiratory drive may allow pH to fall to 7.25 before recovering uneventfully in response to aggressive respiratory therapy. In less obvious situations, the decision to ventilate should be guided by *trends* in pH, arterial blood gases, mental status, dyspnea, and response to therapy.

Once mechanically assisted, a comatose overventilated patient (backup rate set too high) is frequently mistaken for an apneic one. The distinction can generally be made by increasing F_IO_2 to 1.0 for 5 breaths, then reducing the ventilator rate, waiting for 1–2 minutes, and watching for an indication of spontaneous effort (e.g., the assist indicator).

Inadequate Oxygenation

Arterial oxygenation can be raised by supplementing F_IO_2, by increasing mean airway pressure, or by changing the pattern of ventilation. Inspired oxygen fractions < 0.5 are safely and reliably administered to non-intubated patients using masks or nasal cannulas. Without tracheal intubation, delivery of high F_IO_2 can only be achieved with a tight-fitting, non-rebreathing mask, which often becomes displaced or must be intentionally removed for eating or expectoration.

Although positive airway pressure can be applied to spontaneously breathing, non-intubated patients (a mode known as continuously positive airway pressure, CPAP), this technique encourages gastric distention and vomiting. With the airway unprotected, CPAP should be used only in alert patients. Inherently uncomfortable, it is best tolerated at low levels ($\leq$ 7.5 cmH$_2$O) for brief periods. Intubation facilitates the application of PEEP and CPAP needed to avert oxygen toxicity.

Excessive Workload

Although little work is usually expended by normal subjects in breathing quietly, the O_2 demands of the respiratory system account for a high percentage of total body oxygen consumption ($\dot{V}O_2$) during periods of stress. Experimental animals in shock who receive mechanical ventilation survive longer than their unassisted counterparts. Such data strongly suggest the importance of minimizing the ventilatory O_2 requirement during periods of restricted output so that blood flow can be redirected to other O_2-deprived vital organs. Therefore, the physician should intervene early to relieve an excessive breathing workload in patients with compromised cardiac output.

Most patients who need intubation and positive end-expiratory airway pressure (CPAP or PEEP) for oxygenation also expend a great deal of energy to meet ventilatory requirements. Although it is possible to use CPAP alone in many patients, fatigue often sets in. Therefore, most physicians use fully assisted mechanical ventilation in the initial period, adding PEEP as needed to maintain oxygenation.

TYPES OF VENTILATOR

Although of historical interest and potentially useful outside the hospital, *negative pressure* ventilators (e.g., tanks or body suits) are not appropriate for the acute care setting. *Positive pressure inflation* can be achieved with machines which end inspiration according to *pressure, volume,* or *time* limits. The latest generation of positive pressure ventilators enable the physician to select at will among these options.

In their simplest form *pressure-cycled* (pressure limited) machines allow gas to flow continuously until a set pressure limit is reached. A pressurized gas source is all that is required to operate many of these machines, making them immune to electrical failure. Small size and low cost suit them well for portable applications, home use, and respiratory therapy, where they can be used for intermittent delivery of aerosols or deep breathing (intermittent positive pressure, IPPB). However, because they are pressure limited, the delivered tidal volume (V_T) varies with changes in airway resistance and lung compliance. Therefore, they are not satisfactory to sustain ventilation in hospitalized patients who undergo sudden variations in airway resistance or chest compliance—unless V_T *is continuously monitored* and the pressure limit is adjusted to maintain constant exhaled volume. Pressure-limited ventilators are a poor choice to

support patients with decompensated asthma or chronic obstructive pulmonary disease (COPD). Changes in body position, airway secretions, bronchospasm, dynamic hyperinflation, or muscular tone can have an important effect on V_T. High flow capacity pressure limited ventilators (PLVs) compensate well for small air leaks and are therefore appropriate for use with uncuffed endotracheal (ET) tubes in the pediatric patient. Premature pressure limiting (with insufficient delivered volume) is very common in agitated or hyperventilating patients who attempt to exhale prematurely. IPPB cannot be delivered effectively to uncooperative patients for this reason. Furthermore, many PLVs cannot be used in patients with stiff lungs and high ventilatory requirements, because the flow characteristics of such machines limit the amount of gas which can be moved at the required pressures. In adults, hospital use of PLVs is currently restricted to IPPB applications and to continous support of comatose patients with stable and relatively normal thoracic mechanics. More sophisticated ventilators apply and *maintain* a set level of airway pressure throughout inspiration. Unlike PLVs, these units have a number of useful applications in problems of weaning and oxygenation (see pp. 69–72).

Differences between Pressure and Volume-limited Ventilation

PLVs are used in preference to volume-cycled ventilators in neonatal intensive care for several reasons. Volume-cycled machines operating with a fixed inspiratory duty cycle (inspiratory time) cannot *follow the rapid and chaotic breathing rhythms* of the neonate. Furthermore because uncuffed ET tubes are used, *PLVs compensate for air leakage more effectively* than volume-cycled ventilators, delivering adequate tidal volumes in the face of sizeable gas leaks. Gas stored in compressible circuit elements does not contribute to effective alveolar ventilation. In adult patients, such losses ($\approx$ 2–4 ml/cmH$_2$O of peak pressure) constitute a modest fraction of the tidal volume. In infants, however, *compressible losses* may comprise such a high fraction of the V_T that effective ventilation varies markedly with peak cycling pressure. Thus, during volume-cycled ventilation moment-by-moment changes in chest impedance caused by bronchospasm, secretions, and muscular activity can force peak airway pressures and compressible circuit volume to rise and effective tidal volume to fall. Finally, because airway pressure is controlled, *PLVs are somewhat less likely to cause barotrauma*, a major life-threatening problem in this age group.

Time-cycled machines limit the pressure achieved in the system and cause the ventilator to cycle at a preset interval, thereby setting frequency. V_T is varied by adjusting the flow rate and inspiratory time, or by setting minute ventilation ($\dot{V}_e$) and frequency. Many ventilators, expecially those used in neonatology, are pressure limited but time-cycled, allowing the delivered V_T to be highly variable.

Volume-cycled machines (VLMs) provide a pre-set volume unless a specified pressure limit is exceeded. Major advantages are the capacity to deliver unvarying tidal volumes (except in the presence of a gas leak), flexibility of adjustment, and power to ventilate difficult patients. Virtually all ventilators currently used for continuous support in adults use volume cycling as the primary option. Despite their advantages for acute care, it should be noted that VLMs also suffer from a few disadvantages. They cannot ventilate the patient effectively unless the airway is well sealed. Furthermore, once flow rate is set, the inflation time of the machine is fixed and unresponsive to the patient's native cycling rhythm.

STANDARD MODES OF POSITIVE PRESSURE VENTILATION

Controlled Mechanical Ventilation

With the sensitivity adjustment turned off during controlled mechanical ventilation (CMV), the machine provides a fixed number of breaths per minute and remains totally uninfluenced by the patient's efforts to alter frequency. This mode demands constant vigilance to make appropriate adjustments for changes in ventilatory requirement and is usually used only in situations where pH and/or $PaCO_2$ must be tightly controlled. Most patients require sedation to ensure comfort.

Assist-Control Ventilation

During assist-control (or assisted mechanical ventilation, AMV), inspiration is triggered by the patient but powered by the ventilator (Fig. 7.1). Sensitivity to inspiratory effort can be adjusted to require a small or large negative pressure swing below the set level of end-expiratory pressure to initiate gas flow. As a safety mechanism, a "backup rate" is set, so that if the patient does not initiate a breath within the number of seconds dictated by that frequency, a machine cycle is started automatically. A backup rate set high enough to cause alkalosis blunts respiratory drive and terminates

the patient's efforts to breathe at the "apneic threshold". (In normal subjects, this threshold is usually achieved when $PaCO_2$ is abruptly lowered to 28–32 mmHg.) Note that unlike synchronized intermittent mandatory ventilation (SIMV) (see below), changes in set backup frequency during AMV have no effect on $\dot{V}_e$ unless the "backup" frequency is set high enough to terminate the patient's respiratory efforts.

Intermittent Mandatory Ventilation

During intermittent mandatory ventilation (IMV), the intubated patient is connected to a single circuit that allows both spontaneous and mechanical breathing cycles. Ventilator breaths are interspersed to supplement spontaneous ventilation. If breaths from the ventilator are timed to coincide with spontaneous effort, the mode is termed synchronized IMV (SIMV) or intermittent demand ventilation (IDV). Because SIMV can provide any degree of ventilatory support (0 to 100% of the need), it is used both as a full support mode and a weaning mode (see p. 92).

VENTILATOR SET-UP

Ventilator "Circuit"

With the upper airway bypassed, pressurized gas must be warmed and humidified before entering the trachea. Because the warmed, saturated gas cools somewhat in the unheated connecting tubing, condensation should occur (rain-out). If these water droplets are not evident, a humidifier malfunction is likely.

At the start of inspiration, the exhalation valve closes and pressure builds. Expiratory valves are usually of a diaphragm (mushroom) or scissor type, located on the expiratory side of the Y connection that links the ET tube to the ventilator. Tubing inserted between the ET tube and the Y connector serves as an extension of the anatomic deadspace. After the set volume has been delivered, the exhalation valve opens widely, routing gas into a spirometer or through an electronic device (pneumotach) that senses exhaled flow and volume. The spirometer or pneumotach resets when the next ventilator-delivered breath begins. PEEP is applied by causing the exhalation valve to close at a preset pressure level.

Ventilator Settings

The ventilator is a device for delivering conditioned gas and assisting ventilation. Therefore, major decisions to be made concern mode, F_iO_2, tidal volume, and ventilator frequency. No matter what

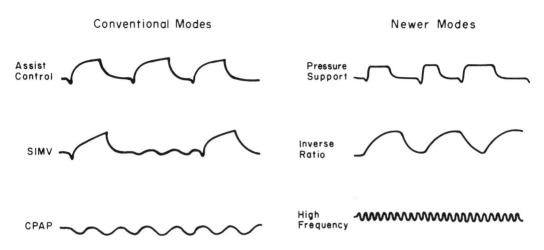

Figure 7.1   Airway pressure tracings of conventional and newer modes of mechanical ventilation.

the initial settings, F_iO_2 and frequency should be adjusted according to the results of arterial blood gases drawn within 15 minutes of initiating ventilation.

Mode

The *AMV mode* is generally the best choice for full support because it allows the patient to control pH and $PaCO_2$, but powers inflation. Trigger sensitivity should be set at the lowest level that avoids auto-cycling (approximately 0.5–1.0 cmH$_2$O below end-expiratory pressure). It should be recognized, however, that effective triggering sensitivity is greatly reduced in the presence of dynamic hyperinflation (auto-PEEP, see pp. 20, 54, 83).

Unresponsive to changes in the patient's requirements and efforts to inspire, the *control* mode transfers responsibility for maintaining appropriate ventilation to the physician. Efforts to assist may be suppressed deliberately with sedation or paralysis in patients who "fight" the ventilator or in those who choose inappropriately high breathing rates.

Although primarily a method to facilitate weaning, *IMV* is useful for other purposes. Compared to other modes of positive pressure ventilation, IMV allows lower mean intrathoracic pressure, minimizing inhibition of venous return. IMV provides an alternative to sedation and control for patients who require some mechanical assistance, but who hyperventilate markedly when allowed to trigger the machine on every cycle (e.g., central neurogenic hyperventilation, anxiety). The venti-

latory workload of IMV increases proportionally to the number of spontaneous breaths.

CPAP alone may be appropriate for those patients who can comfortably maintain ventilation but require airway protection and/or improved arterial oxygenation [e.g., mild forms of adult respiratory distress syndrome (ARDS)]. Newer ventilators provide the *pressure support* option that *selectively* boosts inspiratory airway pressure by an amount set by the physician, while allowing the patient to maintain control of cycle timing and depth (see p. 69).

Inspired Oxygen Fraction (F_iO_2)

Initially, F_iO_2 should be set to err deliberately on the high side, with later adjustment guided by arterial blood gases. After resuscitation, for example, pure oxygen should be given.

Tidal Volume

Delivered tidal volumes of 10–12 ml/kg are usually appropriate. Shallow breaths (< 7 ml/kg) encourage microatelectasis, unless interrupted periodically by larger inflations. If volumes ≤ 7 ml/kg are chosen, one or more sighs (generally 2–3 $\times$ V_T) should be delivered at set intervals.

Some of the set tidal volume is not delivered to the patient but is lost in circuit tubing and compressible elements of the ventilator (internal reservoirs, filters, humidifiers, etc.). With ventilators operating in the range of 40–60 cmH$_2$O peak pressure, a typical value for such compressible losses is 3–4 ml per cmH$_2$O of peak system pressure. However, compression volume (CV) varies with ventilator type, peak cycling pressure, and the length, diameter, and composition of the tubing. (Pediatric circuits use less compliant tubing, $\simeq 1$ ml/cmH$_2$O.) The compression ratio is not a fixed number but varies alinearly with peak pressure. Therefore, much less of any specific set V$_T$ may actually reach the patient if thoracic compliance falls (requiring an increase in peak pressure). "Exhaled" volume measurements usually include CV because decompression occurs as pressure falls. Many modern ventilators compensate for CV on their readout.

Frequency

The initial frequency should be chosen in conjunction with V$_T$ to provide a minute ventilation ($\dot{V}_e$) adequate to maintain pH and patient comfort. In the assist mode, the "backup" rate should be adjusted to a frequency sufficient to provide 70–80% of usual $\dot{V}_e$ in case of complete failure of the patient to trigger. (In the AMV mode, any adjustments in the set frequency—up or down—have no effect on $\dot{V}_e$ or on the level of machine support, so long as the patient triggers each breath.) To avoid paradoxical motion of a flail segment, patients with multiple rib fractures should be maintained at a rate which just suppresses spontaneous efforts, or at a very sensitive trigger setting.

Other Settings

Most volume-cycled ventilators allow the physician to choose *inspiratory flow rate*. Faster rates may cause the distribution of ventilation to worsen marginally in some patients, however the longer exhalation time is a marked advantage in patients with airflow obstruction and in those with marginal cardiopulmonary reserve. Although peak pressure rises as flow rate increases, the mean pressure averaged over the entire ventilatory cycle may remain unaffected or fall. It is mandatory for the peak flow setting of the ventilator to be greater than the patient's inspiratory flow demand. Otherwise, the patient is forced to work against the resistance of the ventilator circuitry, as well as against his own internal impedance to airflow and chest expansion. (Peak flows that exceed flow demand do not influence breathing effort.) Rapid inspiratory flow rates are also desirable in order that the machine completes inflation before the patient's own ventilatory rhythm cycles into its exhalation phase— otherwise the patient "fights the ventilator". As a general rule, the *peak flow setting should be approximately 3.5–4.0 times the minute ventilation requirement*.

Peak airway pressure is influenced by inspiratory flow rate, airway resistance, tidal volume, and total thoracic compliance. To avoid barotrauma, *maximum pressure* (alarm and "pop-off" pressure) should be set 15–20 cmH$_2$O above peak cycling pressure observed during a typical breath.

The *expiratory retard* setting is theoretically useful for patients with airway collapse during exhalation, but its effectiveness is uncertain. The *inflation hold* setting sustains peak chest volume, raises mean inflation pressure, allows calculation of lung mechanics, and may improve gas distribution in some patients. In theory, an inflation hold helps reverse atelectasis and aids the distribution of therapeutic aerosols. (Barotrauma, however, may be increased.)

On some pressure limited time-cycled machines the ratio of inspiratory to expiratory time (*I:E ratio*) can be set directly. However, on volume-cycled ventilators I:E ratio is usually set indirectly by specifying inhaled volume, frequency, and inspiratory flow rate. In general, shorter I:E ratios allow more time for exhalation and lower mean intrathoracic pressure. To avoid gas trapping, most ventilators warn visually or alarm when the I:E ratio exceeds 1.0, provided that the patient is not triggering.

NEW MODES OF VENTILATION

The primary purposes of mechanical ventilation are to achieve adequate alveolar ventilation and to improve oxygen exchange. Until recently, volume limited ventilation, used alone (AMV, CMV) or in conjunction with spontaneous breathing (SIMV), has been the only form of machine assistance commonly used in adults. Similarly, enrichment of F$_i$O$_2$ and the addition of end-expiratory pressure (PEEP, CPAP) have been the primary means of supporting oxygenation for twenty years. Recently, a number of new techniques have been introduced to clinical practice, each with a defensible physiologic rationale, but little objective supporting data to document benefit. Because the majority of these newer modes are pressure cycled, *independent volume monitoring* is highly desirable.

Pressure Support Ventilation

Description

Pressure support (PS) is a method in which *each* breath taken by a spontaneously breathing patient receives a pressure boost. Inspiratory airway pressure is maintained constant at whatever level is set by the physician. Because PS is flow cycled, the patient retains control of cycle length and tidal volume.

Advantages

PS hybridizes machine to spontaneous breathing cycles, providing assistance that ranges from no support to fully powered ventilation. Because the depth, length, and flow profile of the breath are patient controlled, PS adjusted to provide adequate power tends to be extraordinarily comfortable. Adaptability to the vagaries of patient cycle length can prove especially helpful in patients with erratic breathing patterns (e.g., COPD, anxiety). The transition to spontaneous breathing is eased by the *gradual* removal of machine support. Thus, *P_S has its widest application as a weaning mode.* Pressure support is also valuable in *offsetting the resistive work* required to breathe spontaneously *through an endotracheal tube*, as during CPAP or SIMV.

PS should be adjusted to maintain an adequate tidal volume at an acceptable frequency (< 30/min). In theory, PS would provide the entire work of breathing if set to meet or exceed the average inspiratory pressure requirement ($\bar{P}$). For a normal subject breathing at a moderate rate, $\bar{P}$ is amazingly small, seldom > 5 cmH$_2$O. In patients appropriate for weaning ($\dot{V}_e \leq 10$ l/min), $\bar{P}$ does not commonly exceed 10 cmH$_2$O. This explains why patients appear to be "weaning smoothly" until a threshold value is reached, at which point further reductions precipitate sudden deterioration. When PS > $\bar{P}$, the patient performs little work, but rather adjusts frequency and tidal volume to minimize effort.

Problems

PS requires the ventilatory cycle to be patient initiated and cannot adjust itself to changes in the ease of chest inflation. *Therefore, PS is not a mode for patients with unstable ventilatory drive or for those with variable thoracic impedance* (e.g., bronchospasm, copious secretions). Furthermore, the ability of most ventilator systems to provide a true square-wave of airway pressure tends to deteriorate as ventilatory demands increase.

Minimum Minute Ventilation

Minimum (or minimal) ventilation (MMV) *guarantees a certain minute ventilation*, whether or not the patient attempts to breathe. Unlike SIMV, MMV does not provide a fixed number of breaths— no machine cycles are delivered if the patient breathes at an adequate pace. MMV sees its greatest application as a stand alone "automatic" weaning mode (see p. 93). MMV can be provided by *intermittent volume-cycle breaths*, delivered only as required. *Alternatively, a PS level* for each breath can be adjusted to optimize tidal volume or frequency.

Advantages

In principle, MMV provides a nearly ideal backup mode to PS. Although ready to step in if needed, MMV does not obligate the patient to receive machine support.

Disadvantages

MMV guarantees $\dot{V}_e$, but may allow fatigue to occur in the attempt to achieve the targeted value. Indeed, the minute ventilation target can be achieved by shallow tachypnea, even as exhaustion sets in. (Frequency and tidal volume alarms can be added to warn of deterioration.) Modes that adjust PS to accomplish MMV, yet limit maximal frequency and maintain tidal volume, would seem desirable in preventing or compensating for fatigue.

High Frequency Ventilation

The collective term high frequency ventilation (HFV) refers to modes of ventilation in which tidal volumes smaller than anatomic deadspace are moved at frequencies that range from 60 to 3000 cycles/min.

High frequency positive pressure ventilation (HFPPV) is identical in concept to conventional ventilation; however, tidal volumes are very small, and cycling frequencies are very fast (60–100/min).

Jet ventilation (HFJV) works differently. A small diameter injecting catheter positioned in the central airway pulses gas along the luminal axis under high pressure (5–50 psi) at a rapid cycling rate (typically 60–240 cycles/min). The actual period of insufflation, the inspiratory dwell time, is normally set to occupy 20–50% of the total cycling period. Conditioned gas is entrained with the pulse, augmenting the effective tidal volume (V_T). V_T is not a set parameter but varies with jet driving pressure, frequency, and dwell time. Exhalation is passive, with exhaled gas expelled more or less continuously through a valveless port. Although HFJV is the most frequently used form of HFV in adults, there is debate on the mechanism of its action. Most evidence is compatible with modified convective ("bulk") flow. Efficiency is improved by square-wave delivery, placement of the injector close to the carina, and a jet lumen/exhaust lumen ratio of 1:11 to 1:6.

High frequency oscillation (HFO) operates on yet another mechanical principle. A very small volume (1–3 ml/kg) is moved to and fro by a piston at extremely high frequencies (500–3000 cycles per minute). Fresh gas is introduced as a continuous flow, and a narrow gauge venting tube (a "low pass filter") provides egress for waste gas. Delivered tidal volume depends upon the relative resistances for gas flow through the airway and the bias flow lines. CO_2 elimination is a function of tidal volume and, to a lesser degree, vibration frequency. Although fresh gas must access the airway directly, it is not clear that pulsatility must originate in the airway for effective ventilation. In experimental animals, mere vibration of the chest wall has successfully established effective gas exchange. Indeed, pulsatility itself does not seem to be a strict requirement for some alveolar ventilation to occur. A continuous stream of O_2 introduced near the carina can maintain arterial oxygenation and accomplish CO_2 washout in apneic animals, a technique dubbed "apneic diffusion", "continuous flow apneic ventilation", or "tracheal insufflation of oxygen (TRIO)". Although not currently advocated for clinical use, apneic ventilation may have some temporizing utility in emergent settings where standard endotracheal intubation cannot be accomplished.

The mechanism by which these varied forms of HFV establish alveolar ventilation is uncertain and almost certainly differs from one technique to another. Yet, all forms of HFV are characterized by lower *peak* airway pressures than conventional ventilation. *Peripheral airway pressure*, however, is generally higher than measured central airway pressure, and *mean alveolar pressures* may not differ greatly from those observed during conventional ventilation.

Applications of HFV

HFV can silence the normal respiratory rhythm and phasic variations of chest volume. This feature has already proven advantageous during lithotripsy and certain delicate surgical procedures in which gross thoracic motions must be minimized. Because HFJV does not require a cuffed endotracheal tube, it has proven helpful in bronchoscopy and laryngeal surgery. Furthermore, HFJV has been used effectively in the setting of bronchopleural fistulas that are refractory to closure, perhaps because of lower peak airway pressures. (It is also conceivable, however, that the fistula draws less flow at higher frequencies because the time constant of the fistulous pathway is longer than that of alternative routes.)

Jet ventilation synchronized to the heart beat has

been demonstrated to boost the cardiac output of patients with dilated cardiomyopathy, presumably because systolic heart compression decreases left ventricular afterload. Because high airway cycling pressure may be instrumental in causing bronchopulmonary dysplasia, a disease of neonates, HFV may also have a role in preventing this complication.

Despite these specific indications, HFV has proven disappointing. With rare exception, HFV seems to offer little advantage with regard to cardiovascular performance, lung water accumulation, or gas exchange at equivalent levels of end-expiratory alveolar pressure. Indeed, many patients with high ventilation requirements or high thoracic impedance cannot be successfully ventilated by HFV. Finally, although initial problems with inadequate humidification, jet-induced mucosal disruption, and mechanical breakdown have been largely mastered, monitoring alveolar pressure and gas exchange remain vexing clinical problems during HFV.

NEW MODES FOR OXYGENATION

Pressure Control and Inverse Ratio Ventilation

Description

In order to prevent gas trapping, it has been common practice to allow at least as much time for exhalation as for inhalation; however, gas exchange may be markedly improved when the I:E ratio is forced to values > 1:1. First applied in neonates with hyaline membrane disease, *inverse ratio ventilation* (IRV) has now been used in adult patients with refractory ARDS and other forms of hypoxemia.

IRV can be applied by slowing the rate of flow delivery during conventional volume ventilation or, more commonly, by maintaining pressure at a controlled level for a fixed time *(pressure-controlled ventilation)*. Because both methods require a passive patient, sedation, overventilation, and/ or paralysis are usually necessary.

Mechanism of Action

How IRV improves oxygenation is uncertain. However, *raised mean intrathoracic pressure* (and increased lung volume) is almost certainly a primary mechanism. Auto-PEEP is generated in most cases. *Sustained tethering forces* may recruit lung units that would otherwise remain collapsed, and *units with very slow time constants* may be given sufficient time to *ventilate*. IRV is not an appropriate mode of treatment in severely obstructed patients.

Advantages of IRV

The proposed advantages of IRV are *improved oxygenation* and *reduced peak cycling pressure*. Whether the incidence of barotrauma is reduced by the latter is not currently known, as IRV requires *mean* alveolar pressure to increase.

Disadvantages of IRV

Higher mean intrathoracic pressure may impede venous return and contribute to barotrauma. After the same time, alveolar pressure is *imprecisely controlled*. For specific values of cycling pressure and I:E ratio these characteristics fluctuate with inflation impedance. Finally, IRV requires *deep sedation or paralysis* and close monitoring of gas exchange.

Airway Pressure Release Ventilation

Description

Airway pressure release ventilation (APRV) can be thought of as a variant of the IRV concept, intended for use by *spontaneously breathing patients* with poor oxygenation. The idea here is to provide added support for *ventilation* in a patient who needs CPAP for oxygenation and can provide most of the ventilatory power requirement without machine assistance. APRV allows the patient to make ventilatory efforts around an elevated pressure baseline (CPAP) but allows the system to depressurize (partially or completely) for brief periods at a frequency set by the physician. After release, fresh gas enters as CPAP builds to its baseline value.

Advantages

APRV can be viewed as a method to aid ventilation in patients requiring CPAP for oxygenation. Phasic release cycles function in a manner similar to the machine cycles of SIMV insofar as they augment ventilation. The difference is that *high peak cycling pressures are avoided*. As with IRV, sustained high airway pressure may exert traction and improve ventilation in slow time constant units. Unlike IRV, however, maximal alveolar pressures are more readily assessed. The *patient remains conscious* and can adjust alveolar ventilation to the extent he/she is able to do so.

Disadvantages

The efficacy of the pressure release cycle depends on (1) the duration of release, (2) the mechanical properties of the chest; (3) the level to which airway pressure is allowed to fall, and (4) the cycling frequency. As ventilation support increases, mean air-

way pressure falls, dissipating some of the oxygen exchange benefit of CPAP. More importantly, APRV is *a questionable mode of support in patients with significant airflow obstruction or in those with severely reduced compliance*. In the first instance, release cycles are relatively ineffectual. In the second instance, the work of spontaneous breathing may be too great to sustain.

APRV has not undergone rigorous testing and is not available for routine use in patients at the present time. It appears as if APRV will find most use in a relatively small number of unobstructed and CPAP-responsive patients in oxygenation failure with modest ventilatory requirements.

GENERAL APPROACH TO THE VENTILATED PATIENT

The complex interaction of patient and ventilator must be approached in systematic fashion to optimize performance and minimize hazards. A number of important questions must be asked in the daily assessment of the ventilated patient:

Patient status

1. **Are cycling pressures excessively high (>50 cmH$_2$O)?** Have they changed? Are changes attributable to alterations in resistance or compliance? (Or, alternatively, are flow, tidal volume, or PEEP different, with constant mechanics?)
2. **Are there reversible factors impeding airflow (bronchospasm, secretions) or worsening the compliance of the lung (new infiltrate, atelectasis) or of the chest wall (agitation, ascites, pleural effusion, abdominal distention)?** Do secretion volume and character suggest respiratory infection, ongoing aspiration, or pulmonary hemorrhage? Is there any sign of *unaddressed congestive heart failure, volume overload, volume depletion, or sepsis*?
3. **What is the minute ventilation requirement?** To determine whether a high $\dot{V}E$ is related to drive, metabolic requirement, acidosis or iatrogenic hyperventilation, $\dot{V}_e$ must be interpreted in conjunction with PaCO$_2$, pH, and the physical examination.
4. **How hard is the patient working to breathe?** Are there signs of fatigue—elevated respiratory rate, abdominal paradox, irregular breathing rhythm? *What is the drive to breathe?* Is the patient making spontaneous breathing efforts? What are pH and PaCO$_2$? On what mode of ventilation were gases obtained? The implica-

tions of respiratory acidosis, for example, are much different for CMV (underventilation), AMV (reduced drive), or low level SIMV (reduced drive, inadequate strength).

5. **Is the patient still ventilator-dependent?** What is ventilatory requirement? Are cycling pressures high or low? Is patient alert, strong? If unweanable, is dependency likely to change anytime soon? (Should a tracheostomy be scheduled?)

Ventilator status

1. **Are ventilator connections appropriate?** Are connectors tight, the ET tube cuff well-sealed, and the circuit tubing unkinked and water-free?
2. **Is there a need to raise or lower the overall level of machine support for oxygenation or ventilation?** Is there an appropriate PAO_2/PaO_2 ratio? Should PEEP be adjusted? Is a change in ventilation mode or cycling frequency indicated to increase or decrease support?
3. **Are machine adjustments in mode, flow rate, corrected tidal volume, or PEEP required?** Is the patient comfortable? Are airway pressures during ventilator cycles uniform and of expected shape, indicating synchrony of patient and ventilator breathing cycles?

The following checklist is suggested for use in a bedside evaluation of the ventilated patient.

Bedside Evaluation of the Ventilated Patient

Mental status	pH and gas exchange
Spontaneous breathing rhythm	Breath sounds
	Chest x-ray
Minute ventilation requirement	Mode of cycling
	Cycling pressure
Muscular strength	(compliance/
Secretion character and volume	resistance)
	Medications
Breathing effort/ paradox/ coordination	

COMPLICATIONS OF MECHANICAL VENTILATION

Cardiovascular Impairment

Mean intrathoracic pressure rises during mechanical ventilation because of positive inspiratory pressure. PEEP can have a profound additional effect. Since venous return is driven by the difference between mean systemic venous pressure (determined by intravascular volume and venous tone) and intrathoracic vena caval pressure, cardiac output will fall unless mean systemic pressure rises to compensate.

The mechanisms impairing cardiac output during positive pressure ventilation are discussed elsewhere in this volume (see p. 79). Reduction of cardiac output is particularly likely to occur in patients whose mean intrathoracic pressures rise highest and in those who either are volume depleted or fail to venoconstrict. Most evident shortly after mechanical ventilation or PEEP is instituted, output reduction is minimized by slowly adapting compensatory changes in intravascular volume and vessel tone. Profound and abrupt deterioration may occur in patients developing auto-PEEP shortly after the institution of positive pressure ventilation (see p. 83). In general, patients with normal sympathetic reflexes and normal or increased intravascular volume tolerate mechanical ventilation best.

Barotrauma

Barotrauma refers to the consequences of alveolar overdistention and is extensively discussed in Chapter 31. Air can gain access to the pleural space in two ways: (1) a "blow-out" of the visceral pleura, facilitated by obstructed airways, parenchymal inflammation, and necrosis; or (2) overdistention and rupture of individual alveoli, allowing interstitial air to track along bronchi and vessels to the mediastinum, where it migrates into soft tissues and commonly perforates the thin mediastinal pleura to cause pneumothorax. This second mechanism is perhaps the most common and explains why subcutaneous emphysema and pneumomediastinum commonly precede or occur simultaneously with pneumothorax.

Fluid Retention and Redistribution

Extravascular fluid retention tends to develop during positive pressure ventilation for several reasons: (1) Ventilated patients are relatively immobile. (2) As increased intrathoracic pressure limits venous return, stretch receptors located in the atria signal for additional antidiuretic hormone (ADH) release to help replenish central vascular volume. (3) Hypotension induced by positive pressure may curtail renal perfusion, redistribute renal blood flow, reduce glomerular filtration, and promote sodium retention. PEEP may cause similar redistribution of intrarenal blood flow by reflex mechanisms. As positive pressure ventilation is discontinued, these fluid shifts reverse and may precipitate cardiac decompensation in patients with poor reserve, as fluid translocates from extravascular sites to the central vessels.

Fluctuations In H^+ Concentration

The ventilator can have a powerful impact on acid-base balance. When support is initiated, special care should be exercised not to reverse acidosis too quickly or to cause marked respiratory alkalosis. Metabolic alkalosis tends to develop in mechanically ventilated patients because of intravascular volume contraction, nasogastric suctioning, use of steroids, etc. If repletion of KCl or intravascular volume fails to correct it, acetazolamide (Diamox) may prove useful in controlling extravascular fluid retention while dumping excess bicarbonate.

In the assist mode, marked fluctuations in pH and $PaCO_2$ can occur in patients who are alternately agitated and sedated, especially if the backup rate is inappropriately low. Mental status and ventilation mode should always be taken into account when interpreting blood gas values.

Infections

Infections of the lung and upper respiratory tract are exceedingly common during mechanical ventilation. *Endotracheal intubation* prevents glottic closure, disrupts the laryngeal barrier, slows the mucociliary escalator, impedes secretion clearance, and provides an open pathway for large quantities of aspirated pharyngeal bacteria and fungi to inoculate the lung. Oral and nasal secretions continuously gravitate to the lower tract via the cuff interstices, even though cuff inflation prevents massive gastric aspiration. The oropharynx of critically ill patients quickly recolonizes with hospital-prevalent pathogens, e.g., gram-negative bacteria and staphylococci. *Nasogastric tubes* commonly used during mechanical ventilation for gastric decompression or feeding serve as a conduit for enteric bacteria to the pharynx and upper respiratory tract. Furthermore, *bacterial overgrowth is common* when histamine blockers, antacids, or tube feedings buffer the gastric pH to levels > 4.0. Recent evidence suggests that sucralfate, which requires acid production for optimal action, may be preferable to pH-altering regimens for this reason. Duodenal instillation of the liquid feeding reduces the risk of aspiration and avoids acid buffering.

Condensate within corregated tubing allows bacteria to multiply. Therefore, great care should be taken to prevent transfer of the condensate into the trachea during manipulations of the ventilator circuit. Nasotracheal and nasogastric tubes frequently precipitate *sinus infection* by blocking their ostia, preventing drainage. Of itself, occult sinusitis is a frequent cause for febrile episodes in intubated patients. Furthermore, blocked sinuses also provide a seeding focus for infections of the lung and bloodstream. It should be emphasized that occult sino-pulmonary infections are often responsible for the sepsis syndrome in intubated, mechanically ventilated patients, even when organisms cannot be recovered by conventional culturing techniques. Overt pneumonitis, frequently polymicrobial, usually manifests on the 7–12th hospital day.

Deconditioning

Weakening and discoordination of respiratory muscles may occur as the burden, timing, and breathing pattern are machine controlled for prolonged periods. Substantial work is performed in the effort to trigger the ventilator, especially by breathless patients. As a general rule, patients receiving assisted mechanical ventilation expend sufficient effort in triggering the ventilator to prevent disuse atrophy, but it is unclear whether original muscle bulk and strength are preserved. The problem of deconditioning would appear most serious in those patients who must assume a large workload of breathing when mechanical ventilation is discontinued, in those with pre-existing neuromuscular impairment, in those with suppressed ventilatory drive, and in those requiring prolonged sedation or paralysis. Nutritional support, increased spontaneous muscle activity (CPAP, IMV pressure support), and muscle training may be helpful. Periodic "sprints" (or 5 to 10-minute CPAP trials) may help preserve bulk and strength, even during the acute stage.

Specific "Early Phase" Problems

Initial discomfort may be extreme, due to the unfamiliar ET tube, distended hollow viscera, impaired swallowing, pharyngeal or sinus pain, anxiety, disorientation, inability to speak, or discomfort related to recent invasive procedures. Stimulation of bronchial, laryngeal, and carinal irritant receptors triggers bronchospasm and coughing efforts. Furthermore, mechanical ventilators are usually set to deliver higher tidal volumes than the patient would choose spontaneously, whereas inspiratory pattern, flow rate, and cycling frequency differ from those of the pre-support period. Hence, shortly after mechanical ventilation begins, attempts to "fight the ventilator" are the rule in alert, awakening, and mildly obtunded patients.

Initial mismatching usually abates spontaneously (within minutes) as the patient becomes accustomed to the machine. *Constant attendance by trained medical personnel is necessary* throughout this period, however, to calm the patient, adjust the setting to the patient's requirements, and ensure that the agitation neither interferes with gas exchange nor has a more serious origin.

It is extremely important to secure all tubing connectors and *restrain the arms* of an intermittently agitated or rousable patient. Ventilator disconnection or *self-extubation is a potentially lethal and common event.*

When the patient is initially connected, sensitivity should be adjusted so that minimal effort is required to trigger a ventilator breath. Inspiratory flow rate is adjusted to a level commensurate with the vigor and frequency of the patient's efforts. (A flow setting $\simeq 4 \times \dot{V}_e$ usually satisfies flow demands.) Tidal volume may need to be reduced temporarily to achieve an adequate matchup between patient and ventilator frequencies. With the machine properly adjusted, mechanical malfunctioning ruled out, the patient examined, the initial set of blood gases analyzed, and the chest x-ray checked for position of the tube tip and pneumothorax, morphine may be given to assist smooth linking of endogenous respiratory and ventilator rhythms. Intratracheal lidocaine (2–4 ml of 2% concentration) can briefly arrest coughing spasms and reduce pain. A nasogastric tube helps to decompress the gastrointestinal tract and is particularly helpful in patients who swallow air around orotracheal tubes.

Specific "Support Phase" Problems

Smooth interaction between the patient and machine may be interrupted by malfunction of the ventilator system, worsening of cardiopulmonary mechanics, or factors completely unrelated to ventilation. Malfunctions of the ventilator system cause failure to achieve adequate ventilation or oxygenation and usually present as altered states of consciousness (agitation or obtundation), worrisome changes in vital signs, or unexplained deterioration in blood gases.

Diagnostic Approach to Patient Agitation during Mechanical Ventilation

When a sudden crisis develops during mechanical ventilation, the clinician must undertake the diagnosis in an organized (even stereotyped) fashion with "all deliberate speed". Knowledge of the exhaled versus set tidal volume is crucial data. A major difference indicates a circuit leak or machine dysfunction. Checking the airway pressure ma-

nometer and comparing the peak dynamic and static pressures against previous values also provide essential information. A large disparity between P_D and P_S suggests a resistance problem in tube or airways (bronchospasm, secretions). It is useful to classify these problems as those that usually cause elevations of peak cycling pressure (pressure limiting) and those that usually do not (Table 7.1). Three components of the system must be checked carefully: *the patient, the endotracheal tube,* and *the ventilator system* itself.

Patient

The importance of auscultation for signs of pneumothorax, bronchospasm, and pulmonary edema deserves emphasis. Among the most important distinctions to make is the one between massive atelectasis and tension pneumothorax (see p. 178 and Chapter 31). Note that pneumothorax that does not have a tension component (the minority) may not elevate peak pressure noticeably. *Non-pulmonary causes of discomfort (distention of bladder or intestinal tract, unvarying body position, pain, etc.) are easily overlooked.* Pulmonary emboli and cardiac ischemia are exceedingly common.

Agitated patients often oppose the ventilator, causing dyssynchrony and pressure limiting. Once begun, dyssynchrony tends to be self-perpetuating, inasmuch as small (pressure-limited) inflations do not allow adequate ventilation. A vicious cycle is especially likely to develop in patients with airflow obstruction who hyperinflate, causing Auto-PEEP (AP) and associated muscle dysfunction and hemodynamic stress. Both work of breathing and dyspnea escalate markedly as the patient struggles to breathe. Simply disconnecting the ventilator and providing adequate ventilation manually with a re-

Table 7.1
Sudden Crises during Mechanical Ventilation

Pressure Limiting	Non-Pressure Limiting
Central airway obstruction	Cuff deflation/tube withdrawal
Massive atelectasis	Circuit disruption
Tube occlusion	Machine malfunction
Mainstem intubation	Pneumothorax without tension
Tension pneumothorax	Gas trapping (auto-PEEP)
Irritative bronchospasm	Hemodynamic crisis
Decreased chest wall compliance	Pulmonary embolism
Secretion retention	Pulmonary edema

suscitator bag will break the cycle and frequently stop the process. Although agitation often has a trivial origin, it must never be ignored or suppressed with sedatives until possible serious causes are investigated.

Rapidly developing, profound bradycardia is often experienced by patients during temporary machine disconnection for suctioning. Although sudden hypoxemia is occasionally responsible, this phenomenon is usually a reflex effect, blockable by pretreatment with atropine.

Endotracheal Tube

Modern volume ventilators are equipped with audible alarms which sense excessive system pressure, failure to exhale a minimal tidal volume, or disconnection of the patient from the machine. If the cause for distress is not immediately obvious, *listen for cuff leaks* during inflation and *palpate the pilot balloon* to sense the pressure in the cuff. ET tubes often kink, block with secretions, or become constricted by the teeth of a biting patient. *Disconnect* the patient from *the ventilator*, "preoxygenate", and *pass a suction catheter* to check patency of the endotracheal tube and aspirate central airway secretions. Check vital signs and auscultate quickly for evidence of pneumothorax, massive atelectasis, or bronchospasm as the patient is ventilated manually with 100% oxygen. Tubes which are poorly placed or secured may migrate into the larynx or right main bronchus or may rest on the carina, producing cough and bronchospasm.

Ventilator Circuit

The integrity of the ventilator *circuit is then quickly inspected*, with special attention given to tubing *connections* and the *settings* for tidal volume, frequency, trigger sensitivity, and oxygen fraction. *Tubing* is checked for accumulated water, which may increase resistance, causing inadvertent expiratory retard or PEEP.

If all seems intact, the patient can be briefly reconnected to check delivered versus set minute ventilation. If delivered minute ventilation is too low, the therapist should check all connections carefully for leaks, especially around the humidifier and the exhalation valve. If the problem persists and the chest x-ray is negative, judicious doses of morphine can be given, so long as gas exchange remains well maintained as judged by arterial blood gases. Paralysis must never be undertaken until an alert patient is sedated.

Distinction must be made between fighting the ventilator (dysynchrony) and attempting to "breathe around" the ventilator. The first may prevent effective ventilation or signal a serious disorder; the second is usually innocuous. Breathing around the ventilator refers to the patient's ineffective attempts to pull additional breaths during the exhalation phase of the ventilator cycle. With gas exchange uncompromised, sensitivity appropriately set, and the patient not in distress, such a pattern seems to have little detrimental effect. However, a strong tachypneic patient, especially one intubated for purposes of oxygenation, may attempt to pull breaths deeper than the ventilator is set to deliver them. When this happens, gas drawn from the reservoir of the ventilator during inspiration adds to the delivered tidal volume or a second breath is prematurely triggered. As a result, the patient inhales a larger volume of gas than set, but a similar F_iO_2 is maintained.

Special Problems of Patients with High Ventilatory Requirements

Patients with very high ventilatory requirements may overtax the capacity of the ventilator to deliver gas, and hence may work against the machine as well as their intrinsic disease. If a more powerful machine is not effective or available, this is one of the few situations which justifies heavy sedation and use of the control mode.

Hyperpnea strains the capacity of the machine to coordinate with the patient, forcing major deviations between intended and delivered waveforms. Asynchrony markedly elevates the breathing workload and tachypnea accentuates the importance of resistance within the endotracheal tube and other circuit elements.

Active use of the expiratory musculature may cause hypoxemia by combatting the volume recruitment effect of PEEP (see p. 78), altering ventilation-perfusion relationships and desaturating mixed venous blood. Reducing active effort can therefore improve arterial oxygenation. Although deep sedation and paralysis can be helpful, *prolonged immobility encourages regional secretion*, *regional atelectasis*, and *muscle atrophy*. Ventilator disconnections can be rapidly lethal.

In extreme circumstances adequate ventilation is difficult to achieve, even with paralysis and full machine support. A steady infusion of bicarbonate may allow pH to remain compensated as CO_2 stabilizes at a higher level.

It is not commonly realized that the PEEP valves used with most ventilators offer substantial airflow resistance, which increases with the level of PEEP. In part, this is an unavoidable consequence of the fact that such valves are pressure-activated and must sense a pressure difference across the valve in order to block further exhalation at the pre-set level. If exhalation is *passive*, this resistance slows airflow (an "expiratory retard" effect) but does not influence the amount of ventilatory work done by the patient. During *active* exhalation, however, this increased resistance must be overcome by patient effort and adds substantially to the work performed.

SUGGESTED READINGS

1. Boysen PG, Kacmarek RM, eds.: Mechanical Ventilation Symposium (Parts 1 and 2). *Respir Care* 32:(6–7):403–614, 1987.
2. Grum CM, Chauncey JB: Conventional mechanical ventilation. *Clin Chest Med* 9(1):37–46, 1988.
3. Grum CM, Morganroth ML: Initiating mechanical ventilation. *J Int Care Med* 3(1):6–20, 1988.
4. Hudson LD, Hurlow RS, Craig KC, et al: Does intermittent mandatory ventilation correct respiratory alkalosis in patients receiving assisted mechanical ventilation? *Am Rev Respir Dis* 132:1071–1074, 1985.
5. MacIntyre NR: New forms of mechanical ventilation in the adult. *Clin Chest Med* 9(1):47–54, 1988.
6. Marini JJ: Mechanical ventilation. In Simmons DH (ed). *Current Pulmonology*, Vol 9, Year Book Medical Publishers, Chap 6, pp. 164–208, 1988.
7. Marini JJ: Newer concepts in mechanical ventilation. *Pulmonary Perspectives*. American College of Chest Physicians, Vol 5, pp. 3–8, 1988.
8. Marini JJ, Capps JS, Culver BH: The inspiratory work of breathing during assisted mechanical ventilation. *Chest* 87(5):612–618, 1985.
9. Morganroth ML (ed): Mechanical Ventilation Symposium. *Clin Chest Med* 9(1):1–173; 1988.
10. Spicher JE, White DP: Outcome and function following prolonged mechanical ventilation. *Arch Int Med* 147:421–425, 1987.
11. Weisman IM, Rinaldo JE, Rogers RM, et al.: Intermittent mandatory ventilation. *Am Rev Resir Dis* 127:641–647, 1983.
12. Zwillich CW, Pierson DJ, Creagh CE, et al.: Complications of assisted ventilation: a prospective study of 354 consecutive episodes. *Am J Med* 57:161–170, 1974.

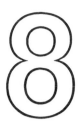

Positive End-Expiratory Pressure

DEFINITIONS

Hypoxemia resulting from alveolar collapse or filling often responds to a higher lung volume maintained by positive airway pressure at end-exhalation. When positive end-expiratory pressure (PEEP) recruits lung volume, it may also reduce the elastic work of expanding the lung. PEEP has no proven prophylactic value in averting the adult respiratory distress syndrome (ARDS) but may help reduce pulmonary complications in the postoperative setting. Although PEEP may improve oxygen exchange and thereby allow reduction of the inspired oxygen concentration (F_iO_2), it has not been shown conclusively to improve survival.

The expressions "assisted ventilation with PEEP" and "continuous positive pressure breathing (CPPB, CPPV)" are synonymous, referring to mechanically delivered tidal breaths with positive pressure maintained at end expiration (Fig. 8.1). The term continuous positive airway pressure (CPAP) refers to spontaneous tidal breathing with a fixed amount of positive pressure applied to the airway throughout the ventilatory cycle (including end-exhalation). If only the exhalation line is pressurized, the terms "spontaneous PEEP" or expiratory positive airway pressure are used. In this mode, the patient works much harder to breathe, because negative inspiratory pressures must be generated from an elevated pressure baseline. Mean intrathoracic pressure, however, is lower than with other modes of end-expiratory pressure.

PATHOPHYSIOLOGIC CONSIDERATIONS

The utility of PEEP stems primarily from its ability to recruit collapsed alveoli and to prevent their re-collapse. PEEP also improves the distribution of alveolar liquid and translocates fluid from alveolar to interstitial spaces, lowering the diffusion distance for oxygen exchange. When PEEP

reduces cardiac output, blood flow through shunt regions may also decline, causing a reduction in venous admixture. Contrary to previous belief, it appears unlikely that PEEP decreases lung water; fluid content may actually increase due to distention of the interstitial space and raised pulmonary venous and lymphatic pressures.

If exhalation is passive (as it is during quiet, unstressed breathing), PEEP achieves its desired effect—an increase in end-expiratory lung volume. However, if the resulting lung expansion is uncomfortable, patients may actively oppose PEEP in attempting to maintain the original lung volume. In this way PEEP or CPAP may provide a mechanism by which the dyspneic or fatigued patient can use the expiratory muscles to accomplish inspiratory work. Active expiration to a volume lower than the equilibrium position stores potential energy. At the onset of inspiration, outward recoil of the chest wall then provides an inspiratory boost as the expiratory muscles relax. Although this reduces the inspiratory work, the cost is a reduction in the volume recruitment effect of PEEP. Sedation or paralysis restores volume recruitment and can markedly improve oxygenation. The total work of breathing may also be reduced as the ventilator assumes the task of powering ventilation.

Assuming exhalation is passive, the volume recruited by PEEP (ΔV) is a function of both lung (C_L) and chest wall (C_W) compliance:

$$\Delta V = PEEP \times C_L C_W / (C_L + C_W).$$

Although most lung recruitment is complete within 3–5 breaths, several hours may be required to realize the full impact of PEEP. On the other hand, desaturation usually occurs quite abruptly upon withdrawal.

Because the beneficial effect of PEEP relates to maintenance of lung volume and not to positive pressure itself, it does not matter whether the lung

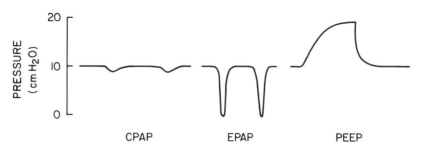

Figure 8.1   Three modes of maintaining elevated pressure at end-exhalation. CPAP and expiratory positive airway pressure (EPAP) require the patient to supply the energy needed to ventilate.

is expanded by internally positive or externally negative pressure. Therefore, it should cause no concern for lost volume when a patient pulls an inspiratory airway pressure lower than the set PEEP level. To generate a lower airway pressure, pleural pressure must have decreased at least as much, so that transpulmonary pressure and lung volume are preserved.

ADVERSE EFFECTS

Cardiovascular Impairment

At end exhalation, pressure within the central airway approximates alveolar pressure, provided that flow has stopped (see ''Auto-PEEP Effect,'' p. 83). Under these static conditions, an increment of pressure applied to the airway (PEEP) distributes across the lung and chest wall according to the formula:

$$\Delta P_{pl} = PEEP \times C_L / (C_L + C_W)$$

where P_{pl} and PEEP refer to pleural and airway pressures, and C_L and C_W denote compliance of the lung and chest wall, respectively. Normally, the lungs and chest wall have similar compliance characteristics in the tidal range; therefore, $\approx \frac{1}{2}$ of the applied PEEP transmits to the pleural space. With abnormally stiff lungs, less is transmitted (typically, $\frac{1}{4}$ to $\frac{1}{3}$). With compliant lungs and a stiff chest wall (e.g., in a patient with emphysema, obesity, or massive ascites), the pleural pressure increment is a higher fraction of applied PEEP.

Because the heart and great vessels are surrounded by pressures similar to P_{pl}, PEEP reduces venous return but tends to raise all intrathoracic pressures. Such pressure changes complicate the interpretation of central venous pressure (CVP) and pulmonary artery wedge pressure (see p. 20).

Although PEEP may raise pulmonary vascular resistance, this effect is relatively unimportant un-

less the right ventricle is already failing or high levels of PEEP are used. Very high levels of PEEP can increase right ventricular (RV) afterload sufficiently to cause RV dilation and reduction of *left* ventricular compliance by the phenomenon of ventricular interdependence. In recent years, PEEP has also been suggested to cause myocardial dysfunction, but such effects, if present at all, must be very minor.

Compensation for PEEP-induced reductions in cardiac output is accomplished by increasing heart rate, raising venous tone, and retaining fluid to raise the pressure driving venous return. These counterbalancing effects are maximized within hours to days. Cardiac output is usually stable when moderate levels of PEEP are used in normovolemic patients with good cardiovascular reflexes and myocardial reserves.

Repletion of intravascular volume, guided by the PEEP-adjusted wedge pressure, should be the primary treatment for depressed cardiac output. Once adequate intravascular volume is assured, vasopressors may also be added to improve the driving pressure for venous return.

Barotrauma

Barotrauma during mechanical ventilation is discussed elsewhere (see Chapter 31). The increased incidence of barotrauma on PEEP appears related to increases of both mean and peak alveolar pressures. These pressures are effectively reduced by lowering tidal volume as end-expiratory pressure is raised and by compensating for the lower tidal volume with periodic sighs.

Reduced Oxygen Delivery

PEEP may exert an adverse effect on oxygen delivery via three mechanisms: (1) *decreased cardiac output*; (2) *increased venous admixture*; and (3) *increased intracardiac or non-capillary shunt*

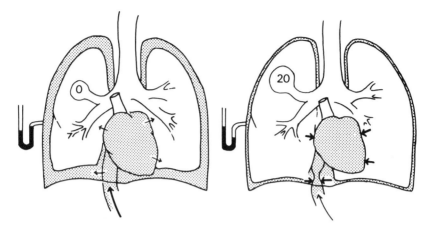

Figure 8.2 Effects of PEEP on cardiovascular function. As PEEP holds the lungs distended, increased pleural pressure tends to compress the heart and great vessels, impeding venous inflow to the thorax while raising intracavitary pressures.

flow. If the drop in cardiac output is greater than the rise in arterial oxygen content, oxygen delivery will fall. Furthermore, provided oxygen consumption remains constant, more oxygen will be stripped from arterial blood, and the O_2 saturation of mixed venous (pulmonary artery) blood will decrease. In turn, reduced mixed venous O_2 saturation adversely affects arterial O_2 content after admixture. Hence, when PEEP is applied it is mandatory to follow cardiac output or arterial-venous oxygen difference $[(a-\bar{v})O_2]$, as well as partial pressure of arterial oxygen (PaO_2).

PEEP may also worsen distribution of blood flow within the lung. Positive pressure has its greatest stretching effect on compliant alveoli. Resistance to blood flow through compliant units increases disproportionately, redirecting blood flow toward stiffer, diseased areas. Fortunately, this effect usually does not outweigh the beneficial effects of alveolar recruitment and hypoxic vasoconstriction in diseased tissues. However, in patients with regional, nonhomogeneous disease (e.g., unilateral pneumonia), PEEP may lower PaO_2 by this mechanism.

PEEP can increase shunt flow by a similar mechanism in patients with intra-pulmonary or intra-cardiac right-to-left communications. Pulmonary arteriovenous malformations, atrial septal defects, and the pulmonary shunt vessels of cirrhosis may receive a larger percentage of flow as PEEP raises pulmonary vascular resistance and right heart filling pressure.

Adverse Effect on CO_2 Elimination

PEEP often impairs CO_2 elimination by reducing lung perfusion and raising intra-alveolar pressure, thereby creating high ventilation/perfusion ($\dot{V} / \dot{Q}$) units. Such effects tend to increase physiologic deadspace, contributing to the ventilation requirement and CO_2 retention of patients with marginal ventilatory reserve.

Alterations in the Work of Breathing

Most PEEP valves offer significant resistance to gas flow during active exhalation. More importantly, although well designed CPAP circuits maintain constant airway pressure throughout the spontaneous breathing cycle, many impose substantial external resistance. PEEP itself may either increase or decrease the work of breathing (W_b). Volume recruitment tends to reduce the W_b, but *overdistention* proves *detrimental* on two counts. First, lung compliance may worsen as additional volume is forced into a fully recruited lung, increasing elastic work. Second, excessive chest distention limits the ability of the inspiratory muscles to perform work by placing them on a disadvantageous portion of their length-tension curve. When the expiratory muscles oppose the volume recruitment of PEEP, the total (inspiratory plus expiratory) W_b tends to increase. As already discussed, however, PEEP may change the distribution of work by forcing the expiratory muscles to work more and the inspiratory muscles to work less (see p. 78).

Impaired Cerebral Perfusion

PEEP increases *cerebral* venous and intracranial pressures (ICP), by raising CVP. This effect is predictably less when the lungs are stiff and transmit less pressure to the pleural space.

The combined effects of lowered arterial pressure (BP) and raised ICP reduce cerebral perfusion pressure (CPP): CPP = BP − ICP (see p. 251). However, in the setting of intracranial hypertension PEEP-related arterial hypotension is a considerably greater risk for precipitating cerebral dysfunction than is central venous hypertension. (When ICP exceeds CVP, increases in CVP caused by PEEP may not transmit to the cerebral veins.)

Abrupt application of PEEP can raise intracranial pressure and precipitate herniation in patients with intracranial mass lesions or seriously elevated ICP. Abrupt withdrawal of PEEP may also be dangerous; PEEP withdrawal can cause a surge in venous return, transiently boosting BP and ICP. Despite its potential dangers, PEEP can safely be used if excessive levels are avoided and if it is applied and withdrawn in small increments.

Hepatic and Renal Impairment

An elevated CVP impedes blood exiting from the liver and thereby reduces hepatic perfusion. As with right heart failure, the resulting passive hepatic congestion can cause mild elevations of bilirubin and hepatic enzymes. PEEP has also been reported to interfere with renal function, even when cardiac output is well-preserved. Although a variety of mechanisms (reflex, humoral) have been proposed, none are generally accepted.

CLINICAL USE

Candidates for PEEP

Good candidates for a trial of PEEP are those who have: (1) hypoxemia despite an $F_iO_2 \geqslant 0.5$; (2) diffuse acute pulmonary disease; (3) poorly compliant lungs; (4) adequate cardiac reserve with normal to increased intravascular volume; (5) a tendency to atelectasis (e.g., following upper abdominal surgery).

Poor candidates have: (1) unilateral or localized lung disease; (2) normally compliant or emphysematous lungs; or (3) cardiovascular compromise (hypotension, intravascular volume deficit). Nonetheless, a cautious *trial* of PEEP should not be withheld from apparently poor candidates with refractory hypoxemia.

Physiologic PEEP

Indeed, there is a good rationale for using at least 3–5 cmH₂O PEEP or CPAP in most patients. Considerable volume loss occurs in moving from the upright to supine position in all but severely obstructed patients. A normal young person loses about 1 liter. Since the compliance of the respiratory system approximates 100 ml/cmH₂O, this would translate into a PEEP effect of ≃ 7.5–10 cmH₂O. Other positional changes are also important to consider. Turning side to side increases the volume of the upper lung as the shifting abdominal contents alter regional chest wall compliance. The prone position is dramatically helpful in some patients with diffuse lung injury, presumably because it causes a regional PEEP effect.

Methods for Choosing the Appropriate Level of Peep

Once the decision has been made do introduce PEEP, the appropriate level must be determined. The effect of PEEP as end-expiratory pressure is raised is neither smooth nor predictable. Some patients show little response until high levels (20–25 cmH₂O) are reached, at which point gas exchange improves remarkably; others respond adequately at 5 cmH₂O or less. Maximal response so a given level of PEEP may require an hour or more.

There is no consensus as to what constitutes an optimal level of PEEP; however, *oxygen saturation*, *oxygen delivery*, *venous admixture*, *lung compliance*, and *volume recruitment* have all been used to guide the selection of PEEP. Despite its effectiveness in improving O_2 saturation, PEEP may prove detrimental if it causes barotrauma or impairs O_2 delivery by reducing cardiac output. Most physicians choose the minimal level of PEEP required to provide *acceptable oxygen saturation* (90%) on an F_iO_2 of ≤ 0.5. O_2 saturation alone, however, does not tell the whole story. Mixed venous oxygen saturation ($S\bar{v}O_2$) can help greatly in determining when reductions in O_2 delivery as a result of lowered cardiac output outweigh the benefits of improved O_2 saturation. ($S\bar{v}O_2$ will fall if O_2 delivery is compromised, even as PaO_2 rises.) A close watch must be kept on peak and mean airway cycling pressures. A marginal boost in PaO_2 or in O_2 delivery may not be worth the increased risk of lung rupture. Many patients with good cardiac function easily compensate for marginal reductions in O_2 saturation, maintaining O_2 delivery by increasing cardiac output.

Two factors are crucial to maintaining adequate tissue oxygenation: a PaO_2 sufficient to maintain an adequate gradient from capillary to mitochondrion and sufficient O_2 flux to satisfy oxygen demand. In patients with a healthy heart and preserved ability to increase oxygen extraction (the (a-v̄) O_2 difference), a rather wide range of oxygen desaturation can be tolerated. However, if either is impaired, the tissues may become oxygen deprived unless O_2 delivery is optimized. In this setting, oxygen consumption (CO times the difference between arterial and mixed venous oxygen contents) can provide useful information in gauging the need for added PEEP.

At some centers, an attempt is made to *maximize oxygen delivery*, even if the airway pressure required is higher than that which achieves 90% saturation. Believing that alveolar inflation improves healing of injured lung, others attempt to reduce the *shunt fraction* below an arbitrary limit, provided that cardiac output can be maintained by fluids and vasopressors. It has also been suggested that the "optimal" PEEP can be selected without the benefit of wedge pressure or $S\bar{v}O_2$ measurements by raising PEEP while monitoring effective "total thoracic compliance". Advocates of this method believe the level of PEEP which *maximizes compliance* coincides with the greatest oxygen delivery, lowest alveolar deadspace, and maximal alveolar recruitment. Although this is an attractive hypothesis, cardiac output may fall independently of changes in total thoracic compliance, and clinical experience suggests that this technique is unreliable. (In some patients, the peak of the compliance curve is not sharp, and in others total thoracic compliance may continue to rise as PEEP is raised to levels which induce hypotension.) Two recently introduced methods are variants of this optimal recruitment concept. The first compares *arterial and end tidal CO_2 tensions*. This difference is minimized at the point of maximal recruitment and widens as overdistention increases deadspace. The second variation uses the *airway pressure curve* as a guide to identify the point of full lung recruitment (see p. 52).

The PEEP Trial

Rationale.   To determine what level of PEEP is most beneficial, a systematic appraisal should be carried out—the PEEP "trial". During the trial, PEEP level should be the only variable. F_iO_2 and all other ventilator settings remain at fixed, safe levels. Infusions of cardiotropic drugs should also be maintained constant.

The trial should be conducted at the lowest F_iO_2 which results in acceptable O_2 saturation at the lowest level of PEEP acceptable to the clinician. (A safe margin of O_2 saturation should be maintained in case of a paradoxical response to PEEP.)

There are two distinct advantages in selecting an F_iO_2 as close as possible to that intended for use with PEEP after the trial is completed. First, it is not possible to predict with certainty what

PaO_2 will do when F_iO_2 is lowered from the trial level to that used for support. (The PaO_2 depends upon the precise fractions of admixture due to shunt, to moderately low $\dot{V} / \dot{Q}$ units, and to very low $\dot{V} / \dot{Q}$ units.) As a very rough guide, the ratio of PaO_2 to F_iO_2 (the "P/F" ratio) can be used to estimate what PaO_2 to expect, but the actual PaO_2 observed is highly variable (see p. 49). Second, if an F_iO_2 of 1.0 is selected for the trial, only shunt contributes to hypoxemia, so that a beneficial effect of lower levels of PEEP on $\dot{V} / \dot{Q}$ mismatching can be missed.

Technique.   Before the PEEP trial is begun, the airway is suctioned free of secretions. The trial is conducted by raising PEEP in 3–5 cmH_2O increments every 10–20 minutes, to an arbitrary "upper end" limit (e.g., 15–20 cmH_2O), or until a clearly beneficial or detrimental response is seen. Airway pressure, thoracic compliance, O_2 saturation, blood pressure, heart and respiratory rates, cardiac output and/or $S\bar{v}O_2$ should be measured at each level. Timing should be precise. (Changes should not be delayed by the tardy return of previous results from the laboratory.) The entire trial should be completed expeditiously to minimize drift in PaO_2 due to factors other than changes in PEEP. However, sufficient time should elapse between increments to allow slow responders to improve. (It should be recognized that the PaO_2 values obtained at 20 minutes may underestimate the final response.)

The level of PEEP selected will depend upon the criterion chosen. Although admittedly arbitrary, one rational method is to adopt the lowest level of PEEP that yields an O_2 saturation > 90% at an acceptable F_iO_2 without depressing cardiac output or chest compliance. Once the PEEP level has been chosen, F_iO_2 must be lowered to the desired level (generally < 0.6), and blood gases or oximetry must be performed to confirm that oxygenation is acceptable at the level of F_iO_2 as well. If PaO_2 is unacceptable, the next higher increment of PEEP yielding improved gas exchange is selected, and the arterial blood gases resampled.

Peep Withdrawal

Clinically unstable patients, i.e., those requiring an F_iO_2 > 0.4, and those with worsening gas exchange are poor candidates for PEEP removal. PEEP should be withdrawn cautiously, with oximetry or arterial blood gases monitored before and after each step change. The final reduction of PEEP (from 5 to 0 cmH_2O) should be done with special caution; failure to move successfully to the next lower level most often occurs in this range. Patients who have shown .ly marginal PEEP response are a possible exception to these guidelines. Abrupt or premature withdrawal of PEEP can cause deterioration of gas exchange, which may respond slowly to reinstitution of PEEP. Sudden termination of PEEP can also cause cardiovascular overload, increase the work of breathing, and precipitate dangerous increases in intracranial pressure.

"Prophylactic PEEP"

Some physicians administer low levels of PEEP (3–5 cmH$_2$O) "prophylactically" to all intubated patients. The rationale for applying PEEP to all intubated patients rests primarily on the belief that such patients have a lower functional residual capacity (FRC), simply because the larynx is bypassed. Although there is documentation of this effect, its physiologic basis is unclear.

The routine application of PEEP to the airway of patients who require intubation after surgery or trauma rests on firmer ground. PEEP could offset the considerable fall in FRC known to occur in the first hours to days following thoracic or upper abdominal incisions (a contributing factor for atelectasis and impaired gas exchange). Thus, so long as intubation is required for other reasons, adding 5 cmH$_2$O PEEP seems defensible. At the present time, there is no convincing proof of benefit or danger from this approach. PEEP (8 cmH$_2$O) has not been shown to protect against adult respiratory distress syndrome (ARDS) (see Ref. 5).

"Super-PEEP"

Occasionally, very high levels of PEEP (> 20 cmH$_2$O) must be applied to achieve acceptable O$_2$ saturation. Although potentially hazardous, this technique is feasible when careful attention is paid to fluid and vasopressor support. Barotrauma is an ever-present, life-threatening risk. Every effort must be made to reduce peak and mean cycling pressures and the minute ventilation requirement. Sedation, paralysis, and reduced tidal volume may prove helpful. Nonetheless, a trial of "super-PEEP" seems justified in some desperately ill patients with oxygenation failure that cannot be compensated for by safe concentrations of inspired oxygen and lower end-expiratory pressures.

"Auto-PEEP" Effect

In patients with severe airflow obstruction and high minute ventilation requirements, hyperinflation develops when ventilator cycling occurs before passive expiratory flow ceases. At normal lung volumes, elastic recoil and expiratory flow are in-

adequate to expel the full tidal volume (V_T) at the set frequency; however, active expiration and/or hyperinflation re-establishes the balance. Patients who trap air above the relaxed volume of the chest must maintain positive pressure in the alveoli and small airways at end-exhalation. Hence, alveolar pressure remains continuously positive throughout the ventilatory cycle, raising intrathoracic pressure and impeding venous return. Monitored pressure in the central airway remains nearly ambient unless expiratory flow is interrupted.

Unsuspected, this "auto-PEEP" (AP) effect can seriously reduce true cardiac filling pressures and confound interpretation of pulmonary artery and wedge pressures, raising them by an amount similar to the pressure transmitted to the pleural space (see Chapter 2). Because AP must be reversed before inspiratory airflow can begin or the ventilator can be triggered, the work of breathing also rises.

Although AP is most predictable in patients with severe airflow obstruction, it occurs anytime the ventilator cycles automatically before the lung returns to its fully relaxed volume. To reduce AP, it is crucial to *reduce minute ventilation requirement* and *improve expiratory flow resistance*. The cardiovascular consequences of AP can be minimized by increasing the rate of fluid or pressor infusion or by increasing the fraction of *spontaneous* efforts (e.g., by reducing intermittent mandatory ventilation frequency or substituting pressure support). The detection, consequences and management of AP are discussed in greater detail in Chapters 2, 5, and 7.

SUMMARY

The following is a list of the benefits and problems associated with the use of PEEP:

Benefits	Problems
Improves oxygenation	Predisposes to barotrauma
Reduces work of breathing	Impedes preload and right ventricular ejection
Improves lung compliance	
Aids the left ventricle	Reduces cerebral perfusion
Splints the chest wall	Weakens the ventilatory pump
Mobilizes distal secretions	
Splints the chest wall	Increases deadspace
Mobilizes distal secretions	Confounds monitoring
	Increases deadspace
	Confounds monitoring

SUGGESTED READINGS

1. Blanch L, Fernandez R, Benito S, et al: Effect of PEEP on the arterial minus end-tidal carbon dioxide gradient. *Chest* 92:451–454, 1987.
2. Gong H, Jr: Positive pressure ventilation in the adult respiratory distress syndrome. *Clin Chest Med* 3(1):69–88, 1982.
3. Kacmarek RM, Pierson DJ (eds): Positive end-expiratory pressure. (Special Issue, Parts 1 and 2), *Respir Care* 33:419–630, 1988.
4. Luce JM: The cardiovascular effects of mechanical ventilation and positive end-expiratory pressure. *JAMA* 252(6):807–811, 1984.
5. Pepe PE, Hudson LD, Carrico CJ: Early application of positive end-expiratory pressure in patients at risk for the adult respiratory distress syndrome. *N Engl J Med* 311:281–286, 1984.
6. Pepe PE, Marini JJ: Occult positive end-expiratory pressure in mechanically ventilated patients with airflow obstruction. The "Auto-PEEP" effect. *Am Rev Respir Dis* 126:160–170, 1982.
7. Rounds S, Brody JS: Putting PEEP in perspective. *N Engl J Med* 311:323–325, 1984.
8. Suter PM, Fairley HB, Isenberg MD: Optimum end-expiratory airway pressure in patients with acute pulmonary failure. *N Engl J Med* 292:284–289, 1975.

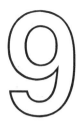

Weaning from Mechanical Ventilation

Many patients tolerate abrupt termination of mechanical assistance without needing to adjust to spontaneous breathing (e.g., post-anesthesia). However, when machine withdrawal proves difficult, a strategy for transfer of the respiratory workload must be developed. Weaning is the graded removal of ventilator support from those patients who will not tolerate sudden conversion to spontaneous breathing. The weaning process actually occurs in several stages: weaning from positive pressure inflation, weaning from positive end-expiratory pressure (PEEP), weaning from the endotracheal or tracheostomy tube, and weaning from supplemental oxygen.

PHYSIOLOGIC DETERMINANTS OF VENTILATOR DEPENDENCE

A continuing need for machine assistance may be dictated by hemoglobin desaturation during spontaneous breathing, cardiovascular instability during machine withdrawal, psychologic dependence, or, most commonly, imbalance between ventilatory capability and demand.

Arterial Hypoxemia

Mechanical ventilation can improve arterial oxygenation by providing large tidal breaths that oppose atelectasis, sealing the airway to allow high inspired oxygen concentrations and PEEP application, reducing or offsetting the effects of pulmonary edema, and improving the balance between tissue oxygen delivery and demand. Under stress, the respiratory muscles consume a substantial fraction of the available oxygen supply. When cardiac output is compromised, the oxygen demand of the respiratory system forces greater O_2 extraction by other vital organs. The resulting desaturation of mixed venous blood contributes to venous admixture. Mechanical ventilation mitigates this problem by relieving the ventilatory workload.

Cardiovascular Instability

Inappropriately low cardiac output often contributes to hypoxemia and weakness of the ventilatory pump. Cardiovascular instability overtly limits the pace of ventilator withdrawal when pulmonary edema or arrhythmias develop during spontaneous breathing. The sudden demands of spontaneous breathing can overwhelm patients with marginally compensated cor pulmonale or left heart compromise. Rhythm disturbances are frequently provoked during the transition to spontaneous breathing by hypoxemia, reflex stimulation, altered cardiac loading, and the stress of resuming the ventilatory burden. In this setting, oxygen administration, improved electrolyte and pH balance, anti-arrhythmic therapy, diuresis, and more gradual conversion to spontaneous breathing may be instrumental to the success of machine withdrawal.

Imbalance of Ventilatory Capability and Demand

Although isolated impairment of ventilatory drive may occasionally cause CO_2 retention, the most common reason for ventilator dependence relates to the inability of the patient to maintain appropriate ventilation without intolerable dyspnea. The total ventilatory workload is determined by the product of minute ventilation requirement ($\dot{V}_e$) and the energy expended per liter of gas flow. Poor ventilatory drive and muscle weakness compromise the ability to meet demand.

Ventilatory Demand—Minute Ventilation Requirement

Three primary factors determine the $\dot{V}_e$ requirement: the CO_2 production, the fraction of wasted ventilation (the deadspace), and the sensitivity of the central drive mechanism (Table 9.1).

Table 9.1
Factors Affecting Ventilatory Demand

CO_2 Production	↑ V_D/V_T	↑ Drive
Fever	Lung disease	Neurogenic
Shivering	Hypovolemia	Psychogenic
Pain/agitation	Vascular	Metabolic
Trauma/burns	occlusion	Acidosis
Sepsis	External	Hypoxemia
Overfeeding	apparatus	Sepsis
	Excessive PEEP	Hypotension

CO_2 Production

Fever, shivering, pain, agitation, increased work of breathing, burns, sepsis, and overfeeding are common causes of increased CO_2 production in the intensive care unit (ICU). CO_2 production is also influenced by underlying nutritional status as well as by the number and composition of the calories administered. The semi-starvation which often precedes critical illness suppresses CO_2 production. Despite the importance of adequate nutrition, patients should not be overfed. Excess calories may be converted to fat, generating CO_2 as a metabolic by-product unrelated to energy production. Burning carbohydrate produces more CO_2 per calorie generated than burning fat or protein. However, even though large carbohydrate loads can precipitate ventilatory failure, the importance of calorie composition to ventilator dependence remains to be convincingly shown.

Ventilatory Deadspace

Virtually all of the diverse processes that damage the lung or airways of the critically ill patient increase the wasted ventilation or "deadspace" (DS) fraction. Certain reversible factors unrelated to underlying lung pathology can also prove important. For example, thromboembolic or vasculitic arterial occlusion or hypovolemia may reduce perfusion to the ventilated lung, creating DS. Tubing interposed between the endotracheal tube and the "Y" of the ventilator circuit adds to the DS and should be minimized in patients who are slow to wean from machine support.

Central Drive

Enhanced central drive (CD) arising from neurogenic, psychogenic, or metabolic stimuli augments ventilatory demand and workload. In conditions such as asthma and acute pulmonary edema, drive stimuli arising from the lung or chest wall reverse after correction of the underlying disorder. Hypoxemia, hypotension, developing sepsis, and acidosis also accentuate CD. Correction of metabolic acidosis is one of the most important ways in which CD can be diminished. It is also important not to force $PaCO_2$ below the patient's normal resting value, as the ensuing bicarbonate diuresis redefines the $\dot{V}_E$ needed to maintain pH homeostasis. In the chronic state, anxiety is the major reversible psychogenic factor influencing ventilatory demand. Clinicians should remain alert to its presence and treat it judiciously by counseling, by co-opting the patient into the weaning plan, and by use of anxiolytics when required.

Ventilatory Demand—Work Per Liter of Ventilation

Intrinsic Factors

Apart from the $\dot{V}_E$ requirement, the other major component determining ventilatory burden is the energy expended by the respiratory system per liter of ventilation. The product of mechanical workload and neuromuscular efficiency defines how much breathing energy is expended. Once tidal volume and inspiratory time are set, the frictional and elastic properties of the thorax determine the pressure that must be required per breath and the external work output per liter of ventilation. The average pressure developed by the respiratory system per breath can be determined by a simple formula: $\bar{P} = R\ (V_T/t_i) + V_T/2C_{rs} + $ auto-PEEP, where R and C_{rs} are the inspiratory resistance and compliance of the respiratory system, V_T is tidal volume, and t_i is the time required for inspiration (see p. 56). Therefore, for the same level of $\dot{V}_E$, more external work must be done if C_{rs} falls or if V_T, auto-PEEP, mean inspiratory flow (V_T/t_i), or R increase. Bronchospasm, secretion retention and mucosal edema are the primary reversible factors that increase R. Secretion retention greatly accentuates the inspiratory workload in patients with already narrowed airways. Infiltrates, high lung volumes, pleural effusions, abdominal distention and poor positioning reduce C_{rs}. Auto-PEEP is discussed elsewhere (see p. 54).

These are not the only factors that determine the energy needed by the respiratory musculature, however. The respiratory muscles consume more oxygen (become less sensitive) when they begin contraction from a mechanically disadvantaged high lung volume or when the pattern of muscle contraction is not well coordinated. For example, patients with diaphragmatic weakness may allow the abdominal contents to be sucked upward with each inspiratory effort so that much of the tension developed by the inspiratory muscles of the chest cage fails to translate into negative pleural pressure. It is easy to see why patients with COPD, who combine hyperinflation with narrowed airways and a tendency to retain secretions, often have difficulty in sustaining spontaneous ventilation during T-piece trials.

Extrinsic Factors

The external properties of the ventilator circuit can also play an important role in determining the ventilatory workload. Endotracheal tube resistance exceeds the normal resistance of the upper airway. Frictional pressure losses increase rapidly when high flows are driven through small caliber tubes. Kinking and secretion encrustation may encroach on an otherwise adequate lumen. In some instances, it may be wise to replace a nasotracheal, an orotracheal tube, or tracheostomy in order to reduce resistance and improve secretion clearance. Occasionally, extubation facilitates ventilator withdrawal, especially when the patient bites the tube or shows extreme discomfort, or when a narrow bore tube hinders airflow and impedes (rather than assists) secretion hygiene. Tracheostomy may often be helpful because larger tube diameter, shorter axial length, and improved secretion clearance minimize resistance.

The resistance of other circuit components varies widely and can add significantly to the ventilatory burden. Considerable effort may be needed to draw conditioned gas through the ventilator during the spontaneous breaths of synchronized intermittent mandatory ventilation (IMV) or continuous positive airway pressure (CPAP). (On the other hand, the addition of low-level CPAP can compensate for microatelectasis, thereby improving thoracic compliance and the work of breathing.) The flow resistance offered by exhalation valves and PEEP devices can provoke a sense of dyspnea. Largely for these reasons, direct extubation or T-piece weaning is better tolerated than low level IMV by many patients.

Ventilatory Capability

The ability to maintain acceptable effort is determined by respiratory drive and muscle performance.

Central Drive

Multiple interacting factors can suppress the output of the ventilatory drive center. As a general rule, old and debilitated patients are the most susceptible. Sedatives and neurological impairment

generally receive the most clinical attention. However, other reversible causes are important. For example, chronic loading of ventilation (as during a severe bout of asthma) can condition the ventilatory center to tolerate higher $PaCO_2$—presumably an adaptive response to prevent neuromuscular fatigue. Metabolic alkalosis, hypothyroidism, and sleep deprivation are commonly overlooked as causes of drive center impairment. Because the output of the ventilatory center tends to parallel metabolic rate and caloric intake, *nutritional status* profoundly affects drive. Starvation impairs hypoxic, and to a lesser extent, hypercapnic sensitivity. Interestingly, drive is rapidly restored within a day or two of reinitiating adequate feeding. The composition of the calories ingested may also be influential: amino-acid infusion evokes a particularly prompt and convincing enhancement of hypercapnic drive. The administration of pharmacologic stimulants such as doxapram or progesterone has been advocated when depressed drive impedes weaning. However, these drugs are not usually helpful.

Muscular Performance

Strength. Given normal drive, retention of carbon dioxide is uncommon when a patient can generate more than 25% of maximal predicted inspiratory pressure. The strength of the respiratory muscles is determined by muscle bulk, the intrinsic properties and loading conditions of the contractile fibers, and the chemical environment in which the muscle contracts. Poor nutrition causes muscle wasting, thereby limiting maximal respiratory pressures. As overall body weight diminishes, the mass and strength of the diaphragm decrease proportionately. Glucocorticoids greatly accelerate the rate of protein catabolism. Optimal concentrations of calcium, magnesium, potassium, phosphate, H^+, chloride and carbon dioxide are each important in maximizing muscle performance. Hypoxemia has a greater detrimental effect on endurance than on muscle strength itself. Certain commonly used drugs (e.g., aminoglycosides) also contribute to weakness in the setting of myasthenia gravis or other underlying neuromuscular impairment. Conversely, aminophylline and beta sympathomimetic drugs may produce modest improvement in contractility and endurance. Intriguing experimental data suggest that the resting potential of the skeletal muscle membrane may be abnormal for several days following sepsis, and perhaps other forms of critical illness. (Such data may help to explain the apparently profound muscle weakness observed in many of these patients.)

Contractile Fiber Properties. As discussed in depth in *Respiratory Medicine for the House Officer* (Ref. 4), the contractile force developed by a stimulated muscle fiber relates directly to its resting length at the onset of contraction, and inversely to its speed of contraction. Force output is therefore compromised when a patient inhales rapidly from high lung volume, as so often occurs in breathless, hyperinflated patients with chronic obstructive pulmonary disease (COPD) or asthma.

Endurance. Endurance, the ability of a muscle to sustain effort, is determined by the balance between energy supply and demand. Because working muscles must receive a constant flow of oxygenated blood for optimal performance, hypoxemia, anemia, and ischemia are especially important to correct. Although the respiratory muscles receive adequate blood flow under normal circumstances and possess a large recruitable reserve, even this luxuriant supply may be insufficient under conditions of high stress and a failing cardiac pump. Spontaneously breathing experimental animals placed in cardiogenic shock quickly succumb to respiratory failure, whereas mechanically ventilated animals subjected to similar stresses survive for extended periods.

Insufficiency of the energy supply becomes increasingly likely at high work rates. As the workload increases, forceful contraction persists for a progressively greater fraction of the total respiratory cycle. The forcefully contracting muscle may compress the vascular network of the diaphragm, limiting nutrient flow. Studies of patients in acute respiratory failure indicate that spontaneous breathing routinely consumes $\simeq 25\%$ of the oxygen used by the entire body, and more during flagrant respiratory distress. (Normal resting percentage value for respiratory oxygen consumption is $\simeq 1\%$.) Even in the non-acute phase of ventilatory support, recent work suggests that many patients who fail weaning do so because of inadequate delivery of oxygen to the respiratory muscles.

Over the years there have been many attempts to gauge endurance by comparing spontaneous breathing cycles with maximal voluntary efforts. For example, the ability to voluntarily double $\dot{V}_E$ or tidal volume has been used as a positive sign. Unfortunately, voluntary indices require patient cooperation. Recently, however, indices that do not require patient cooperation have moved from the physiology laboratory to the bedside. Two such measures are the ratio of average inspiratory pressure to maximal inspiratory pressure ($\bar{P}/P_{max}$) and the inspiratory effort quotient (IEQ)—the product of $\bar{P}/P_{max}$ and the inspiratory time fraction (t_i/t_{tot}). $\bar{P}/P_{max}$ ratios > 0.4 and IEQs > 0.15 indicate that the patient is working near the limits of fatigue. $\bar{P}$ can be estimated as already described, and P_{max} is the maximal inspiratory pressure generated during airway occlusion.

Fatigue recognition is facilitated by observing the respiratory pattern. The respiratory rate (f) is the most sensitive but least specific indicator of developing problems. Early in the course of respiratory muscle fatigue, f increases. Preterminally, the f diminishes—a harbinger of approaching apnea. The respiratory rhythm tends to lose regularity as the fatigue threshold is approached.

Other components of the respiratory pattern, although harder to quantitate, provide equally valuable diagnostic clues. At moderate levels of exertion, pressure in the abdomen rises as the diaphragm contracts, displacing the abdominal contents downward and outward. Vigorous activity recruits the thoracic musculature, elongating the chest, expanding the rib cage, and lifting the diaphragm. If diaphragmatic contraction is not forceful enough, it will rise rather than fall during inspiration and the abdomen retracts paradoxically. During expiration the thoracic muscles relax and the abdominal contents return to their original position. When observed in the supine position, this phenomenon, known as *paradoxical abdominal motion*, indicates a high level of exertion relative to the capability of the diaphragm. Some clinicians view this finding as an indicator of established muscle fatigue, but it is more likely a sign only of high stress (that may or may not be tolerable). Much less commonly, the ribcage and abdomen alternate primary responsibility for inspiratory activity, a pattern known as *respiratory alternans*. (Teleologically, this pattern might allow one muscle group to rest while the other works.) Overt respiratory alternans is much less commonly observed than paradoxical abdominal motion and when seen often has a neuropathological origin.

Importance of Muscle Rest. To reverse fatigue, the primary intervention is to *rest the muscle*. Complete rest is certainly not required, but a substantial fraction of the imposed workload must be relieved. Assisted mechanical ventilation, optimally adjusted to meet patient demands, usually allows the patient to rest sufficiently to achieve this purpose. As a general rule, the support level is adequate if the patient is made comfortable.

How long a skeletal muscle must be rested before it is fully recovered from fatigue is not known with certainty. However, physiologic evidence of subnormal performance can be detected for 12–24 hours after an acutely fatiguing load is applied. Furthermore, the resting electrical potential of skeletal muscle membrane remains subnormal for days after the onset of systemic injuries, such as sepsis. Therefore, a rest period of at least 12–24 hours seems appropriate after acute decompensation.

PREDICTING WEANABILITY

As already indicated, many predictive indices have been suggested to forecast the outcome of the weaning trial (Table 9.2). If the patient is ventilator dependent for reasons unrelated to muscle strength (e.g., hypoxemia), such indices are of little use. Even when poor ventilatory endurance is responsible, no single index has been universally successful, perhaps because multiple factors cause the patient to remain ventilator dependent. One widely used panel of indicators tests $\dot{V}_E$, muscle strength, muscle reserve, and respiratory impedance. Patients who successfully wean from mechanical support generally have a $\dot{V}_E < 10$ l/min, a maximum negative inspiratory pressure (MIP) exceeding -20 cmH$_2$O, and an ability to double the baseline $\dot{V}_E$ upon command. In practice, the problem with such criteria is two-fold: only selected components can be measured in uncooperative patients, and the outcome is uncertain when only one or two indices lie within the acceptable range. Thus, although these time honored criteria are predictive when all are satisfied, they are of questionable assistance in difficult cases.

Involuntary Measures

Minute Ventilation

In current practice the most reliable measures of ventilatory requirement and patient capability are $\dot{V}_E$ and the maximal inspiratory pressure (MIP)

generated against an occluded airway. Although $\dot{V}_E$ is easy enough to measure, it should be corrected for body habitus, metabolic rate, and pH. For example, a 50 kg patient whose pH at the time of $\dot{V}_E$ measurement is 7.25 with a PCO$_2$ of 60 mmHg, may have a minute ventilation of 10 l/min and be unable to wean. Conversely a patient weighing 100 kg with respiratory alkalosis may wean easily at the same level of $\dot{V}_E$. However valuable $\dot{V}_E$ may be, it only tells half the story of ventilatory demand. Work per liter of ventilation ($\bar{P}$) is equally important.

Maximal Inspiratory Pressure

MIP must be carefully measured to be of real value (see p. 59). Although highly negative numbers encourage a weaning attempt, low values may reflect defective measurement technique rather than patient weakness. In poorly cooperative patients airway occlusion must start from a low lung volume and continue for at least 8–10 efforts before the value is recorded. The MIP, a good measure of isometric muscle strength, does not itself yield information regarding endurance. The IEQ holds promise as an integrative index of capability and demand (see p. 88).

Spontaneous Breathing Pattern

Patients who are well compensated to the ventilatory workload usually choose tidal volumes $\geq$ 5 ml/kg of body weight and breathing frequencies $<$ 30/min. Although each breath taken with a shallow tidal volume is less energy costly than a deeper breath, the total energy expenditure necessary to maintain a given $\dot{V}_E$ may be greater, inasmuch as anatomic deadspace occupies a larger percentage of each breath during shallow breathing. Hence, patients who must breathe at frequencies $>$ 35/min usually do so because they are too weak or fatigued to inspire to an appropriate depth. (Some patients with neurological disease assume rapid

Table 9.2
Predictors of Weanability

	Measured Values			Clincal Observations	
Ventilation	Strength	Endurance		Neuromuscular	Other
$\dot{V}_E \leq$ 10 l/min	MIP > -20 cmH$_2$O	MVV $> 2 \times \dot{V}_E$		Absence of scalene or abdominal muscle activity	F$_I$O$_2 \geq$ 0.40
$\dot{V}_E \leq$ 175 ml/kg/min	V$_t \geq$ 5 ml/kg V$_t \geq$ 5 ml/kg VC $\geq$ 10 ml/kg	IEQ $<$ 0.15 P$_{0.1} <$ 6 cmH$_2$O f $<$ 30/min		Asynchrony Irregular breathing	70 $<$ pulse $<$ 120 pH $>$ 7.30 BP $>$ 80 mmHg

shallow patterns because of disordered ventilatory control and may effectively wean at frequencies $\geq 40/\text{min}$.) The pattern assumed during a brief (5-minute) trial of spontaneous breathing under direct observation proves an excellent integrative test of endurance.

Other Data

In attempting to discontinue mechanical ventilation, some investigators have found that observations unrelated to standard indices of lung mechanics correlate well with an adverse weaning outcome. Pulse rates < 70 or > 100 beats per minute, respiratory rates > 30 per minute, forceful abdominal contractions, or accessory muscle activity, ataxic breathing patterns, and coma are all negative prognostic factors. Non-respiratory factors often predominate in the most difficult weaning cases.

WEANING TRIAL

Preparations for Weaning from the Ventilator

The great majority of patients are easily discontinued from mechanical ventilation. Those who fail require optimal preparation before another weaning trial is undertaken. The inability to discontinue mechanical support often results from failure to correct one or more of the factors that adversely affect strength, capacity for responding to stress, ventilatory requirement, gas exchange, or lung mechanics. The patient should be in good electrolyte, pH, and fluid balance. Infection, arrhythmias, and heart failure must be well under control. Airways should be optimally dilated and cleared of secretions. Balanced nutritional support is essential. Administration of excessive calories or high carbohydrate diets can increase respiratory quotient and carbon dioxide output. Gaseous distention of the abdomen must be relieved. Care should be taken not to ventilate patients with chronic CO_2 retention to an artifically normal $PaCO_2$ before the attempt. Should this happen, the patient may not be able to maintain the lower CO_2 level during spontaneous breathing, allowing acute acidosis to develop.

Weaning Sequence

The steps involved in removing mechanical support are:

1. Estimation of the likelihood of success (''parameter'' measurement)
2. ''T-piece trial'' of spontaneous ventilation

3. Weaning, if the T-piece trial is poorly tolerated.

While favorable weaning parameters may support a decision to undertake a weaning attempt, poor parameters should not preclude a carefully observed T-piece trial or attempts to wean if clinical judgment otherwise suggests a favorable outcome.

T-Piece Trial

A T-piece trial is a brief but stringent test of the ability to sustain spontaneous ventilation. It is generally undertaken when clinical judgment suggests that the patient should be able to breathe spontaneously without ventilator support. In such patients passing the trial justifies an attempt to withdraw the ventilator quickly; failing such a trial indicates that weaning is necessary. One reasonable method for conducting the T-piece trial is the following:

1. Initial T-piece trials should be undertaken in the morning when the patient is well rested and a full staff is available. If the patient is alert, explain the purpose of the procedure.
2. Place the patient in the sitting or semi-upright position for maximal mechanical advantage.
3. Unless PaO_2 is high enough to provide a comfortable margin, increase F_iO_2 by at least 10%, because microatelectasis and retained secretions may develop during shallow spontaneous breathing.
4. Suction the airway and oropharynx.
5. Monitor pulse, blood pressure, tidal volume, respiratory rate and level of comfort before starting and every 5 minutes for the first 20 minutes. If the outcome is in doubt, arterial blood gases are analyzed. Blood gas analysis may be unnecessary if the patient is monitored continuously by end-tidal capnometry and oximetry.
6. If the patient appears to be doing well, continue. However, if there is any question of tolerance, resume mechanical ventilation immediately.
7. Terminate the trial if the patient indicates *intolerable dyspnea* or if *diastolic blood pressure* falls or rises by more than 20 mmHg, *pulse* rises or falls more than 30 per minute, *respiratory rate* increases by more than 10 per minute over the initial spontaneous value, *mental status deteriorates*, *arrhythmias* develop, or *arterial blood gases* return unacceptable. (Remember that moderate disturbances of vital signs can be seen in successful trials).

During trials longer than 15 minutes, periodic suctioning and hyperinflation should be performed. Prolonged T-piece trials are discouraged in patients having no need for the airway, inasmuch as the intubated patient cannot cough effectively and the tube may increase airway resistance. In general, the duration of the T-piece trial should parallel the duration of pre-trial mechanical ventilation and vary inversely with the confidence of the physician in the extubation outcome. It should be noted that the first minutes to hours off the ventilator are often the most stressful because tidal volume and functional residual capacity (FRC) may decrease, and changes occur in central vascular volume, respiratory work, and pattern of breathing. Once the patient has comfortably sustained spontaneous ventilation for 1–2 hours, acute deterioration is unlikely and extubation should be considered if no contraindication exists and the patient appears strong. Special caution is indicated in patients who have undergone a prolonged period of ventilatory support. Patients with potentially unstable respiratory drive centers (e.g., after cerebrovascular accident, CVA) should be watched for a longer period before removing the tube. Despite all precautions, it is distressingly common for marginal patients who are apparently weaned successfully to require reintubation 12–48 hours after extubation. Therefore, recently extubated patients must be watched very closely for signs of decompensation.

WEANING STRATEGIES AND METHODS

General Principles

A failed T-piece trial in an otherwise viable candidate indicates that weaning is necessary. Key to the success of the weaning effort is careful attention to optimize the physiologic determinants of ventilator dependence described above. Reversal of heart failure, electrolyte imbalance, hypoxemia, anemia, nutritional deficiencies, and bronchospasm are of particular importance. It should be emphasized that patients undergoing prolonged weaning regimens (of whatever type) should receive *full ventilator support at night to allow sleep*. Forcing the patient to work continuously may cause fitful sleep and compromise the weaning effort. The patient must be kept fully informed of the weaning plan and be given "veto power" to terminate the trial if he/she experiences intolerable discomfort. Panic reactions must be avoided, especially in patients with chronic obstructive pulmonary disease (COPD) who experience a self-reinforcing cycle of dyspnea, hy-

perinflation, and compromised muscle function during these episodes. Tracheostomy should be considered in all patients who prove difficult to wean. Tracheostomy provides a more stable airway than an endotracheal tube, allows ambulation and oral feeding, decreases the work of breathing, and improves secretion clearance.

Methods of Weaning

There are three weaning methods in widespread use at the current time: progressive T-piece trials, intermittent mandatory ventilation (IMV), and pressure support (PS) ventilation. Very recently, another mode, mandatory (or minimum) minute volume (MMV), has been introduced to clinical practice.

T-Piece Wean

Using the intermittent "T-piece" or "blow by" method, the duration of independent breathing is progressively lengthened, according to patient tolerance. T-piece weaning provides stress periods punctuated by recovery periods of total rest. Although traditional, this approach remains highly attractive, based on recently acquired knowledge of fatigue and muscle reconditioning. Furthermore, the T-piece generally provides conditioned gas at negligible resistive work cost.

The main disadvantages of this method are that it requires significant staff time to implement and monitor, and abrupt transitions occur between periods on and off the ventilator. The latter can prove problematic in patients who must assume a high-impedance workload, anxiety-prone patients, and patients with congestive heart failure. Unlike IMV, no apnea alarm is provided during periods of spontaneous breathing on a T-piece. Although the "zero-CPAP" option of many ventilators is suboptimal in terms of resistive work, allowing the patient to breathe spontaneously while attached to the ventilator circuit provides an apnea alarm, enables the application of positive end-expiratory pressure, and facilitates interconversions between no support and full support modes.

During the T-piece trial the patient is disconnected from the ventilator and attached to a blow-by source of humidified oxygen ≃ 10% more concentrated than that delivered by machine. If well tolerated, periods of spontaneous ventilation are progressively lengthened. Failure to progress to the next interval mandates reinstitution of continuous ventilator support for 12–24 hours and a search for correctable problems. If the patient remains comfortable while breathing on the T-piece for 30–60 minutes, shows no sign of hemodynamic instability or respiratory decompensation, and maintains acceptable blood gases (pH > 7.30, PaO_2 > 50 mmHg), spontaneous breathing may continue, punctuated by periodic hyperinflations and suctioning. The time that a patient must be observed during T-piece breathing before the ventilator is discontinued entirely should be governed by the length of time the patient has received mechanical ventilation and the apparent level of tolerance. In many centers, a modified "sprint" trial has supplemented or replaced the traditional t-piece trial. During sprint periods the patient breathes spontaneously through the machine circuit, with or without low-level pressure support (see p. 69) or CPAP applied. Even before a serious weaning effort is under way, such episodes may provide muscle conditioning and allow assessment of breathing reserve.

Intermittent Mandatory Ventilation

During IMV the machine provides a selected number of positive pressure breaths to furnish 0–100% of the total ventilatory requirement. Machine-delivered breaths are interspersed among spontaneous breaths taken by the patient, and can be delivered at arbitrary time (IMV) or in synchrony with patient effort (SIMV). IMV provides a method to gradually transfer the work of breathing from the machine to the patient without repeated manipulation of the circuit tubing, thereby reducing the potential for technical error while saving nursing time. It is potentially advantageous for patients with congestive heart failure or obstructive lung disease who cannot withstand sudden increments in venous return or in the work of breathing, and for those who experience anxiety when machine support is abruptly withdrawn. IMV provides periodic hyperinflations automatically and may allow the patient to re-train and re-strengthen long rested muscles. Furthermore, low levels of positive end expiratory pressure can be applied more easily during IMV than during T-piece breathing.

Used improperly, however, IMV can increase the work of breathing, prolong the weaning period unnecessarily, or worse, endanger the life of the patient. Inefficient valving of the IMV circuit can markedly increase the work of spontaneous breathing, a problem that can be countered by judicious use of pressure support. One of the greatest dangers of IMV is that the patient will not be watched vigilantly for signs of deterioration at a low assist rate because "he/she is on the ventilator". It should be remembered that hypoventilation and respiratory acidosis can develop without any ventilator alarm sounding, especially when low levels of IMV support are used. In addition, because the respiratory muscles are continuously active during IMV, it is at least theoretically possible that fatigued muscles may never rest sufficiently to enable full recovery, even though blood gases and pH remain within acceptable limits. (Respiratory frequency, expressed dyspnea, and clinical signs are the best guides to fatigue.) It is especially important for patients who are stressed by the level of IMV used during daylight hours to receive full support with assisted mechanical ventilation (AMV) or a significantly higher IMV level at night. An insidious problem relating to IMV is the tendency for clinicians to reduce the machine rate so cautiously that the weaning process is prolonged well beyond the time when machine support can be discontinued.

Pressure-Support Ventilation

Two newer modes of ventilation, pressure support and mandatory minute ventilation, offer attractive options for the weaning patient. *Pressure support* (PS) applies a set level of airway pressure throughout the inspiratory cycle (see p. 69).

At low levels, PS provides enough of a pressure boost to help overcome the extra resistance of the endotracheal (ET) tube. When set high enough, PS resembles assisted mechanical ventilation. Each breath is aided by the ventilator to the pressure level set by the physician. Because every breath is machine assisted, tidal volumes and respiratory rhythms are less variant and more natural than during IMV weaning (Fig. 9.1). Most importantly, however, inspiratory duration, cycling frequency, and timing of respiratory cycles are set by the patient, not by the machine. In allowing the patient to determine the timing characteristics of the inspiratory cycle, synchrony and patient comfort can improve markedly. Finally, PS may be a method of training the muscles for endurance or the respiratory center for improved coordination.

Unfortunately, each breath taken during PS must be patient initiated. It is also quite common for patients to adapt to decreasing PS by increasing frequency, thereby taking maximal advantage of machine power. It is only when PS falls below some critical value that the patient works actively to maintain tidal volume (V_T). Furthermore, the level of support offered by PS varies with the impedance to chest inflation. Therefore, patients

I MV

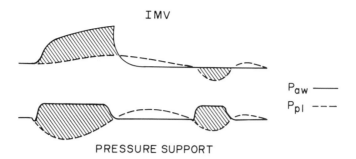

P_{aw} ——
P_{pl} - - -

PRESSURE SUPPORT

Figure 9.1   Intermittent mandatory ventilation (IMV) versus pressure support (PS). Unlike IMV, in which the entire transpulmonary pressure ($P_{aw} - P_{pl}$, hatched areas) is sporadically provided by volume-cycled breaths of fixed duration, PS partially supports every patient-initiated breath. The depth and timing of each PS breath remain under patient control.

with variable inflation impedance (e.g, those prone to accumulate secretions or experience bronchospasm during the weaning trial) *are poor candidates* for its use. As with any pressure-limited mode, the *tidal volume must be monitored closely*. Obviously, patients with unstable ventilatory drive centers are also at major risk, unless PS defaults to an automatic cycling mode when spontaneous efforts cease.

Mandatory minute volume (minimum minute ventilation, MMV) may provide an excellent, if not ideal, backup mode to PS (see p. 70). MMV is based on the concept of supporting the spontaneously breathing patient at a minimal level of minute ventilation ($\dot{V}_E$), but not to intervene until needed. MMV repeatedly examines a time window for the amount of spontaneous ventilation that has occurred within it (Fig. 9.2).

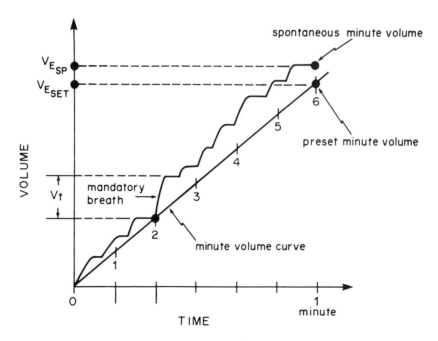

Figure 9.2   Principle of mandatory minute volume. At intervals, the ventilator compares accumulated volume with that needed to achieve the preset minimum volume ($\dot{V}_{E_{SET}}$). Mandatory breaths are given only as needed to ensure that spontaneous minute ventilation ($\dot{V}_{E_{SP}}$) meets the targeted value.

If the observed $\dot{V}_E$ falls below the expected level, the machine delivers a pressurized breath of fixed volume to achieve this goal or, alternatively, amplifies the PS level until an acceptable tidal volume is achieved. MMV is not equivalent to synchronized IMV (SIMV). During SIMV a fixed number of breaths are delivered by the machine under all conditions. During MMV no assistance is provided until the $\dot{V}_E$ declines below the target level, and then support is only added to bring the patient up to the desired $\dot{V}_E$. Within the time window (typically 8–10 seconds), minor fluctuations in ventilatory rate can be offset by the patient without activating the support mechanism.

Unfortunately, a guaranteed minute volume does not ensure adequate alveolar ventilation. Rapid, shallow breathing with inadequate tidal volumes will inhibit the backup mechanism. Furthermore, the deficiency in ventilation must develop at a steady rate to ensure optimal function of ventilator circuitry. Its purpose can be defeated by patients with highly irregular breathing rhythms (e.g., Cheyne-Stokes ventilation). The availability of microprocessor technology and servo feedback may enable future systems to intervene with added pressure support when tidal volume falls too low or frequency increases excessively.

THE UNWEANABLE PATIENT

The need for continued ventilatory support is often a psychological as well as physiological problem. To ensure patient cooperation a few points are important to keep in mind.

1. The *patient must be "co-opted"* into the effort as part of the team and kept fully advised of the treatment plan.
2. The *patient must be given full veto power* to terminate an overly taxing trial.
3. *"Panic" reactions are especially detrimental in patients with chronic airflow obstruction*. At such times patients experience discoordinated breathing, hyperinflation, increased CO_2 generation, hypoxemia, and extreme dyspnea. The setback can be mental as well as physical.
4. A *non-sedating anxiolytic* may be highly beneficial in selected patients.
5. Before a weaning attempt has any hope of success, the patient must be *fully rested*. This can best be assured by 10–12 hours of assist control ventilation and a full night of sleep prior to the trial.
6. *Hidden problems* such as diastolic dysfunction, coronary insufficiency, endocrinopathy (hy-

poadrenalism, hypothyroidism), or Parkinson's disease may explain protracted ventilator dependence and must be aggressively sought in puzzling cases.
7. *Mobilization and exercise* are keys to the weaning effort as well as to general rehabilitation. Prolonged bed rest is attended by multiple adverse physiologic changes related to the changed vector of gravitational forces. These include depression of vascular tone, reduced extravascular volume, loss of red cell mass, electrolyte shifts, calcium depletion, aberrations of hormonal balance, and depletion of skeletal muscle mass. Prevented from weight bearing, the lower extremities undergo disproportionate atrophy in patients continually at bed rest. Standing, leg exercises in bed, and ambulation help greatly in the rehabilitation effort. Chronically ventilator-dependent patients demand less attention than other ICU patients. Immobilized and deprived of sensory stimulation, they often become passive, discouraged, or poorly cooperative. Efforts to *provide sensory stimulation* and physical and occupational therapy may improve mental outlook, strength, and prospects for recovery.

MUSCLE TRAINING

It makes good physiologic sense to deliberately stress the ventilatory musculature for brief periods several times daily, encouraging spontaneous breathing (CPAP or T-piece), just as soon as the crisis period has passed. After being fully rested, such "wind sprints" may help strengthen and condition the ventilatory muscles, in a fashion similar to athletic training for limb muscles.

Many patients with marginal reserve do best when extubated directly rather than being weaned with low levels of machine support. This is particularly true when a highly resistive endotracheal tube is in place—e.g., a small caliber nasal tube. A small amount of pressure support (3–5 cmH$_2$O) helps to overcome tube resistance and should be used in most patients. In like fashion, low level PEEP is desirable for most patients (see p. 81). Those who cannot be extubated may benefit from tracheostomy, a procedure that lowers airway resistance, improves secretion hygiene, and allows mobilization.

TRACHEOSTOMY

The optimal timing for tracheostomy is still unsettled. Some patients in ventilatory failure should receive early tracheostomy, (e.g., those with slowly reversible neurological problems). For patients with acute lung disorders that are expected to reverse, there is no ironclad rule as to when tracheostomy should be performed. As a general guideline, tracheostomy may be appropriate any time after the first 7–10 days. The decision to undertake tracheostomy should consider the pace of improvement; if the patient is progressing sufficiently to be ready for extubation within 3–5 days, tracheostomy can be reasonably deferred. It should be emphasized that some patients keep endotracheal tubes in place for longer than 3 weeks without suffering permanent laryngeal or tracheal injury. In a patient whose primary problem is ventilatory mechanics (and not respiratory drive), it may be worthwhile to allow $PaCO_2$ to rise slowly over several days, maintaining oxygenation and pH balance. Higher $PaCO_2$ enables each breath to eliminate CO_2 more efficiently. Furthermore, the higher bicarbonate levels buffer fluctuations in $PaCO_2$ more effectively.

For chronically ventilated patients improvement in general health and increased activity level may prove the key interventions. Preparation of the patient is of prime importance. Rehabilitative programs that include physical therapy and ambulation may prove the difference between success and failure. It is important to encourage the patient to assume as much normal activity as possible; a useful technique is to have the patient walk (using a walker or a stroller) for 10–15 minutes, one or more times daily. During ambulation ventilation is provided manually or with a pressure cycled ventilator.

A multifactoral approach based on the answer to the question "What limits withdrawal?" offers the best hope of ventilator removal at the earliest possible time (Table 9.3). Keeping the patient fully informed and involved in the weaning attempt will help to assure a successful outcome.

WEANING FROM THE ENDOTRACHEAL TUBE

Once the patient is weaned from the ventilator, the need for continued endotracheal intubation should be assessed independently. Although virtually all patients have disordered swallowing transiently after extubation, those likely to have a persisting problem of airway protection after tube removal (e.g., deep coma) should not be extubated. Because airway protection reflexes (pharyngeal gag and laryngeal closure) are lost earlier than cough triggered deep within the airway, a patient who fails to cough vigorously on tracheal suctioning is not likely to protect the airway efficiently when the tube is removed.

Patients with copious airway secretions and ineffective cough should retain the tube to facilitate suctioning. Vital capacity > 20 ml/kg, MIP more negative than −40 cmH$_2$O, a vigorous expulsive effort on tracheal stimulation, and an expiratory pressure generated against an occluded airway > 60 cmH$_2$O predict effective coughing post-extubation.

Table 9.3
Therapeutic Measures for Factors that Limit Weaning Progress

Hypoxemia	Impedance	↑ $\dot{V}_E$
Positioning	Positioning	Sedation
↓ Secretions	↓ Secretions	↓ Fever
Bronchodilation	Bronchodilation	↓ Pain
Diuresis	Diuresis	↓ V_D/V_T
CPAP	↓ $\dot{V}_E$	Correct acidosis
↑ F$_I$O$_2$	↓ Circuit resistance	Allow PaCO$_2$ ↑
↓ Drive	Endurance	Psychologic Factors
↑ Nutrition	Rest periods	Reassure patient
↓ Loading	Positioning	Convey plan
↓ Alkalosis	Correct electrolytes, hgb, and blood	Anxiolytics
↓ Sedatives	gases	Encourage normal activity
↑ Sleep	↑ Calories	Ambulation/PT
↑ Thyroid	Steroid replacement	

↑, increased; ↓, decreased.
PT, physiotherapy.
hgb, hemoglobin.

WEANING FROM TRACHEOSTOMY

Consideration should be given to removal of the tracheostomy tube when the patient no longer requires suctioning for secretion removal, high fractions of inspired oxygen, or periodic reconnection to the ventilator.

Replacement of the standard tracheostomy tube with a fenestrated one facilitates talking and allows easier assessment of true cough effectiveness. There are essentially three methods for gradually discontinuing a tracheostomy: use of partial plugs, use of progressively smaller tracheostomy tubes, and use of stomal buttons.

Plugs that progressively occlude a standard sized tracheostomy orifice (e.g., ½ and ¾ plugs) can be used in an attempt to assess the need for continued intubation. (The cuff on the endotracheal tube *must* be deflated during orifice occlusion.) However, it should be remembered that an occluded tracheostomy tube severely narrows the effective tracheal lumen, thereby increasing the work of breathing and the tendency toward secretion retention. For this reason many physicians prefer to replace the original tracheostomy with progressively smaller uncuffed (or uninflated) endotracheal tubes. Unfortunately, the stomal orifice rapidly adapts to the smaller caliber tube as well, so that effective ventilation through the tracheostomy may not be possible should an acute need arise. If the ability to sustain spontaneous ventilation, clear secretions, or protect the airway is questionable, a tracheostomy button will maintain the stoma over several days to weeks to allow tube reinsertion, emergency ventilation, suctioning, and effective administration of inhaled bronchodilators, without adding substantially to airway resistance.

SUGGESTED READINGS

1. Greenleaf JE, Kozlowski S: Physiological consequences of reduced physical activity during bedrest. *Exerc Sport Sci Rev* 10:84–119, 1982.
2. LeMaire F, Teboul JL, Cinotti L, et al: Acute left ventricular dysfunction during unsuccessful weaning from mechanical ventilation. *Anesthesiology* 69:171–79, 1988.
3. MacIntyre NR: Respiratory function during pressure support ventilation. *Chest* 89:677–683, 1986.
4. Marini JJ: Respiratory medicine for the houseofficer, 2nd ed. Baltimore, Williams & Wilkins, 1987.
5. Marini JJ: The physiologic determinants of ventilator dependence. *Respir Care* 31(4):271–282, 1986.
6. Marini JJ: The role of the inspiratory circuit in the work of breathing during mechanical ventilation. *Respir Care* 32(6):419–430, 1987.
7. Perel A: Newer ventilation modes—temptations and pitfalls. *Crit Care Med* 15:707–709, 1987.
8. Pierson DJ: Weaning from mechanical ventilation in acute respiratory failure. Concepts, indications and techniques. *Respir Care* 28:646–662, 1983.
9. Pingleton SK: Nutritional support in the mechanically ventilated patient. *Clin Chest Med* 9(1):101–112, 1988.
10. Rochester DF, Arora NS: Respiratory muscle failure. *Med Clin N Am* 67:573–597, 1983.
11. Roussos C, Macklem PT: The respiratory muscles. *N Engl J Med* 307:786–797, 1982.
12. Rubin M: The physiology of bed rest. *Am J Nursing* 88:50–56, 1988.
13. Sahn SA, Lakshminarayan S, Petty TL: Weaning from mechanical ventilation. *JAMA* 235:2208–2212, 1976.
14. Sporn PHS, Morganroth ML: Discontinuation of mechanical ventilation. *Clin Chest Med* 9(1):113–126, 1988.
15. Tobin MJ, Peres W, Guenther SM, et al: The pattern of breathing during successful and unsuccessful trials of weaning from mechanical ventilation. *Am Rev Respir Dis* 134:1111–1118, 1986.

10 Radiology in the Intensive Care Unit

Conventional and specialized radiographic techniques often play key roles in the care of the critically ill. For example, computed tomography (CT) scanning is indispensable for neurologic, abdominal, and sinus evaluation. Ultrasound facilitates cardiac, nephric, and gallbladder diagnosis, and nuclear medicine techniques help to confirm embolic diseases, gastrointestinal (GI) bleeding, and fistulous communications. These and other specialized applications are discussed elsewhere in this volume with the specific diseases they help define. The present chapter concentrates on the two studies that are applied almost universally in the critical care setting—the chest radiograph and the abdominal plain film.

CHEST RADIOGRAPHY

Importance of Filming Technique and Timing

The usefulness of the portable anterior-posterior (AP) chest x-ray (CXR) is largely determined by positioning and exposure technique. Orientation of the patient with respect to the radiographic beam is of critical importance. Kyphosis, lordosis, and rotation around the body's longitudinal axis have a dramatic impact on the apparent dimensions of intrathoracic structures as well as on the detectability of pathology. Film penetration may emphasize or diminish parenchymal lung markings. A properly exposed CXR should reveal vertebral interspaces in the retrocardiac region. Films on which these interspaces are not visualized are underpenetrated, exaggerating parenchymal markings and making visualization of air bronchograms difficult.

The AP technique magnifies the anterior mediastinum and great vessels. When x-rays are obtained with the patient in the supine position, cardiovascular structures also appear enlarged, due to augmented venous filling and reduced lung volume. Conversely, pneumothoraces (PTXs) and

pleural effusions often become imperceptible. Changes in lung volume also influence the appearance of parenchymal infiltrates, most notably in mechanically ventilated patients or in those receiving positive end-expiratory pressure (PEEP). To facilitate comparison, serial films should be exposed during the same phase of the respiratory cycle and with comparable tidal volume and end-expiratory pressure.

To assure proper position and exclude complications, chest radiographs should be obtained within 60 minutes of such invasive procedures as endotracheal intubation, transvenous pacemaker insertion, thoracentesis, pleural and transbronchial biopsy, and central vascular catheter placement. A CXR must also follow failed attempts at catheterization via the subclavian route, especially before contralateral placement is attempted.

Placement of Tubes and Catheters

Endotracheal or Tracheostomy Tube Position

Radiographic confirmation of tube placement is crucial; positioning the endotracheal (ET) tube in the right main bronchus often results in atelectasis or barotrauma. (Left main intubations are uncommon because the left main bronchus is smaller and angulates sharply from the trachea.) Conversely, if the tube tip lies too high in the trachea (above the level of the clavicles), accidental extubation is likely. When the head is in a neutral position, the tip of the ET tube should rest in the mid-trachea, ≈ 5 cm above the carina. In adult patients the T5–7 vertebral level is a good estimate of carinal position if it cannot be directly visualized. ET tubes move with flexion, extension, and rotation of the neck. Contrary to what might be expected, the ET tube tip moves caudally when the neck is flexed, whereas head rotation away from the midline and

97

neck extension elevate the ET tube tip. Total tip excursion may range over 4–5 cm.

The normal ET or tracheostomy tube occupies ½ to ⅔ of the tracheal width and does not cause bulging of the trachea in the region of the tube cuff. Gradual dilation of the trachea may occur during long-term positive pressure ventilation, but every effort should be made to prevent this complication by minimizing ventilator cycling pressure and cuff sealing pressures.

After tracheostomy a chest radiograph may detect subcutaneous air, PTX, pneumomediastinum, or malposition of the tube. The T3 vertebral level defines the ideal position of the tracheostomy site. Sharp anterior angulation of the tracheal tube is associated with the development of tracheo-innominate fistulas, whereas posterior erosion can produce a tracheoesophageal fistula. Lateral radiographs are necessary for evaluation of AP angulation.

Central Venous Pressure Lines

For accurate pressure measurement the tip of the central venous pressure (CVP) catheter must lie within the thorax, well beyond any venous valves. These are commonly located in the subclavian and jugular veins, ≃ 2.5 cm from their junction with the brachiocephalic trunk (at the radiographic level of the anterior 1st rib). Because CVP catheters positioned in the right atrium or ventricle may cause arrhythmias or perforation, the desirable location for these lines is in the mid-superior vena cava, with the tip directed inferiorly. Stiff catheters, particularly those used for temporary hemodialysis using the subclavian route, may impinge on the lateral wall of superior vena cava, potentially resulting in vascular perforation. Complications resulting from vascular puncture include fluid infusion into the pericardium or pleural space, hemopneumothorax, and tamponade.

Pacing Wires

When transvenous pacing wires are inserted emergently they are often malpositioned in the coronary sinus, right atrium, or pulmonary artery outflow tract. On an AP view of the chest, the pacing catheter tip should overlie the shadow of the right ventricular apex. However, it is often difficult to assess the position of the pacing wire on a single film. On a lateral view, the tip of the catheter should lie within 4 mm of the epicardial fat stripe and point anteriorly. (Posterior angulation suggests coronary sinus placement.) In patients with permanent pacemakers, leads commonly fracture at the entrance to the pulse generator, a site that should be checked routinely.

Chest Tubes

The most appropriate position for a chest tube depends upon the reason for its placement. Posterior positioning is ideal for the drainage of free-flowing intrapleural fluid, whereas anterior placement is preferred for air removal. Placement may appear appropriate on the AP film, although the tube actually lies within subcutaneous tissues or lung parenchyma. Oblique or lateral films are often necessary to confirm an intrapleural location. A clue to the extrapleural location of a chest tube is the *inability to visualize both sides* of the catheter. Most chest tubes are constructed with a "sentinel eye", an interruption of the longitudinal radioopaque stripe that delineates the opening of the chest tube closest to the drainage apparatus. This hole must lie within the pleural space to achieve adequate drainage and assure that no air enters the tube via the subcutaneous tissue. After removal of the chest tube, fibrinous thickening stimulated by the presence of the tube may produce lines (the *tube track*), which simulate the visceral pleural boundary, to suggest PTX (see chapter 31).

Intra-aortic Balloon

The intra-aortic balloon (IAB) is an inflatable device placed in the proximal aorta to assist the failing ventricle. Diastolic inflation of the balloon produces a distinct, rounded lucency within the aortic shadow, but in systole the deflated balloon is not visible. Ideal positioning places the catheter tip just distal to the left subclavian artery. Placed too proximally, the IAB may occlude the carotid or left subclavian artery. Placed too distally, the IAB may occlude the lumbar or mesenteric arteries and produce less effective counterpulsation. Daily radiographic assessment of the aortic contour for evidence of IAB-induced dissection is prudent.

Swan-Ganz Catheter

Each of the insertion-related complications of central venous catheterization, including PTX, pleural entry, and arterial injury, can result from the placement of the pulmonary artery catheter. Unique complications of Swan-Ganz catheter placement include knotting or looping and entanglement with other catheters or pacing wires. The most common radiographic finding is distal catheter tip migration, with or without pulmonary infarction. With an uninflated balloon, the tip of the Swan-Ganz catheter should overlie the middle third of a well-centered AP chest radiograph (within 5 cm of the midline). Distal migration is common in the first hours after insertion as the catheter softens and loses slack. If pressure tracings suggest continuous wedging, it is important to look for a catheter folded upon itself across the pulmonic valve or a persistently inflated balloon (appearing as a 1 cm rounded lucency at the tip of the catheter). The width of the mediastinal and cardiac shadows should be assessed following placement of the catheter because perforation of the free wall of the ventricle may result in pericardial tamponade. Temporary phrenic nerve paralysis due to the lidocaine used in catheter placement has been reported to cause hemidiaphragm elevation.

Specific Conditions Diagnosed by Chest Radiography

Atelectasis

Acute atelectasis is a frequent cause of infiltration on intensive care unit chest radiographs. The wide spectrum of radiographic findings ranges from invisible *microatelectasis*, through *plate and segmental atelectasis*, to *collapse of an entire lung*. The radiographic differentiation between segmental atelectasis and segmental pneumonia is often difficult, particularly since these conditions often coexist. However, marked volume loss and rapid onset and reversal are highly characteristic of acute collapse.

Atelectasis tends to develop in dependent regions and, more commonly, in the left rather than the right lower lobe by a 2:1 margin. Radiographic findings of atelectasis include: hemidiaphragm elevation, infiltration or vascular crowding (especially in the retrocardiac area), deviation of hilar vessels, ipsilateral mediastinal shift, and loss of the lateral border of the descending aorta or heart. Contrary to popular belief, the "silhouette sign" is not always reliable on portable films, particularly in the presence of an enlarged heart or on a film obtained in a lordotic projection. Air bronchograms extending into an atelectatic area suggest that collapse continues without total occlusion of the central airway and that attempts at airway clearance by bronchoscopy or suctioning are likely to fail.

Pleural Effusion and Hemothorax

Recognition of pleural effusions requires proper patient positioning. On the supine AP CXR, large effusions redistribute, causing a hazy density to overlie the entire hemithorax without loss of vascular definition. Apical pleural capping is another radiographic sign of large collections of pleural fluid in the supine patient. Upright or lateral decubitus x-rays may help confirm the presence of pleural fluid (Fig. 10.1). If a large collection of pleural fluid obscures the lung parenchyma, a contralateral decubitus film may be helpful. Pleural fluid is not ordinarily visible until several hundred milliliters have accumulated. On lateral decubitus films, 1 cm of layering fluid indicates a volume that can usually be tapped safely. Occasionally, subpulmonic or loculated fluid may be difficult to recognize.

Hemidiaphragm elevation, lateral displacement of the diaphragmatic apex, abrupt transitions from lucency to solid tissue density, and increased distance from the upper diaphragmatic margin to the gastric bubble (on an upright film) are all signs of a subpulmonic effusion (Fig. 10.2). Ultrasound is a useful adjunct in detecting the presence of pleural fluid and in guiding thoracentesis.

Extra-alveolar Gas

Extra-alveolar gas can manifest as interstitial emphysema, cyst formation, PTX, pneumomediastinum, pneumoperitoneum, or subcutaneous emphysema (see Chapter 31). Although long recognized in neonates and young children, radiographic signs of gas in the pulmonary interstitium have only recently been described in adults. These include lucent streaks that do not conform to air bronchograms and cysts at the lung periphery, usually at the bases. These signs, best seen when the parenchyma is densely infiltrated, portend the development of PTX.

Pneumothorax

Positioning assumes great importance in the detection of PTX. On supine films or in patients with pleural adhesions, gas may collect exclusively in the anterior regions of the thorax. Thus, gas may outline the minor fissure or may move anteriorly over the heart, mimicking pneumomediastinum or pneumopericardium. Radiographic signs of PTX on the supine CXR include a "deep sulcus sign" and lucency over the upper portions of the spleen or liver (see p. 264). An upright expiratory CXR is the best film for detecting a PTX. This view confines a fixed amount of intrapleural air within a smaller volume, accentuating the proportion of thoracic volume it occupies and the separation of lung from chest wall.

The visceral pleura provides a specific marker: a radiodense thin stripe of appropriate curvature with lucency visible on both sides and absent lung

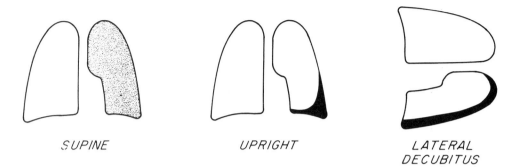

SUPINE   UPRIGHT   LATERAL
                                    DECUBITUS

Figure 10.1   Appearance of a mobile pleural effusion in three positions. In the supine position, a "ground glass" lateralized diffuse density (with preservation of vascular markings) may be the only sign of layered pleural fluid. A changing appearance with position confirms the diagnosis.

markings beyond. Skin folds often mimic the pleural edge but can be distinguished by certain features: lucency present only on one margin, poorly defined limits, and extension beyond the confines of the rib cage. Because PTX reduces blood flow to the collapsed lung, lung density may be surprisingly normal, even with an extensive gas collection.

PTXs are often characterized by the percentage of the hemithorax they occupy. This practice is highly imprecise, both because the CXR is only two-dimensional and because apparent percentage changes occur with variations in breathing depth and position. As with pleural fluid, *precise* estimation of the size of a PTX is neither possible nor necessary. A tension PTX (of any size) and a "large" PTX both require drainage—the former because of its immediate physiologic effects, the latter because it creates a pleural pocket that is unlikely to reabsorb spontaneously over an acceptable time. The reabsorption rate of a PTX has been estimated to be "1–2% per day", a crude

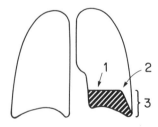

Figure 10.2   Radiographic signs of a subpulmonic effusion (1) hemidiaphragm elevation with separation of lung from gastric bubble, (2) lateralization of the diaphragmatic dome, (3) abrupt transition from lucency to soft tissue density.

rule of thumb that emphasizes the slowness of this process. Thus, a 15% PTX would require 1–2 weeks to reabsorb.

Tension Pneumothorax.   The diagnosis of *tension* PTX must be made on clinical grounds if serious morbidity and mortality are to be prevented. Delaying therapy for radiographic confirmation significantly increases mortality. Radiographically, tension PTX often shifts the mediastinum and flattens or inverts the hemidiaphragm ipsilateral to the PTX. Yet, tension is usually difficult to diagnose with confidence on a single film; infiltrated or obstructed lungs fail to collapse completely, and an unyielding mediastinum may not shift noticeably, despite a marked pressure gradient. A comparison of serial films with clinical correlation is most often required.

PTX occurs in up to 50% of patients receiving mechanical ventilation with peak inflation pressures > 60 cm H_2O, and a large fraction of these are under tension. PTX commonly complicates the course of patients with necrotizing pneumonias, secretion retention, or expanding cavitary or bullous lesions.

Pneumomediastinum

After gaining access to the mediastinum, gas normally decompresses into adjacent soft tissues. Thus, unless gas trapping occurs, pneumomediastinum rarely produces important physiologic effects. Mediastinal gas may arise from neck injuries, from rupture of the trachea or esophagus, or (most commonly) from alveolar rupture and retrograde dissection of air along bronchovascular bundles. Pneumomediastinum appears radiographically as a lucent band around the heart and great vessels caused by gas within the space separating the parietal pleura from the mediastinal contents. On the heart's inferior border, this lucency can extend across the mediastinum, linking the two sides of the chest with a "complete diaphragm sign." An unnaturally sharp heart border is the first indicator of pneumomediastinum, a sign that must be distinguished from the "kinetic halo" often seen at the heart border or diaphragm. The mediastinal pleura, defined by gas on both sides of a thin radiodense line, can often be detected. On a lateral film, pneumomediastinum usually appears as a thin crescent of gas outlining the ascending aorta. Not uncommonly, extrapleural gas extends from the mediastinum, lifting the parietal pleura off the diaphragm or outlining the inferior pulmonary ligament.

Subcutaneous Gas

In the adult, subcutaneous gas (SG), also known as subcutaneous emphysema, normally has important diagnostic but limited physiologic significance. SG produces lucent streaks or bubbles in the soft tissues that outline major muscle groups. During mechanical ventilation, generalized SG usually results from alveolar rupture and medial dissection. SG indicates an increased risk of PTX. Once PTX has occurred, progressive accumulation of gas in the subcutaneous tissue suggests the presence of a bronchopleural fistula or a malfunctioning chest tube, especially if SG is bilateral. Small amounts of SG detected shortly after chest tube placement frequently enter via the tube track itself. SG detected immediately after blunt chest trauma should raise the possibility of tracheo-bronchial or esophageal disruption (see Chest Trauma, Chapter 30).

Pulmonary Edema

Certain CXR findings may be helpful in determining the etiology of lung water accumulation. Fluid overload, cardiogenic pulmonary edema, and noncardiogenic pulmonary edema (adult respiratory distress syndrome, ARDS) have characteristic radiographic features. These forms of edema are distinguished by three features: size of the heart and great vessels, distribution of vascular markings, and the pattern of infiltration. Cardiac edema and volume overload are characterized by a widened vascular pedicle, an even or inverted pattern of vascular markings, and a tendency toward a gravitational distribution of edema ("bat wing" or basilar). Kerley's lines are common in established congestive failure (usually of several days to weeks duration), whereas crisp air bronchograms are unusual. Conversely, the immobile infiltrates of ARDS

are widely scattered, patchy, and often interrupted by distinct air bronchograms (see Ref. 4).

Although edema is usually bilateral and symmetric, it may collect unilaterally in the presence of massive thromboembolism to the contralateral lung or with unilateral aspiration, re-expansion pulmonary edema, or extensive bullous disease. Gravity may redistribute edema fluid to dependent lung regions over brief periods, a mechanism for shifting unilateral edema after decubitus positioning.

Mediastinal Widening

Mediastinal widening (particularly following chest trauma) provides a clue to aortic disruption. Obtaining an upright posterior-anterior CXR, although highly desirable, is frequently not possible because of injuries or hypotension. Radiographic clues to aortic disruption include a widened superior mediastinum (the most sensitive sign), a blurred aortic knob, rightward deviation of the nasogastric tube or aortic shadow, and tracheal deviation to the right and anteriorally. Inferior displacement of the left main bronchus, left-sided pleural effusion (with or without apical capping), and displacement of intimal calcifications of the aorta provide other signs suggestive of aortic disruption (see p. 258). Mediastinal widening with vascular injury is frequently associated with traumatic fractures of the first two ribs and clavicle. Widening of the cardiac shadow should prompt careful review of the aortic contour, because blood may dissect from the aorta into the pericardium. If aortic disruption is suspected, angiography (not CT scanning) is the procedure of choice to delineate the disruption.

Pericardial Effusion

Pericardial effusion is recognized radiographically by enlargement of the cardiac shadow. The classic "water bottle configuration" of the cardiac silhouette, although highly characteristic, is unusual. An apparent epicardial fat pad wider than 2 mm on the lateral view provides CXR evidence for the presence of a pericardial effusion, as does splaying of the tracheal bifurcation. Echocardiography is the procedure of choice for the detection and evaluation of pericardial effusions and simultaneously affords the opportunity to assess heart chamber size, vena caval diameter, and contractile function (see p. 26).

Air-Fluid Levels (Lung Abscess versus Empyema)

Several guidelines help to decide whether an air-fluid level lies within the pleural space or within the lung parenchyma. On an AP film, pleural fluid collections generate wide, moderately dense air-fluid levels, whereas intrapulmonary collections are usually smaller, more dense, and rounded. Lung abscesses and liquid-filled bullae tend to project similar diameters on both AP and lateral films. The air-fluid level of pleural fluid collections must abut the chest wall on either AP or lateral film (Fig. 10.3).

Fluid collections that cross a fissure line on upright films are associated with a pleural location. Lung abscesses generally have thick, shaggy walls with irregular contours, unlike liquid-filled bullae and pleural fluid collections. As position is altered, pleural fluid collections frequently undergo marked changes in shape or contour. CT scanning is the technique of choice for sorting out difficult cases.

Post-Thoracotomy Changes

After pneumonectomy, fluid accumulates in the vacant hemithorax over days to months. Whereas the absolute fluid level is of little significance, *changes* in the level of fluid are important. A rapid decline in the fluid level should prompt concern for a bronchopleural fistula (BPF), a complication that most commonly develops within 8–12 days of surgery. If a BPF develops within the first 4 postoperative days, mechanical failure of the bronchial closure should be suspected, prompting consideration of reoperation. BPFs occurring post-thoracotomy may be confirmed by instilling a sterile tracer into the pleural space and inspecting the expectorated sputum immediately afterward, or, alternatively, by the inhalation of radioactive gas, followed by imaging of thorax. A BPF tends to displace the mediastinum to the contralateral side,

an unusual occurrence during uneventful postoperative recovery. Small residual air spaces may remain for up to a year following pneumonectomy and do not necessarily imply the presence of a BPF. Very rapid postoperative filling of the hemithorax suggests infection, hemorrhage, or malignant effusion.

Fistulous Tracts

Fistulas between the trachea and innominate artery occur most frequently when a tracheal tube angulates anteriorly and to the right in patients with low tracheostomy stoma, persistent hyperextension of the neck, or asthenic habitus. An anteriorly directed tracheostomy or ET tube should be repositioned.

Fistulas also may form between the trachea and esophagus during prolonged ET intubation. These usually occur at the level of the ET cuff, directly behind the manubrium. Predisposing factors include cuff overdistention, simultaneous nasogastric intubation, and posterior angulation of the tube tip. The sudden occurrence of massive gastric dilation in a mechanically ventilated patient provides an important clue. A radiographic contrast agent may be introduced into the esophagus after cuff deflation or tube removal in an attempt to confirm the presence of the fistula.

Pulmonary Embolism

Although the plain CXR rarely helps to diagnose pulmonary embolism, large emboli may give rise to highly suggestive findings: ipsilateral hypovascularity, enlargement of the pulmonary arteries, and (rarely) abrupt vascular cutoff. Local oligemia (Westermark's sign) may be seen early in the course of pulmonary embolism, usually within the first 36 hours. "Hampton's hump", a pleural-based triangular density due to pulmonary infarction, is seldom seen. About 50% of patients with pul-

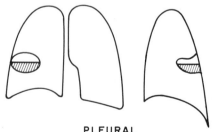
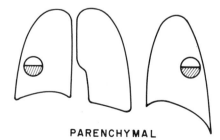

PLEURAL   PARENCHYMAL

Figure 10.3   Intra-parenchymal versus intra-pleural fluid collections.

monary emboli have an associated pleural effusion.

The rarity of normal CXRs diminishes the value of ventilation/perfusion scanning in the critically ill. Nonetheless, normal perfusion scans are very helpful, and abnormal scans help guide the angiographic search for pulmonary emboli. In the absence of a normal perfusion scan, angiography is the only way to confirm or rule out embolic disease. Angiography can be safely undertaken in critically ill patients, provided that care is used in transport and that pulmonary artery pressures are not excessive at the time of contrast injection. For patients who cannot be moved to the angiography suite, bedside angiography through a flow-directed catheter offers a less satisfactory option. Septic pulmonary embolism should be considered in patients with multifocal cavitary lesions of varying size.

Pneumonitis

Although bacterial infection often supervenes, *gastric aspiration* initially produces a sterile chemical pneumonitis. Massive aspiration, although somewhat position- and volume-dependent, typically appears as bilateral diffuse alveolar and interstitial infiltrates of rapid onset. Aspiration in the supine position usually affects the perihilar regions and superior and basilar segments of the lower lobes. Patients who aspirate in a decubitus position often develop unilateral infiltrates. Foreign objects (teeth, dental appliances) are occasionally aspirated in patients undergoing resuscitation, trauma, or ET intubation.

Although the CXR is never diagnostic, it may give a clue to the organism producing bacterial pneumonia. Common bacterial pathogens typically produce patchy or lobar involvement. Bulging fissures, although uncommon, suggest *Klebsiella pneumoniae*. A diffuse, patchy, "ground glass" appearance suggests *Legionella, mycoplasma,* or *pneumocystis.* Small, diffusely scattered nodular densities suggest *Mycobacterium tuberculosis* as the etiological organism. Larger nodular densities are associated with *actinomycosis* or *nocardiosis. Aspergillus* often gives rise to a peripheral wedge-shaped infiltrate caused by vascular invasion and secondary infarction. Frank cavitation suggests tuberculosis, fungal infection (histoplasmosis, cryptococcosis, coccidiomycosis), lung abscess, or septic pulmonary embolism.

Pneumonitis that develops in pre-existing areas of bullous emphysema often produces air-fluid levels that can be confused with lung abscess. The thinner contour of the cavity wall, the more rapid pace of development and resolution, and premorbid CXRs demonstrating bullae help to identify this problem.

Intra-Abdominal Conditions

The upright CXR also helps to diagnose acute intra-abdominal problems. Midline or paraesophageal hiatal hernias usually pose little diagnostic problem. Diaphragmatic disruption may allow abdominal contents to herniate into the chest following abdominal trauma, often displacing a gas containing viscus into the left chest. Oral contrast studies aid in the diagnosis, as does CT scan, injection of a sterile contrast agent into the pleural space, or diagnostic pneumoperitoneum. The upright CXR also provides the most sensitive method of detecting free air within the abdominal cavity. (A cross-table film of the abdomen taken at least 5 minutes after decubitus positioning serves a similar purpose.) Intubated patients frequently swallow air, producing gastric dilation. In the appropriate setting, massive gastric dilation can suggest the possibility of esophageal intubation or a tracheoesophageal fistula.

ABDOMINAL RADIOGRAPH

Screening Film

Standard examination of the abdomen includes supine [kidney-ureter-bladder (KUB) or "flat plate"] and upright views. If an upright film cannot be taken, a lateral decubitus view may be substituted. (Cross-table *supine* x-rays are of little value except to demonstrate calcification in aortic aneurysms.) Systematic review of the abdominal film may furnish important information, especially after trauma. Fractures of the lower ribs on the left suggest the possibility of a ruptured spleen or lacerated kidney. Fractures of the lower ribs on the right suggest the possibility of renal or hepatic damage. Fractures of the lumbar spine, pelvis, and hips may be seen as "incidental" findings on plain abdominal radiographs in trauma patients. A ground glass appearance, displacement of the properitoneal fat stripe, or centralization of gas shadows suggests intra-abdominal ascites or blood. Free air usually indicates a ruptured viscus, gas producing infection, barotraumatic pneumoperitoneum, or post-operative change.

Occasionally, the KUB view is useful in the setting of undiagnosed coma. Ingested tablets are frequently radio-opaque. In hydrocarbon ingestion upright or decubitus films of the abdomen may show a characteristic "fluid-fluid" level of hydrocarbon floating on the gastric contents (see p. 231).

The KUB view is a poor indicator of liver size and should not supplant careful physical examination. The gallbladder is poorly defined on the KUB view unless it is very distended or partially calcified. Less than 15% of gallbladder calculi are visible. Gas appearing spontaneously in the biliary ducts is highly suggestive of cholangitis. Hepatic calcifications, although rare, may be due to healed infection, hemangioma, or metastatic carcinoma. Films taken in different positions may help to sort out the location of right upper quadrant calcifications. Calcifications within the kidney or liver maintain a relatively fixed position, whereas stones within the gallbladder are usually mobile. Use of the KUB view in the diagnosis of the "acute abdomen" is discussed on page 286.

Findings Relevant to Specific Organs

Kidneys and Ureters

The visibility of the nephric shadows on the KUB view depends on the amount of perinephric fat and bowel gas. The combination of kidney enlargement and calcification suggest urinary tract obstruction or polycystic kidney disease. If nephrolithiasis is suspected, the renal outlines and course of both ureters should be carefully inspected for calculi (visible in up to 85% of cases). Gas-producing infections of the bladder are also seen occasionally.

Pancreas and Retroperitoneum

Asymmetric obliteration of the psoas shadows or retroperitoneal fat lines suggests a retroperitoneal process (most commonly pancreatitis or a ruptured aorta). Although the pancreas is not normally seen on the plain radiograph, calcifications may occur in chronic alcoholic pancreatitis. Localized areas of ileus over the pancreas, such as the "colon cut-off sign" and the "sentinel loop", may also help in the diagnosis of pancreatic inflammation.

Stomach and Bowel

The stomach normally contains some fluid and air, but massive gastric dilation suggests gastric outlet obstruction, gastroparesis, or esophageal intubation. The small bowel normally contains little air; its presence indicates ileus or small bowel obstruction. Air-fluid levels of *different heights* within the same loop of small bowel on an upright film indicate *mechanical* small bowel obstruction and imply residual peristaltic activity. Fluid levels at the *same height* in a loop of bowel do not neces-

sarily indicate mechanical obstruction. Absence of colonic or rectal gas in patients with small bowel air-fluid levels strongly suggests complete obstruction of the small bowel with distal clearing of gas. Conversely, the presence of gas in the colon (except for small amounts of rectal gas) all but excludes the diagnosis of complete small bowel obstruction. (Incomplete obstruction may be present, however.)

Colonic obstruction due to a sigmoid volvulus may be diagnosed via a KUB view that shows massive sigmoid dilation; the sigmoid forms an inverted "U" whose limbs rise out of the pelvis. Apposition of the medial walls of these bowel segments produces a midline soft tissue density whose inferior extent approximates the site of torsion.

Peritoneal Cavity

On the supine abdominal radiograph, ascites is demonstrated by diffuse haze, indistinctness of the iliopsoas stripes, centralization of small bowel segments, and abnormal separation of bowel loops. Increased pelvic density characterizes ascites on the upright film.

Abnormal gas collections are recognized by their non-anatomic location. Therefore, all gas densities on supine and erect films require explanation. Each must be assigned to an anatomic segment of bowel. Gas may collect under the diaphragm or overlie the liver on erect or lateral decubitus films, respectively. Free air also allows visualization of both sides of the walls of gas-filled bowel. "Bubbly", curvilinear, or triangular gas collections between segments of bowel suggest abdominal abscess. Bowel ischemia may produce a characteristic pattern known as pneumatosis cystoides that represents gas within the bowel wall. Rarely, pneumatosis may rupture to produce free intraperitoneal air, simulating a perforated viscus.

SUGGESTED READINGS

1. Federle MP (ed): Symposium on CT and ultrasonography in the acutely ill patient. *Radiol Clin N Am* 21(3):423–606, 1983.
2. Goodman LR, Putnam CE: *Intensive Care Radiology: Imaging of the Critically Ill*, ed 2. Philadelphia, WB Saunders, 1983, vol. 20.
3. Marini JJ: *Respiratory Medicine for the House Officer*, ed 2. Baltimore, Williams & Wilkins, 1987.
4. Milne EN, et al: The radiologic distinction of cardiogenic and noncardiogenic edema. *Am J Roentgen* 144:879–894, 1985.
5. Putman CE (ed): Symposium on cardiopulmonary imaging. *Radiol Clin N Am* 21(4):607–826, 1983.

11

Acid-Base Disorders

ARTERIAL BLOOD GASES

Methods of Obtaining Blood Gases

Arterial blood gases (ABGs) are only valuable if properly obtained and carefully measured. Patients should have a *stable* F_iO_2 for at least 10 minutes before sampling to allow the PaO_2 to equilibrate. *Patient position should be noted* because PaO_2 may change significantly with varying body position. (Saturation is usually worst in the supine position.)

When sampling from the radial site, it is important to accurately assess collateral blood flow to the hand. Patency of the alternate blood supply, the ulnar artery, is confirmed by the *Allen test*, performed by elevating the hand, occluding both ulnar and radial arteries, and releasing compression of the ulnar artery. If adequate collateral circulation is present, the hand should flush pink within 5–7 seconds.

For arterial puncture, the wrist is positioned in mild extension and the skin cleansed first with an iodophor solution, followed by alcohol. Lidocaine ($\simeq 0.5$ ml of 1% solution) may be used, but is rarely necessary; excessive volumes may obliterate normal landmarks and arterial pulsations. Heparin-coating a 3-ml syringe tipped with a 21-gauge needle provides sufficient anticoagulant. The artery is approached from a 45° angle. Immediately upon vessel entry, pulsatile blood will fill the syringe. Aspiration is not necessary for obtaining samples in most cases. Blood flow will cease if the needle penetrates the posterior arterial wall, but flow may often be re-established merely by retracting the needle. After sampling is complete, the needle should be removed and firm pressure applied to the puncture site for 5 minutes—longer if coagulation disorders exist. The syringe should be capped or the needle inserted into a cork and the blood

and heparin mixed by a rolling motion. Prompt analysis is required to obtain accurate results.

Risks

Risks of arterial puncture are very low for single sticks, but increase greatly when persistent cannulation is used (see p. 27). Infection is very rare unless abnormal or infected skin is traversed enroute to the artery. Arterial occlusion can be avoided by varying sampling sites, using the smallest needle that produces good blood flow, and confirming collateral flow before puncture. (Approximately 3% of hospitalized patients have inadequate collateral circulation.) Occult bleeding into large adjacent soft tissue spaces may occur following femoral or brachial arterial punctures. Nerve trauma is usually due to direct nerve puncture by an inexperienced phlebotomist, but also may result from a compressive hematoma if coagulopathy is present or if inadequate pressure is held at the puncture site.

Basic Concepts

Normal Values

Normally, arterial pH, the negative common logarithm of the hydrogen ion (H^+) concentration, varies between 7.35 and 7.45. When breathing room air, normal $PaCO_2$ varies between 35 and 45 mmHg, and PaO_2 values > 80–90 mmHg are considered normal, depending on age. Venous blood gases have a lower pH than arterial gases (normal $\simeq 7.35$), a lower PaO_2 (normal $\simeq 40$ mmHg), and an increased $PaCO_2$ (normal $\simeq 45$ mmHg). $PaCO_2$, PaO_2, and pH are directly analyzed in most laboratories. However, HCO_3^- concentration is not *measured* but rather calculated from pH and $PaCO_2$, using a nomogram. Direct automated determinations of serum HCO_3^- (total CO_2 content) are more accurate than nomograms for determining HCO_3^- content.

Gas Tension versus Saturation and Content

The partial pressure of a gas—its "tension"—reflects the rapidity with which gas molecules move in the serum. *Gas content depends not only on its partial pressure but also on the storage capacity for that gas in blood.* CO_2 is carried in dissolved form as well as bound to hemoglobin and other protein buffers. CO_2 content parallels its tension across a wide range. However, transport of O_2 is more complex, so that the relationship between tension and saturation (O_2 content) is highly alinear.

Oxygen Tension versus Saturation

Oxygen content of blood is predominately determined by the quantity of O_2 bound to hemoglobin (Hgb), with a minor contribution from dissolved O_2. The O_2 carried in a volume of blood (ml/dl) is influenced by PaO_2 (mmHg), Hgb concentration (gm/dl), pH, and by the characteristics of the Hgb itself:

$$O_2 \text{ content} = 0.0134 \text{ (Hgb)(\%Sat)} + .0034 \text{ } PaO_2$$

ABG analysis determines the partial pressure of dissolved O_2 directly but provides only an indirect (and not always accurate) indicator of O_2 *content.* Anemia has a direct and obvious impact on this relationship. More subtly, *abnormal hemoglobins* (e.g., methemoglobin, carboxyhemoglobin) may bind O_2 with lower affinity than normal, or they may have their O_2-binding sites occupied, producing a lower O_2 content than the relationship between PaO_2 and normal Hgb would predict.

Pitfalls in Interpretation of Blood Gases

Mixed Venous Samples

Systemic arterial blood has a uniform PaO_2. Conversely, the O_2 saturation of venous blood sampled at different sites varies greatly as a result of differential O_2 extraction by various organ systems. For this reason, mixed venous oxygen saturation must be measured using thoroughly mixed pulmonary artery blood, not blood from a peripheral vein, the vena cava, or the right ventricle.

Timing of Analysis

Accuracy depends upon prompt analysis. Under most circumstances, the $PaCO_2$ rises $\simeq$ 3–10 mmHg/hr in un-iced specimens, causing a modest fall in pH. Conversely, the PaO_2 is usually stable in an iced sample for 1–2 hours. Samples of body fluids that do not contain as much hemoglobin or other protein buffers as blood (pleural or joint fluid) demonstrate more rapid pH changes if analysis is delayed.

Pseudohypoxemia

The PaO_2 may be significantly decreased if significant O_2 is consumed after the blood is removed for sampling—a problem most common with marked *leukocytosis* or *thrombocytosis*. Leukocyte counts > 100,000/mm^3 or platelet counts > 10^6/mm^3 are usually required to produce significant changes. Addition of cyanide to ABGs and/or immediate icing of the sample decreases the likelihood of "pseudohypoxemia". Plastic syringes are more permeable than glass to oxygen (particularly at high O_2 tensions). Therefore in a patient with a very high PaO_2, diffusion of O_2 out of the syringe may lead to false reductions in PaO_2. Less commonly saturation is affected.

Pseudoacidosis

"Pseudoacidosis" may occur when incubating leukocytes generate CO_2, causing an acidosis. This problem is most likely to occur with delayed analysis of warm samples containing high numbers of leukocytes. Excessive amounts of acidic heparin remaining in the sampling syringe may also cause pseudoacidosis by diluting serum bicarbonate. (The potential magnitude of heparin related change is small, however.)

Breath Holding

Changing breathing patterns (breath holding or hyperventilation) may alter the $PaCO_2$ and cause *mild* acute changes in the PaO_2. Therefore, abnormal respiratory patterns should be recorded to allow more accurate ABG interpretation.

Temperature Corrections

For any given O_2 content, the measured PaO_2 will increase if blood is warmed because of rightward shifts in the oxyhemoglobin dissociation curve and a decrease in solubility of gases in warmer fluids. Hypothermia shifts the oxyhemoglobin dissociation curve leftward, and as cold blood is warmed to analysis temperature (37°C), O_2 solubility increases. The $PaCO_2$ will also rise as blood is warmed, producing modest declines in the pH. Thermal correction of ABG is usually unnecessary except at temperature extremes, and the physiologic relevance of temperature "correction" remains debatable (see Appendix, p. 300).

Air Bubbles

The PO_2 of room air is $\simeq$ 150 mmHg and the PCO_2 is $\simeq$ 0 mmHg. Therefore, when large air

$\uparrow P_aO_2 \downarrow PCO_2$

bubbles are mixed with arterial blood, the PaO_2 rises and the $PaCO_2$ falls. A small air bubble in a relatively large sample usually has little effect, but when the ratio of bubble-to-blood volume is large, increases in PaO_2 of 30 mmHg may occur. It is uncommon for bubbles to significantly reduce the $PaCO_2$ unless the baseline CO_2 tension is very high.

Oxygen

Hypoxemia

With regard to tissue nutrition, both the quantity of oxygen delivered per unit time (the product of cardiac output and oxygen content per unit volume) and the arterial partial pressure of O_2 (PaO_2) are important.

Tolerance for hypoxemia depends not only upon the extent of desaturation but also upon compensatory mechanisms and the sensitivity of the patient to hypoxia. Apart from *increased O_2 extraction*, the major mechanisms of compensation are *increased cardiac output*, *improved perfusion* (due to capillary recruitment and changes in distribution of resistance), and manufacture of red cells (*erythrocytosis*). Other adaptations, such as improved unloading of O_2 by tissue acidosis and increased anaerobic metabolism, assume importance when failure of the primary methods calls them into action (e.g., circulatory arrest).

If an individual without cardiac limitation or anemia is made hypoxic *over a short period of time*, no important effect will be noted until PaO_2 falls to < 50–60 mmHg. At that level, malaise, lightheadedness, mild nausea, vertigo, impaired judgment, and incoordination are generally the first symptoms noted, reflecting the extreme sensitivity of cerebral tissue to hypoxia. Although minute ventilation increases, little dyspnea develops unless hyperpnea uncovers underlying mechanical lung problems, as in chronic obstructive pulmonary disease (COPD). Confusion resembling alcohol intoxication appears as PaO_2 falls into the 35- to 50-mmHg range, especially in older individuals with ischemic cerebrovascular disease. (Such patients are also prone to heart rhythm disturbances). As PaO_2 falls below 35 mmHg, *renal blood flow decreases*, *urine output slows*, and *atropine-refractory bradycardia* and conduction system blockade develop. Lactic acidosis also appears at this level, even with normal cardiac function. The patient becomes lethargic or obtunded and minute ventilation is maximal. At $\simeq$ 25 mmHg the normal individual unadapted to hypoxemia loses consciousness, and minute ventilation begins to fall due to respiratory center depression.

This sequence of events occurs at higher O_2 tensions if any of the major compensatory mechanisms for hypoxemia is defective. Even mild decreases in O_2 tension are poorly tolerated by anemic patients with impaired cardiac output or coronary insufficiency. In addition, critically ill patients may have impaired autonomic control of perfusion distribution, due to either endogenous pathology (e.g., sepsis) or vasopressor therapy. Because the pulmonary vasculature constricts when alveolar O_2 tension falls, hypoxemia may provoke decompensation of the right ventricle in patients with preexisting cor pulmonale.

Hyperoxia

At normal barometric pressures, venous and tissue O_2 tensions rise very little when pure O_2 is administered to healthy subjects. Hence, non-pulmonary tissues are little affected. However, high concentrations of O_2 eventually replace nitrogen in the lung, even in poorly ventilated regions, causing collapse of poorly ventilated units as O_2 is absorbed by venous blood faster than it is replenished. Atelectasis and diminished lung compliance result. More importantly, high O_2 tensions may accelerate the generation of free radicals and other noxious oxidants, injuring bronchial and parenchymal tissue.

Carbon Dioxide

Hypercapnia

Apart from its key role in regulation of ventilation, the clinically important effects of CO_2 relate to changes in cerebral blood flow, pH, and adrenergic tone. Hypercapnia dilates cerebral vessels, and hypocapnia constricts them, a point of importance for patients with raised intracranial pressure. Acute increases in CO_2 depress consciousness, probably a result of intraneuronal acidosis. Slowly developing hypercapnia is better tolerated, presumably because buffering has time to occur. Nonetheless, a higher $PaCO_2$ signifies alveolar hypoventilation, which tends to decrease alveolar and arterial PO_2. Patients with renal insufficiency tolerate hypercapnia poorly because of their inability to adequately buffer carbonic acid.

The adrenergic stimulation that accompanies acute hypercapnia causes cardiac output to rise and peripheral vascular resistance to increase. During acute respiratory acidosis these effects may partially offset those of H^+ on cardiovascular function, allowing better tolerance of low pH than of metabolic acidosis of a similar degree. Constriction of glomerular arterioles may produce oliguria in some patients. Muscular twitching, asterixis, and seizures can be observed at extreme levels of hypercapnia in patients made susceptible by electrolyte or neural disorders.

Hypocapnia

The major effects of acute hypocapnia relate to alkalosis and diminished cerebral perfusion. Abrupt lowering of $PaCO_2$ reduces cerebral blood flow, raises neuronal pH, and reduces available ionized calcium, causing disturbances in cortical and peripheral nerve function. Light-headedness, circumoral and fingertip paresthesia, and muscular tetany can result. Sudden reduction of $PaCO_2$ (e.g., shortly after initiating mechanical ventilation) can produce life-threatening seizures.

Hydrogen Ion Concentration

For mammalian cells to function optimally, hydrogen ion concentration (as reflected in pH) must be rigidly controlled. The widest range compatible with life is $\simeq 6.8$–7.8 pH units.

Acidemia

Although all organs malfunction to some extent during acidemia, *cardiovascular function is among the most impaired*. Myocardial fibers contract less efficiently, systemic vessels react sluggishly to vasoconstrictors, vasomotor control deteriorates, blood pressure falls, and arrhythmias develop. Because H^+ ions are readily exchanged for K^+ across cell membranes, hyperkalemia frequently accompanies acidosis unless K^+ is lost concurrently (e.g., diabetic ketoacidosis). As a result of these cardiovascular and electrolyte abnormalities, defibrillation and cardiopulmonary resuscitation are difficult in an acidotic patient. In addition, acidemia impairs neuronal conduction and *mental status*, acts synergistically with alveolar hypoxia to cause pulmonary vasoconstriction, and blunts the action of adrenergic bronchodilators. Each of these effects accelerates in severity as pH falls below 7.20. *Respiratory* acidosis has particularly profound effects on mental status; perhaps because of the independent central nervous system (CNS) effects of hypercapnia (e.g., increased intracranial pressure) and the direct effects of accompanying hypoxemia.

Between 7.20 and 7.40, pH itself is not a major concern and should not prompt therapy aimed solely at pH correction. (In fact, the rightward shift of the oxyhemoglobin curve may improve tissue O_2 delivery if cardiovascular performance remains ad-

equate.) However, the pH scale is logarithmic; hence when pH falls below 7.20, H^+ rises dramatically. Mild acidemia is less alarming for its physiologic effects than for what it signifies—seriously decompensated ventilatory, metabolic, or cardiovascular systems in need of urgent attention.

Alkalemia

Alkalemia causes less apprehension among physicians than acidemia of a similar degree because its etiology is usually less life threatening. Elevated pH does not exert the dangerously depressing influence on myocardium and blood vessels seen with similar degrees of acidemia. Furthermore, unless very abrupt and severe, the effects of raised pH on the brain are limited to confusion and encephalopathy. The major risks of extreme alkalosis appear to relate to *lowering of the seizure threshold* and *provocation of cardiac arrhythmias*, effects caused in part by electrolyte shifts (Ca^{2+}, K^+) and diminished oxygen delivery. Alkalosis exerts detrimental effects with regard to release of O_2 to the tissues, shifting the oxyhemoglobin dissociation curve leftward. As a general rule, a pH > 7.60 warrants vigorous measures for reversal. Metabolic alkalemia may cause compensatory CO_2 retention that, when severe, may result in alveolar hypoxemia.

Generation and Excretion of H^+ Ion

Free hydrogen ion (H^+) has a potent impact on tissue enzyme systems. To keep H^+ within narrow limits, generation and elimination rates must be equal. H^+ ion is generated in two ways: (1) by hydration of CO_2 to form "volatile" acid according to the reaction

$$CO_2 + H_2O \rightleftarrows H_2CO_3 \rightleftarrows H^+ + HCO_3^-$$

and (2) by production of "fixed" acids (sulfates and phosphates) as chemical by-products of metabolism. Ventilation eliminates volatile acid while the kidney excretes the bulk of the fixed acid load. If excretion of CO_2 speeds or slows inappropriately when compared to its rate of production, the result is a *respiratory* derangement of acid-base balance. If the excretion rate of fixed acid speeds or slows disproportionately in relation to its production rate, or if abnormal metabolic loads of acid or alkali develop, *metabolic* acidosis or alkalosis occurs. In clinical practice, the concentration of free H^+ ion $[H^+]$ is tracked by the pH $= -\log [H^+]$.

Buffer Systems

Carbonic Acid

Chemical and protein buffer systems oppose changes in free $[H^+]$. The CO_2/HCO_3^- (carbonic acid) and hemoglobin systems are quantitatively the most important. Clinical attention is focused on the carbonic acid system because each of its components is readily measured and because CO_2 and HCO_3^- determinations allow clinical judgments to be made concerning the respiratory or metabolic origin of the problem at hand. To maintain pH at 7.40, the ratio of HCO_3^- to (.03 $\times$ $PaCO_2$) must remain in the 20:1 proportions dictated by the Henderson-Hasselbach equation:

$$pH = 6.1 + \log [(HCO_3^-)/(.03 \times PaCO_2)]$$

Noncarbonic (Protein) Buffers

Hemoglobin and other protein buffers also bind or release H^+ ion, minimizing pH changes while allowing the hydration reaction for CO_2 to continue to run in either direction.

$$CO_2 + H_2O \rightleftarrows H^+ + HCO_3^-$$
$$\hookrightarrow + Hgb \rightleftarrows H^+ \cdot Hgb$$

For this reason, if $PaCO_2$ changes acutely, there will be a small associated change in HCO_3^- in the same direction ($\simeq$ 1 mEq/l per 0.1 pH unit). Such automatic changes in HCO_3^- do *not* imply a metabolic disturbance, and the "base excess" (BE) attributable to this mechanism is zero (see below). Anemic blood fails to buffer fluctuations in H^+ concentration with normal efficiency.

Base Excess

Clinically, it is important to recognize and quantitate metabolic acid-base derangements. At pH 7.40, simple inspection of the HCO_3^- suffices to detect a metabolic component, whether primary or compensatory, for a chronic respiratory disturbance. However, as pH deviates from 7.40, the presence of noncarbonic buffers complicates interpretation.

The "base excess" is a number that quantitates the metabolic abnormality. It hypothetically "corrects" pH to 7.40 by first "adjusting" $PaCO_2$ to 40 mmHg, thus allowing a comparison of the "corrected" HCO_3^- with the known normal value at that pH (24 mEq/l). As a quick rule of thumb, base excess can be calculated from the observed values for HCO_3^- and pH as

$$BE = HCO_3^- + 10 (pH - 7.40) - 24 \text{ (mEq/l)}$$

A "negative" base excess means that HCO_3^- stores

are depleted. However, the BE does not indicate whether retention or depletion of HCO_3^- is pathologic or compensatory for long-standing respiratory derangements; *that* judgment must be made by an analysis of the clinical setting. Likewise it does not dictate the need for bicarbonate administration. Calculation of BE is especially helpful when the observed HCO_3^- is nearly normal (24 $\pm$ 3 mEq/l). The BE calculation is unlikely to provide new insights at more extreme HCO_3^- deviations.

Compensatory Mechanisms

As physiologic stresses on pH balance persist, adjustments in the excretion rate of CO_2 and H^+ counterbalance the effect of these disturbances on pH. In general, renal compensation for a respiratory disturbance is slower (but ultimately more successful) than respiratory compensation for a metabolic disturbance. Thus, although quick to respond, the respiratory system will not eliminate sufficient CO_2 to completely offset any but the mildest metabolic acidosis. Furthermore, the respiratory compensatory response is not fully developed until 24–48 hours after initial activation.

The lower limit of sustained compensatory hypocapnia in a healthy adult is $\simeq$ 10–15 mmHg. Once that limit is reached, even small additional increments in H^+ ion have disastrous effects on pH (and survival). Patients with disordered lung mechanics, such as those with COPD or neuromuscular weakness, are highly vulnerable to metabolic acid loads because they lack the normal ability to compensate by hyperventilation. CO_2 retention in response to alkalosis is very limited— only rarely exceeding 60 mmHg. The hypoxemia associated with hypoventilation helps limit the rise in CO_2 by triggering increased ventilatory effort.

Although the kidney cannot respond effectively to *abrupt* respiratory acidosis and alkalosis, renal compensation may eventually (3–7 days) totally counterbalance a respiratory alkalosis of moderate severity. The kidney also does relatively well with chronic respiratory acidosis, but does not compensate completely for a $PaCO_2$ above 65 mmHg unless another stimulus for HCO_3^- retention is present.

Rules of Compensation

Empiric rules of compensation have been derived for each acid-base disorder based on the usual response in an otherwise healthy individual. Deviations from these values suggest superimposed acid-base disturbances (Table 11.1).

Table 11.1
Compensation for Acid-Base Disorders[a]

Primary Disorder	Primary Change	Compensatory Change	Expected Compensation
Metabolic acidosis	↓ HCO_3^-	↓ $PaCO_2$	$\Delta PaCO_2 = 1.2\ \Delta HCO_3^-$
Metabolic acidosis	↑ HCO_3^-	↑ $PaCO_2$	$\Delta PaCO_2 = 0.9\ \Delta HCO_3^-$
Respiratory acidosis	↑ $PaCO_2$	↑ HCO_3^-	Acute $\Delta HCO_3^- = 0.10\ \Delta PaCO_2$
			Chronic $\Delta HCO_3^- = 0.35\ \Delta PaCO_2$
Respiratory alkalosis	↓ $PaCO_2$	↓ HCO_3^-	Acute $\Delta HCO_3^- = 0.2\ \Delta PaCO_2$
			Chronic $\Delta HCO_3^- = 0.5\ \Delta PaCO_2$

[a] ↓, decreased; ↑, increased.

ACID-BASE DERANGEMENTS

Terminology of Acid-Base Disorders

The terms acidemia and alkalemia refer to blood pH. Systemic pH < 7.35 defines *acidemia*. A pH >7.45 defines *alkalemia*. In contrast, *acidosis* and *alkalosis* do not refer to pH, but rather to basic pathophysiologic *processes* or tendencies favoring the development of acidemia or alkalemia. For example, a patient with diabetic ketoacidosis (the prototypic metabolic acidosis) and hypocapnia stimulated by pneumonia (a respiratory alkalosis) may exhibit *acidemia, alkalemia* or a *normal* p*H* depending upon the relative changes in $PaCO_2$, and HCO_3^-.

Uncomplicated *metabolic acidosis* is characterized by a decline in HCO_3^-, while a primary increase in HCO_3^- denotes *metabolic alkalosis*. Conversely, *respiratory acidosis* is defined as a primary increase in $PaCO_2$, whereas *respiratory alkalosis* occurs when the central feature is a decrease in $PaCO_2$.

Simple Acid-Base Disorders

Metabolic Acidosis

Mechanisms

Metabolic acidosis (MAc) is the consequence of *bicarbonate loss or consumption* (decreased H^+ excretion, increased H^+ production).

Bicarbonate Consumption. H^+ is normally excreted renally as titratable acid (phosphates and sulfates) and ammonia. Renal failure, hypoaldosteronism, and distal renal tubular acidosis (DRTA) all impair this excretion. In DRTA proximal tubular HCO_3^- reabsorption is normal, but distal tubular H^+ secretion is impaired. Hypoaldosteronism also impairs H^+ excretion and may be recognized by the association of MAc, hyponatremia, and hypercalcemia.

Hydrogen Ion Load and the Anion Gap. An *increased H^+ load* may also cause MAc. In such cases, the disparity between the measured concentrations of serum cations and anions—the anion gap (AG)—will widen: normal AG = 9–13 mEq/l. Knowledge of the

$$AG = (Na^+ - Cl^- + HCO_3^-)$$

may be quite valuable in distinguishing the etiology of MAc. Only the addition of *unmeasured* anions can elevate the AG (e.g., HCl administration does not increase the AG since Cl^- is a measured anion). The most common causes of an elevated AG can be recalled by the mnemonic "S.L.U.M.P.E.D." as listed below.

Etiology of Anion Gap Acidosis

Salicylates
Lactate
Uremic toxins
Methanol
Paraldehyde
Ethanol / ethylene glycol
Diabetic ketoacidosis

Lactic acid generated by anaerobic glycolysis is the most common cause of an elevated AG. In high doses, *salicylates* raise the AG by interfering with carbohydrate metabolism and O_2 utilization. Very high serum levels of anionic salicylate molecules may directly elevate the AG. Uremia may lead to accumulation of titratable acids, producing an AG-MAc. Four toxins that commonly produce an AG acidosis include *methanol, ethylene glycol, paraldehyde*, and *ethanol* (see Chapter 27). *Diabetic ketoacidosis* also produces an AG-MAc by increasing unmeasured ketones and lactate (see p. 226).

Bicarbonate Loss. *Bicarbonate loss* may produce MAc but *does not elevate the AG* because *HCO_3^- loss results in compensatory hyperchlo-*

remia. Although renal failure usually impairs H^+ excretion, renal failure may also induce direct HCO_3^- loss. In renal failure, the HCO_3^- usually plateaus at 12–20 mmol/l as further H^+ accumulation is blunted by tissue (bone) buffers. Three conditions decrease HCO_3^- disproportionately to reductions in glomerular filtration rate: *renal medullary disorders* (tubular problems, e.g., proximal renal tubular acidosis, PRTA), *low renin/aldosterone* states, and *renal failure* in which there is decreased HCO_3^- resorption (due to a constant filtered Na^+ load and an increased filtration fraction through a few remaining nephrons). The mild MAc of PRTA is usually an incidental finding. PRTA, a self-limiting disorder, results from an inability to fully resorb filtered HCO_3^-. The limited reabsorptive capacity for HCO_3^- renders pH correction difficult and produces an alkaline urine. In such patients, exogenous $NaHCO_3$ increases the filtered HCO_3^- load, raising urine pH. Apart from MAc and alkaline urine, four ancillary features characteristic of PRTA are decreased serum urate, decreased PO_4^{3-}, glycosuria, and amino aciduria.

The *gastrointestinal (GI) tract* provides a route for HCO_3^- loss in patients with chronic diarrhea or laxative abuse. Cholestyramine may also cause MAc by exchanging HCO_3^- for Cl^-. Because the ileum and colon have ion pumps that reabsorb HCO_3^- in exchange for Cl^-, ureterosigmoidostomy patients frequently develop hyperchloremic acidosis.

Signs and Symptoms

Unlike those with respiratory acidosis, patients with MAc are usually *tachypneic*, unless ventilatory drive is depressed. If the acidosis is severe, lethargy or coma may occur. Neurologic changes are less prominent with metabolic than with respiratory acidosis, perhaps because hypercapnia and hypoxemia of respiratory acidosis exert independent effects. In the most severe cases, hypotension may result from cardiovascular depression.

Compensation

There are *four compensatory mechanisms* for MAc. Initially, *extracellular buffers* blunt the falling pH. Rapidly thereafter, the *respiratory system* increases minute ventilation to reduce $PaCO_2$. The $PaCO_2$ declines $\simeq$ 1.2 mmHg per mEq/liter reduction in serum HCO_3^- but rarely falls below 10 mmHg. The $PaCO_2$ expected in response to an established MAc may be predicted from the equation below:

$$\text{expected } PaCO_2 \simeq 1.5 \times \text{measured } HCO_3^- + 8$$

As a rule of thumb, in *chronic MAc, the expected $PaCO_2$ approximates the last 2 digits of the pH value* (e.g., the expected $PaCO_2$ for a pH of 7.25 is 25). Although respiratory compensation is relatively prompt (fully developed within 24 hours), it is rarely complete. If the $PaCO_2$ is above that expected for a given HCO_3^-, either the time for compensation has been too short, or respiratory acidosis is present. If the $PaCO_2$ is less than that expected, respiratory alkalosis is present. *Buffering* of H^+ by intracellualar protein and fixed buffers in bone (calcium salts) represents a third major mechanism for blunting the pH fall. Finally, the kidney may enhance H^+ excretion, but this function requires the active excretion of H^+ in combination with phosphate and ammonium. Such losses of H^+ are limited to $\simeq$ 50–100 mEq/day, a rate that approximates the normal pace of mineral acid production.

Treatment

If pH disturbances are severe, temporizing measures may be necessary to alter the PCO_2 or bicarbonate content directly. However, the treatment of acid-base disorders should usually be directed at the underlying cause. Major indications for immediate and direct treatment of MAc are:

1. pH < 7.20
2. overt physiologic compromise attributable to acidosis
3. excessive work of breathing required to maintain acceptable pH (> 7.25).

Calculation of the HCO_3^- dose assumes a distribution into total body water. Total body water (in liters) $\simeq$ 0.6–0.7 lean body weight (in kg). The expression:

$$D = (\text{total body water}) \times (24 - HCO_3^-)$$

approximates the HCO_3^- deficit (D) in mEq. Because $NaHCO_3^-$ has potentially adverse effects and because the effectiveness of a given dose is not entirely predictable, it is customary to *replace one-half the calculated HCO_3^- deficit and follow the pH response closely.* $NaHCO_3$ partially equilibrates in total body water within 15 minutes of administration; however, cellular equilibration requires $\simeq$ 2 hours to complete.

$NaHCO_3$ administration entails many potential problems. In large doses *hypertonic hypernatremia* and *fluid overload* may occur. An ampule of $NaHCO_3$ contains approximately as much Na^+ as ½ liter of normal saline. Bolus injection of HCO_3^-

may elicit a biphasic ventilatory response. Immediately after $NaHCO_3$ administration, peripheral pH rises and the drive to breathe falls. However, soon thereafter, rising CO_2 (due both to metabolic load and buffered H^+ ion) diffuses across the blood brain barrier to reduce intracerebral pH and stimulate breathing ("paradoxical CNS acidosis").

Rapid bolus injection of $NaHCO_3$ is potentially dangerous—it may cause a rapid leftward shift of the oxyhemoglobin dissociation curve, alter cerebral hemodynamics, or induce life-threatening hypokalemia. A pH > 7.10 is usually sufficient to maintain near normal vascular tone and myocardial contractility and can almost always be obtained using small doses of $NaHCO_3$. Furthermore, some types of acidosis (e.g., PRTA) are very difficult to correct with exogenous bicarbonate. In organic acidosis (diabetic ketoacidosis, DKA, or lactic acidosis) $NaHCO_3$ may eventually lead to an alkalosis as the organic acids (ketones, lactate) are recycled to HCO_3^- by the liver. (There is no loss of *potential* bicarbonate in these disorders.)

Metabolic Alkalosis

Metabolic alkalosis (MAl) is usually generated and maintained by different pathophysiologic mechanisms. *MAl is always due to the gain of HCO_3^- or loss of H^+ ions.* Exogenous base may accumulate when bicarbonate, citrate, carbonate, lactate, or acetate are administered. H^+ is most commonly lost in gastric juice (e.g., nasogastric suction, vomiting) and less commonly through renal excretion. Increased renal H^+ loss may be mediated by *excess mineralocorticoids, increased distal tubule Na^+ delivery,* or *excessive filtration of non-reabsorbable anions* (e.g., calcium, penicillin).

Renal mechanisms almost never generate MAl but are almost always responsible for its perpetuation. The normal kidney rapidly excretes an alkaline urine in response to a HCO_3^- load, provided that serum Cl^- and K^+ are normal. However, *hypokalemia* and *hypochloremia* both inhibit the excretion of excess HCO_3^-. Hypokalemia augments proximal tubular HCO_3^- resorption and increases distal tubular H^+ secretion. Both effects perpetuate alkalosis. The volume depletion that almost always accompanies Cl^- deficiency stimulates renin and aldosterone secretion, promoting H^+ excretion. Hypermineralocorticoidism increases H^+ secretion, an effect potentiated by high tubular flow rates, the presence of non-reabsorbable anions, and K^+ deficiency. Any disease that stimulates aldosterone secretion (e.g., volume de-

pletion, Mg^{2+} deficiency) promotes HCO_3^- retention.

Diagnostic Criteria

MAl is characterized by an elevated pH, elevated HCO_3^-, and a compensatory increase in $PaCO_2$ if the disorder is chronic. The anion gap may increase because of the increased "charge equivalency" of albumin and stimulation of organic anion synthesis (see Ref. 1).

Signs and Symptoms

MAl impairs neural transmission and muscular contraction, especially when accompanied by hypokalemia and hypophosphatemia—two abnormalities that commonly coexist. Indeed MAl mimics hypocalcemia in its symptomatology (see p. 123). Changes in mental status and thirst due to volume depletion are common.

Precipitants of Metabolic Alkalosis

Severe *hypokalemia* (K^+ < 2.0) causes generalized intracellular acidosis, an effect that impairs the function of the renal tubule. This effect favors HCO_3^- retention and perpetuates MAl. *Nasogastric suctioning or vomiting* depletes circulatory volume (H^+ and Cl^-). In replacing these H^+ losses, HCO_3^- is generated and retained. Volume depletion causes hyperaldosteronism, (HCO_3^- retention, K^+ loss). Aldosterone also promotes maximal Na^+ resorption, leading to high rates of tubular Na^+ for $H^{+'}$ exchange which further worsens the alkalosis.

Relief of long-standing respiratory acidosis (e.g., after institution of mechanical ventilation) results in a rapidly evolving MAl from the HCO_3^- previously retained in compensation. For unknown reasons, chronic respiratory acidosis promotes urinary Cl^- wasting, which helps to perpetuate alkalosis in this setting. *Mineralocorticoid excess* (primary or secondary) is commonly accompanied by K^+ loss and impaired renal tubular HCO_3^- excretion. When loop diuretics are given to volume depleted patients, increased amounts of Na^+ are presented to the distal renal tubule, and the resulting intensified exchange of Na^+ for H^+ perpetuates MAl. If Na^+ is administered along with a non-resorbable anion (e.g., penicillin) in volume depleted patients, the Na^+ will be reabsorbed in the renal tubule and H^+ will be secreted to maintain electroneutrality.

The weak aldosterone-like properties of glucocorticoids may cause MAl in Cushing's syndrome or with exogenous administration of cortisone derivatives. Excess HCO_3^- retention may occur following therapeutic administration, but if circulating volume and K^+ are normal, the kidney has a remarkable ability to excrete excess HCO_3^-. *Iatrogenic* MAl often complicates therapy of acidosis due to DKA or lactate because HCO_3^- is regenerated in the recovery period. *Blood transfusion* delivers citrate, an HCO_3^- equivalent; however, MAl is rare unless > 8–10 units of blood are given. Overt alkalosis rarely complicates antacid administration because most such agents are non-absorbable. *Contraction alkalosis* is a state in which losses of intravascular volume, K^+, and Cl^- act in conjunction with hyperaldosteronism to deplete extracellular fluid around a near-constant amount of HCO_3^-. This effect is to shrink the volume of distribution of bicarbonate, increasing its concentration. Renal exchange of Na^+ for K^+ (under the effects of aldosterone) also leads to excessive H^+ excretion.

Maintenance of the Alkalosis

MAl can be maintained by the same 4 mechanisms responsible for its development: Cl^- deficiency, mineralocorticoid excess, and depletion of circulating volume or K^+. However, in a given patient MAl is often maintained by a different mechanism from that which established it. For example, nasogastric removal of Cl^- and H^+ generate an MAl, but it is the volume depletion and chloride depletion that maintain it, even when nasogastric (NG) suction is discontinued. Cl^- and volume must be administered for reversal. Given a choice, the body chooses to maintain circulating volume status at the expense of Cl^- and pH homeostasis.

Compensation for Metabolic Alkalosis

In MAl the $PaCO_2$ normally rises $\simeq 0.6$ mmHg per mmol increase in HCO_3^-. (Lower $PaCO_2$ values indicate a superimposed respiratory alkalosis.) It is rare to see a compensatory increase in $PaCO_2$ > 60 mmHg when breathing room air, because at this level of hypercarbia the PaO_2 falls to $\simeq 60$ torr and hypoxemia begins to drive respiration.

Diagnostic Techniques

As already indicated, the *clinical history*, the *medication profile*, *serum chemistries*, and *intravascular volume studies are keys to the differential diagnosis. Urine electrolytes* may also be useful in diagnosing the cause of MAl, provided that they are not obtained within 24 hours of diuretic administration. Urine Na^+ and $Cl^- < 10$ mEq/l sug-

gest *volume depletion* and *post-hypercapnic alkalosis* as potential mechanisms. If the urine Cl^- and Na^+ exceed 20 mEq/l, *mineralocorticoid excess*, *early diuretic use*, and *severe hypokalemia* are common causes. Marked disparity between urinary Cl^- and Na^+ strongly suggests mineralocorticoid excess.

Treatment

MAl is often considered in two general categories—"salt" (NaCl)-responsive or salt-unresponsive (Table 11.2). NaCl frequently reverses volume contraction and 2° hyperaldosteronism. NaCl also provides Cl^- ions for reabsorption with Na^+, obviating the need for H^+ secretion. (The effectiveness of NaCl replacement may be determined by *measuring urinary pH*—if Na^+ replacement is sufficient, urinary pH will rise above 7.0.) *Chloride*, the only absorbable anion, is the critical factor in NaCl administration (Table 11.2). Sodium sulfate administration will not improve MAl, even though Na^+ is provided and volume is corrected. Because K^+ depletion contributes to maintenance of MAl, K^+ replacement aids in HCO_3^- excretion.

Chloride-resistant alkaloses (adrenal disorders, corticosteroid administration, excess alkali ingestion, or administration) are usually due to mineralocorticoid excess. Therefore, in most such disorders hypokalemia is a predictable feature. Therapy of mineralocorticoid excess may be directed at removal of the hormonal source (tumor control, withdrawal of steroids) or blockade of mineralocorticoid effect (spironolactone). K^+-sparing diuretics or the combination of Na^+ restriction and K^+ supplementation are also effective.

Rarely, MAl is sufficiently protracted or severe to warrant the administration of intravenous HCl. HCl may be infused as a 0.1–0.2 M solution but must be given directly into a central venous catheter at a rate not exceeding 0.2 mEq/kg/hr. The

Table 11.2

A Classification of MAl Based on Chloride Responsiveness

Cl^- Responsiveness	Cl^- Resistant
Volume depletion	1° Hyperaldosteronism
Vomiting/diarrhea	Exogenous steroids
NG suction	Glucocorticoids
Diuretics	Mineralocorticoids
Post-hypercapnia	Cushing's syndrome
Cationic drugs	
(e.g., penicillin)	

appropriate HCl dose may be approximated from the product of the desired change in HCO_3^- and 50% of the total body weight. Ammonium chloride may be used instead of HCl but should not be administered to patients with renal or hepatic failure.

Respiratory Alkalosis

Inciting Mechanisms

Respiratory alkalosis (RAl) is defined by *primary hypocapnia*. Hypocapnia implies alveolar hyperventilation. Central neurologic disorders, agitation, inappropriate mechanical ventilation, hypoxemia, and alterations in thoracic and lung compliance may all produce RAl.

Symptoms

Acute RAl is usually manifest by tachypnea; however, when chronic, this disorder may be associated with large tidal volume breaths at near-normal respiratory rates. The symptoms of RAl, "the hyperventilation syndrome", vary only in intensity from those of any alkalosis—most notably impaired neuromuscular function (e.g., parasthesias, tetany, tremor). A constellation of symptoms have been described with RAl; these include chest pain, circumoral paresthesias, carpopedal spasm, anxiety, and light-headedness.

Compensatory Mechanisms

Protracted RAl induces renal HCO_3^- wasting to offset hypocapnia. When the stimulus for hyperventilation is removed, hyperpnea tends to continue, driven by CNS acidosis until intracerebral HCO_3^- and pH are corrected.

Mixed Acid-Base Disorders

Complex (mixed) acid-base disorders most frequently occur when there is concurrent lung and renal disease, when compensatory mechanisms are rendered inoperable, or when mechanical ventilation is used. For example, narcotics can blunt the compensatory hyperpneic response to metabolic acidosis, and acetazolamide too aggressively given to patients with chronic hypercapnia can promote bicarbonate wasting and induce a complex acid-base disorder. Even by itself aspirin overdosage can cause a combined respiratory alkalosis and metabolic acidosis.

SUGGESTED READINGS

1. Brenner BE: Clinical significance of the elevated anion gap. *Am J Med* 79:289–296, 1985.
2. DuBose TD: Clinical approach to patients with acid-base disorders. *Med Clin N Am* 67:799–813, 1983.
3. Garella S, Chang BS, Kahn SI: Dilution acidosis and contraction alkalosis: review of a concept. *Kidney Int* 8:279–283, 1975.
4. Hruska KA, Ban D, Avioli LV: Renal tubular acidosis. *Arch Intern Med* 142:1909–1913, 1982.
5. Kreisberg RA: Pathogenesis and management of lactic acidosis. *Ann Rev Med* 35:181–193, 1984.
6. Laski ME: Normal regulation of acid-base balance: renal and pulmonary response and other extrarenal buffering mechanisms. *Med Clin N Am* 67:771–780, 1983.
7. Mitchell JH, Wildenthal K, Johnson RL: The effect of acid-base disturbances on cardiovascular and pulmonary function. *Kidney Int* 1:375–389, 1973.
8. Narins RG, Emmett M: Simple and mixed acid-base disorders: a practical approach. *Medicine* 59:161–187, 1980.
9. Riley LJ Jr, Ilson BE, Narins RG: Acute metabolic acid-base disorders. *Crit Care Clin* 5(4):699–724, 1987.

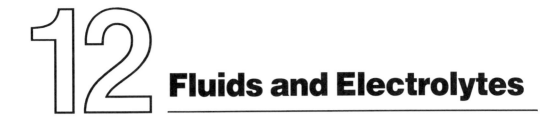

Fluids and Electrolytes

DISORDERS OF SODIUM AND OSMOLALITY

Hyponatremia

In approaching disorders of sodium (Na^+) and osmolality (Osm), the clinician must systematically address seven questions:

1. What is the intravascular volume status?
2. What are the serum concentrations of Na^+, albumin, and lipids?
3. What is the serum Osm?
4. What is the urinary volume, Osm, and electrolyte composition?
5. What medications and fluids is the patient receiving?
6. Is there evidence of renal disease?
7. Is edema present?

Laboratory Evaluation

In combination with a thorough history and physical examination, the urine Na^+, serum glucose, and the serum and urine osmolality provide essential data to determine the etiology of hyponatremia.

Because Na^+ is the predominant osmotically active extracellular cation, serum osmolality is determined largely by the relative proportions of water and Na^+. Measurements of serum osmolality help to separate the hyponatremias into three distinct categories, thereby guiding appropriate intervention. Apart from disturbances in Na^+/H_2O balance, marked elevations of glucose, blood urea nitrogen (BUN) or exogenous substances (alcohols and complex carbohydrates) can elevate serum osmolality. Conversely, reductions in osmolality virtually always are reflected in the Na^+ concentration. The serum osmolality can be approximated by using the following equation:

$$osmolality = 2\,[Na^+] + glucose/18 + BUN/3 + (\text{``unmeasured'' osmoles})$$

Subclasses of Hyponatremia

Isotonic Hyponatremia

Hyponatremia with *normal serum osmolality* occurs when osmotically active solutes expand the plasma volume, diluting $[Na^+]$ (e.g., myeloma, Waldenstrom's macroglobulinemia). Serum protein concentrations $> 12–15$ gm/dl are usually required to produce noteworthy hyponatremia. Dilution of serum Na^+ results not only from the osmotic drag of the serum proteins but also from the need to maintain electroneutrality. As positively charged proteins enter the circulation, chloride is retained and sodium is excreted to prevent charge imbalance. (Hyperlipidemia may also artifactually increase apparent serum volume, decreasing the measured $[Na^+]$. However, lipid removal before analysis normalizes the $[Na^+]$.) Isotonic hyponatremia may also occur during the administration of *isotonic*, non-salt containing solutions (glucose, Hetastarch, mannitol, glycine). Before their solutes are metabolized or excreted, these fluids are restricted to the extracellular space, where they expand the circulating volume and dilute $[Na^+]$. (After solute excretion or metabolism, free water distributes proportionally among intracellular and extracellular sites.)

Hypertonic Hyponatremias

Hypertonic hyponatremia results from the *infusion or generation of (non-sodium) osmotic substances* predisposed to extracellular partitioning. Nonketotic hyperglycemia and therapeutic administration of *hypertonic* glucose, mannitol, or glycine can cause hypertonicity as they depress $[Na^+]$. (Although urea also increases osmolality, it fails to affect $[Na^+]$ because it easily traverses cell membranes, dissipating any osmotic gradient.) Extracellular hypertonicity draws cellular water to the extracellular space in an attempt to reduce the osmotic gradient. This effect partially corrects the hyperosmolality, but it lowers the $[Na^+]$ and causes cellular dehydration. The cause of hypertonic hyponatremia can usually be diagnosed by measuring serum glucose concentration and by reviewing a list of the patient's drugs. When hyperglycemia is the etiology, $[Na^+]$ falls $\simeq 1.6$ mEq/l per 100 mg/dl rise in serum glucose.

Hypotonic Hyponatremias

Hypotonic hyponatremia is the most common category of hyponatremia. Knowledge of the patient's circulating volume status is key to determining etiology and treatment. Hypotonic hyponatremia almost never develops unless the patient has unlimited access to water or is administered a hypotonic fluid.

Hypovolemic Hypotonic Hyponatremia. Hypovolemic hyponatremia with low serum osmolality results from replacing losses of salt-containing plasma with hypotonic fluid. Volume depletion is a potent stimulus for antidiuretic hormone (ADH) release that overwhelms competing osmotic stimuli (hypotonicity) for ADH suppression. Intake of hypotonic fluid, when combined with the decreased free water clearance that results from ADH release, causes hyponatremia. Physical examination reveals signs of volume depletion. Thirst and postural hypotension (the hallmark of hypovolemia in patients with intact vascular reflexes) are more objective and reliable signs than are skin turgor, absence of axillary sweating, sunken orbits, or mucous membrane dryness.

Causes. Hypovolemic hypotonic hyponatremia may result from renal or non-renal causes. *Bleeding*, *diarrhea*, and *vomiting*, common non-renal mechanisms of circulating volume loss, are usually apparent. *Third space losses* (pancreatitis, gut sequestration, or diffuse muscular trauma) are less obvious.

Renal causes of volume depletion and hyponatremia include *salt wasting nephropathy*, *diuretic use*, *mineralocorticoid deficiency*, and *osmotic diuresis* from ketones, glucose, urea, or mannitol. Partial *urinary tract obstruction* and *bicarbonaturia* from renal tubular acidosis or metabolic alkalosis may also deplete volume and produce hyponatremia.

Laboratory Examination. Because hypovolemia reduces renal blood flow and slows tubular flow, urea may "back-diffuse" into the bloodstream. Conversely, because creatinine (Cr) cannot back-diffuse, Cr excretion is less severely impaired, and the BUN/Cr ratio rises. In patients

with functioning kidneys and normal levels of mineralocorticoid hormones, *small volumes* of *hypertonic urine* with *very low* $[Na^+]$ reflect intense conservation of Na^+ and water. If *urine sodium is high* and *urine osmolality normal*, *renal salt wasting is the likely etiology* of volume depletion. In primary adrenal insufficiency, the urine $[Na^+]$ is high, and the urine osmolality is elevated.

Hypervolemic Hypotonic Hyponatremia. *Edema* is the hallmark of hypervolemic hypotonic hyponatremia, a syndrome in which water is retained in excess of Na^+. Because $\simeq 70\%$ of total body water is intracellular, a 12–15 liter excess of total body H_2O must be present before sufficient interstitial fluid accumulates to cause detectable edema (unless hypoalbuminemia or vascular injury is present). Despite increases in both total body water and Na^+, *effective intravascular volume is usually decreased*.

Causes. *Non-renal causes* include conditions which decrease effective renal perfusion (congestive heart failure) and diseases characterized by hypoproteinemia and decreased colloid osmotic pressure (cirrhosis, hepatic failure, and nephrotic syndrome). *Renal causes* can include almost any form of acute or chronic renal failure.

Laboratory Examination. If the cause is extrarenal, there is intense conservation of salt and water with very *low urinary* $[Na^+]$ (< 10 mEq/l), *low urine volumes*, and *high urine osmolality*. Urine electrolytes and osmolality are more variable (and less helpful) in renally induced hypervolemic hyponatremia. Because diuretics impair the ability to conserve Na^+ and water, *at least* 24 hours must elapse between the last dose of diuretic and reliable determinations of urinary electrolytes and osmolality.

Isovolemic Hypotonic Hyponatremia. Isovolemic hypotonic hyponatremia is a misnomer. Such patients maintain a slight (undetectable) excess of total body fluid ($\simeq 3$–4 liters). When renal function is normal and ADH can be inhibited, free water loads are rapidly cleared (> 1 l/hr). Because of this impressive capacity, most cases of H_2O intoxication occur in patients with impaired ability to clear free water or ADH excess. For example, H_2O intoxication occurs with increased frequency in renal disease (decreased clearance) and schizophrenia (increased ADH and increased H_2O intake).

Diuretics commonly cause isovolemic hyponatremia. When normal circulating volume is maintained by diuretics, natriuresis impairs free water clearance and sensitizes to ADH. A "reset" of the serum osmostat may be seen in patients with a variety of underlying problems. (For example, cirrhosis and tuberculosis frequently cause chronic hyponatremia by this mechanism.) The "reset" phenomenon may be distinguished from inappropriate ADH secretion by normal responses to water loading or deprivation, despite hypo-osmolality.

Inappropriate ADH.   Inappropriate ADH syndrome (SIADH) is often misdiagnosed in hospitalized patients. *A diagnosis of exclusion, SIADH requires normal volume status, normal cardiac and renal function, and a normal hormonal environment (exclusive of ADH)*. SIADH is most frequently associated with malignant tumors, particularly of the lung; however, central nervous system (CNS) or pulmonary infections, drugs, and trauma may also be the cause.

SIADH is characterized by an *inappropriately concentrated urine*, with urinary excretion of Na^+ that matches the daily intake. Urine osmolality usually exceeds plasma osmolality. *Urine $[Na^+]$ is > 20 mEq/l*, and the urine cannot be diluted appropriately in response to H_2O loading. (When water-challenged, patients with most other types of hyponatremia completely suppress ADH release and excrete maximally dilute urine < 100 mOsm/l.) Excessive ADH or ADH-like compounds decrease free H_2O clearance, resulting in modest expansion of the extracellular and intravascular volumes. Volume expansion increases cardiac output and glomerular filtration rate (GFR), eventually depleting the stores of total body Na^+. (Because a constant *fraction* of filtered Na^+ is resorbed, there is obligatory renal loss of Na^+.) Serum values of Na^+, Cr, and uric acid are all subnormal because of the expanded circulating volume and increased GFR. The treatment of SIADH is to restrict free water and correct the underlying disorder.

Complications of Hyponatremia

Hyponatremia primarily affects the CNS. As $[Na^+]$ drops below 120 mEq/l, changes in cognition and motor function are common. *Confusion and seizures* often occur at serum $[Na^+]$ < 120 mEq/l, particularly if the fall in $[Na^+]$ occurs acutely. Half of all patients with severe hyponatremia ($[Na^+] < 105$ mEq/l) die. Unfortunately, rapid correction of hyponatremia is also associated with serious neurologic sequelae. *Central pontine myelinolysis* may result from overzealous correction. Most hyponatremic patients should have the $[Na^+]$ corrected to a value slightly > 120 mEq/l

over a 12–24–hour period, at a rate not to exceed 2 mEq/l/hr.

Treatment of Hyponatremia

The treatment of hyponatremia depends upon cause and severity. In *hypervolemic hyponatremia, salt and fluid restriction* are the mainstays of therapy. However, diuretics or dialysis may be required when renal function is impaired. In *hypovolemic hyponatremia, normal or hypertonic saline* should be used to restore circulating volume. In *isovolemic hyponatremia, free water restriction* and *treatment of the underlying disorder* are preferred. Patients with severe hyponatremia may require hypertonic saline and diuretics to achieve a safe serum $[Na^+]$ with adequate speed. In less acute cases of SIADH, hyponatremia may respond to demeclocycline or lithium. The diagnostic categories, and causes of hyponatremia are summarized in Table 12.1.

Hypernatremia

Hypernatremia is rare in patients with intact ADH secretion, a sensitive thirst mechanism, and access to free water. Although hypernatremia may theoretically result from water loss or sodium gain, water loss or deprivation is by far the most common mechanism. Hypernatremia is primarily a disease of patients unable to obtain and drink water, particularly those sustaining simultaneous water losses. Furthermore, because many elderly patients have defective osmoregulation, they are more likely to develop hypernatremia when faced with a provocative stimulus. It is therefore relatively common in the intensive care unit (ICU) setting. *Hypernatremia implies hyperosmolarity*, the major mechanism of toxicity.

Dehydration may result solely from increased insensible losses due to burns, tachypnea, or hyperthermia (high fever, heat stroke, neuroleptic malignant syndrome, malignant hyperthermia; see Chapter 22). Tachypnea does not cause dehydration in mechanically ventilated patients, however, because fully humidified gas is employed. Yet even with increased water losses, hypernatremia usually requires water deprivation. Renal losses of free water may occur from intrinsic kidney diseases or from deficient or ineffective ADH. Osmotic diuretics such as glucose, mannitol, or glycerol may exaggerate free water clearance. Salt loading (primary hyperaldosteronism, hypertonic NaCl, or oral sodium ingestion) rarely produces hypernatremia.

Treatment of hypernatremia consists of the replacement of free water, usually as D5W, with

Table 12.1
Hyponatremia: Diagnostic Categories and Causes[a]

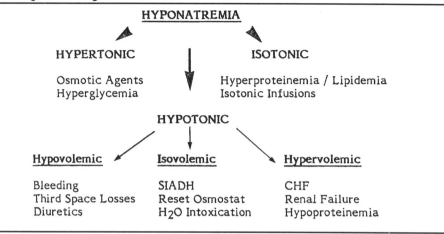

[a]CHF, congestive heart failure.

frequent evaluation of electrolytes and osmolality. If ADH is deficient or defective, it may be replaced with DDAVP, an ADH analog.

POTASSIUM DISORDERS

Hypokalemia

Because obligatory potassium (K^+) losses are only 5–15 mEq/day in healthy patients with normal kidneys, *potassium depletion occurs only when there are excessive K^+ losses or impaired K^+ intake.* Once hypokalemia becomes manifest, the average K^+ deficit approximates 250–300 mEq ($\simeq$ 5–10% of the total body K^+ stores). However, systemic pH influences extracellular $[K^+]$; during acidosis, hydrogen ions move into cells in exchange for potassium, raising extracellular $[K^+]$. Therefore, *hypo*kalemia in the face of acidosis suggests a large total body deficit. Ninety-five percent of total body K^+ is intracellular. Despite the small size of the extracellular compartment, its $[K^+]$ critically influences neuromuscular conduction. As a general rule, the large intracellular pool effectively maintains serum $[K^+]$ until total body K^+ depletion occurs. Conversely, hyperkalemia does not always signify excess total body K^+. Even relatively small K^+ loads may induce hyperkalemia as slow cellular uptake of K^+ occurs from the small intravascular space.

Etiology

Hypokalemia may result from *decreased intake*, *increased losses*, or *redistribution* of K^+. Hypokalemia rarely results from decreased intake be-

cause the healthy kidneys can reduce K^+ excretion to < 10 mEq/day, a level almost always less than dietary intake.

A number of mechanisms may facilitate K^+ entry into cells to produce hypokalemia. *High insulin levels*, whether exogenous or induced by continuous alimentation (e.g., total parenteral nutrition (TPN) or tube feedings), increase cellular uptake. *Metabolic alkalosis* also causes K^+ to enter cells in exchange for H^+. In turn, hypokalemia increases renal bicarbonate absorption, perpetuating the alkalosis. Hypokalemia often occurs within 48 hours of treating *B_{12} or folate deficiency*, as K^+ is massively incorporated into newly formed red cells and platelets. Such patients routinely experience reduction in serum $[K^+]$ of $\simeq$ 1 mEq/l—a potentially life-threatening change.

Renal losses provoked by diuretic use constitute the most common cause of hypokalemia. *Diuretics* increase distal tubular flow and the exchange of Na^+ for K^+ (an effect that may be profound in patients with edema). Simultaneous use of two or more diuretics having actions at different sites in the nephron (usually a thiazide/loop diuretic combination) can produce massive K^+ losses. Volume-depleted patients with metabolic alkalosis secrete high levels of *aldosterone*, accelerating both renal and gastrointestinal (GI) K^+ losses. Patients with *high NaCl intake* are also predisposed to develop hypokalemia because high filtered sodium loads accentuate the tubular exchange of Na^+ for K^+. Although the $[K^+]$ of *liquid stool* may reach 60 mEq/l, stool K^+ losses are rarely severe enough to produce symptomatic hypokalemia. Conversely, *vomiting* induces hypokalemia not through direct losses but by promoting renal K^+ wasting as a result of a newly generated metabolic alkalosis.

Pathophysiology

Hypokalemia impairs muscle contractility and, when severe ($[K^+] < 2.5$ mEq/l), may cause profound, life-threatening respiratory muscle weakness. The severity of the muscular effects of a given $[K^+]$ depends upon *pH, calcium,* and the *rapidity* with which hypokalemia developed. Hypokalemia increases the resting membrane potential of neuromuscular tissue, reducing excitability. The muscles of the lower extremities are usually the first to be affected by hypokalemia, followed by those of the trunk and respiratory system. Even moderate degrees of hypokalemia may impair smooth muscle function, producing ileus, pseudoobstruction, or decreased ureteral motility. Severe hypokalemia also impairs the vascular smooth muscle response to catecholamines and angiotensin, influencing blood pressure stability by this mechanism.

Hypokalemia may cause polyuria and polydypsia by injuring the renal tubular epithelium or diminishing responsiveness to ADH. Although focal neurologic findings rarely result from hypokalemia, lethargy and confusion are common in severe K^+ depletion.

Virtually any arrhythmia may surface during hypokalemia, especially in the presence of digitalis. Hypokalemia doubles the incidence of life-threatening arrhythmias in patients with acute myocardial ischemia, lowers the threshold for ventricular fibrillation, and promotes the re-entry phenomenon. Mild hypokalemia delays ventricular repolarization and is manifested by ST segment depression, diminished or inverted T waves, heightened U waves, and a prolonged Q-U interval. When hypokalemia is severe ($[K^+] < 2.5$ mEq/l), P wave amplitude, PR interval, and QRS duration increase (Fig. 12.1).

Treatment

Total body deficits of K^+ frequently exceed 200 mEq in patients with hypokalemia. Yet, because the intracellular space must be accessed via the small extracellular compartment, K^+ replacement must be cautious and closely monitored to avoid potentially lethal *hyper*kalemia. Special care must be exercised when replacing K^+ in patients with *renal disease* or *diabetes* and in those receiving *drugs that block renin, angiotensin, or prostaglandin activity* (e.g., angiotensin-converting enzyme (ACE) inhibitors, non-steroidal anti-inflammatory agents). Hypomagnesemia aggrevates the physiologic effects of hypokalemia and renders deficit correction difficult. As a general rule, K^+ should never be infused more quickly than 40 mEq/hr and then only in dire emergencies.

Hyperkalemia

It is difficult for healthy subjects to develop hyperkalemia because even minimally functional *kidneys efficiently excrete excess K^+. In addition, adaptation to chronic K^+ administration* increases the ability of the kidney to excrete it. Furthermore, when renal clearance decreases, the colon may increase $[K^+]$ excretion. *Cellular buffering* (particularly by muscle and liver) acutely blunts the impact of a K^+ load while the kidneys eliminate the excess. *Insulin* deficiency inhibits cellular buffering, whereas excretion requires functioning kidneys. Therefore, K^+ handling is greatly impaired in patients with *diabetes and renal insufficiency.*

Diagnosis

Pseudohyperkalemia may occur if venous blood is analyzed following exercise or prolonged tourniquet application. Hemolysis may also cause artifactual elevation of K^+, especially when blood is rapidly withdrawn through a small needle ($<$ 22 gauge). Serum $[K^+]$ is normally 0.5 mEq/l higher than plasma $[K^+]$, because K^+ is released from platelets during clotting. However, severe leukocytosis ($> 100,000/mm^3$) or thrombocytosis ($> 10^6/mm^3$) may also raise the K^+ of the clotted specimen to extraordinary levels. The diagnosis of clot-related "pseudohyperkalemia" is confirmed by a disparity between simultenous determinations of plasma and serum $[K^+]$.

Mechanisms

Three basic mechanisms contribute to hyperkalemia: (1) *increased K^+ intake*; (2) *translocation of K^+* from the intracellular to the extracellular compartment; and (3) *decreased K^+ excretion.*

Increased Potassium Intake

Potassium overloading is often iatrogenic in patients with limited excretory power. The K^+ source may be an unmodified *standing order for K^+ replacement* or other unsuspected therapy (e.g., K^+ containing intravenous fluids, potassium penicillin G, blood products, or salt substitutes). *Ringer's lactate* contains 4 mEq/l of K^+ per liter and should

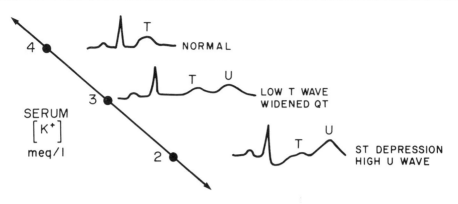

Figure 12.1   ECG manifestations of hypokalemia.

not be administered to patients with renal insufficiency. *Potassium penicillin G* contains 1.6 mEq/10^6 units and may constitute a significant $[K^+]$ load in patients receiving high doses. *Packed red cells*, stored for long periods, may deliver as much as 7 mEq/unit. *Renal transplant* recipients receive significant intraoperative K^+ loads when donor kidneys are perfused with Collins' solution (140 mEq of K^+ per liter) are implanted.

Potassium Shifts

Catacholamines and beta-adrenergic agonists increase the serum K^+—an effect preventable by beta blocking drugs. *Acidosis* is the most common cause of shift-related hyperkalemia. Changes in serum $[K^+]$ are more sensitive to changes in $[HCO_3^-]$ than to pH itself. Therefore, respiratory acidosis has relatively little effect on K^+ distribution, whereas *acute metabolic acidosis exerts a potent effect*. A 0.1-unit decrease in pH produces an average 0.6-mEq/l increase in K^+ (range: 0.4–1.3 mEq/l). K^+ shifts are more marked when mineral acids (e.g., HCl) rather than organic acids (e.g., lactate) are the etiology of acidosis.

Hypertonic solutions (mannitol or hypertonic saline) may also increase the serum K^+, by uncertain mechanisms. Hyperkalemia may follow the *breakdown of red blood cells* in large hematomas or injury that produces extensive *tissue necrosis* with subsequent K^+ release (particularly crush injuries, burns, and tumor lysis). *Digitalis toxicity* poisons the cellular Na^+/K^+ pump and may produce severe refractory hyperkalemia. (K^+ levels exceeding 5.5 mEq/l are associated with poor survival in digitalis toxicity.) Hemolytic *transfusion reactions* and other forms of acute *hemolysis* also cause life-threatening hyperkalemia. *Succinylcholine* (a depolarizing neuromuscular blocker) frequently produces a small, predictable rise in $[K^+]$ (≈ 0.5 mEq/l), but may precipitate a striking rise in patients with burns, tetanus, or other neuromuscular diseases. These effects are minimized by pretreatment with curare.

Decreased Potassium Excretion

Even though 80–90% of renal function must be lost before the kidney fails noticeably to excrete K^+, severe renal insufficiency remains the most common cause of hyperkalemia. Renal failure-induced acidosis further impairs the ability of the kidney to excrete K^+ and promotes the shift of K^+ from cellular stores into the circulation. In renal failure of abrupt onset, serum $[K^+]$ tends to rise before the BUN or Cr, especially when exogenous K^+ is given; low tubular flow rates immediately prevent exchange of Na^+ for K^+, whereas Cr and BUN require time to build to noteworthy concentrations. (However, even when complete renal shutdown occurs, the serum $[K^+]$ seldom rises by more than 0.5 mEq/l/day in response to natural loads.)

Aldosterone is required to maintain circulating volume and to enable tubular Na^+/K^+ exchange. Therefore, serum $[K^+]$ may rise in primary adrenal failure. Adrenal insufficiency should be considered strongly in cases of hyperkalemia in which fluid deficits are prominent. Elevations in K^+ are usually not significant in the absence of another confounding factor (e.g., increased K^+ intake or renal failure). For similar reasons, drugs that interfere with the formation or action of aldosterone (e.g., K^+-sparing diuretics and heparin) may produce overt hyperkalemia.

Signs and Symptoms

Hyponatremia, hypocalcemia, hypermagnesemia, and acidosis potentiate the neuromuscular effects of hyperkalemia. Hence their levels should be evaluated and corrected concurrently. Obvious functional impairment of skeletal muscle rarely occurs at $[K^+] < 7.0$ mEq/l. Proximal lower extremity weakness is the most common symptom. Hyperkalemia usually spares the respiratory muscles, cranial nerves, and deep tendon reflexes. The most devastating effects of hyperkalemia are *cardiac arrhythmias*. The pump-impairing and vasodilatory effects of severe hyperkalemia may cause *refractory hypotension*.

Electrocardiogram

An electrocardiogram (ECG) should be obtained for every patient with a $[K^+] > 5.5$ mEq/l (Fig. 12.2). Widening of the QRS complex (due to delayed depolarization) follows early narrowing and peaking of T waves and QT interval shortening. Atrial activity is usually lost shortly before the characteristic sine wave hybrid of ventricular tachycardia/fibrillation appears.

Treatment

When an elevated $[K^+]$ is discovered, a repeat *serum* sample and a separate *plasma* specimen should both be drawn slowly through a large needle. Leukocyte and platelet counts should also be obtained, and an ECG should be recorded. If the

ECG is normal, elective treatment may await repeat confirmatory $[K^+]$ determinations. If the ECG is abnormal, muscle weakness is present, or the reported $[K^+]$ exceeds 7 mEq/l, immediate action is likely indicated. Continuous ECG monitoring should be initiated, followed by specific treatment on five fronts: (1) *stop all K^+*; (2) administer drugs to *shift K^+ into the cellular compartment*; (3) stabilize neuromuscular and cardiac function with *calcium*, if indicated; (4) *remove K^+ from the body*; and (5) *replenish circulating volume* in dehydrated patients.

Shifting K^+ from serum into muscle rapidly lowers the serum concentration, but this maneuver only temporizes. Sodium bicarbonate (HCO_3^-) causes an exchange of H^+ for K^+ across all membranes, lowering the serum $[K^+]$ within 1 hour. (This effect may last for 12 hours.) Two ampules of HCO_3^- (88 mEq) are usually sufficient. However, in the face of ongoing acidosis, sufficient HCO_3^- should be given to correct the pH. The hypertonicity of bicarbonate solution may lower $[K^+]$ independently of its pH effect. *Insulin* also enhances cellular uptake. Hyperglycemic patients require only insulin; patients with normal blood sugar levels should receive *glucose* concurrently to prevent hypoglycemia (2–3 gm of glucose are required for each unit of regular insulin). Insulin produces a reduction in serum $[K^+]$

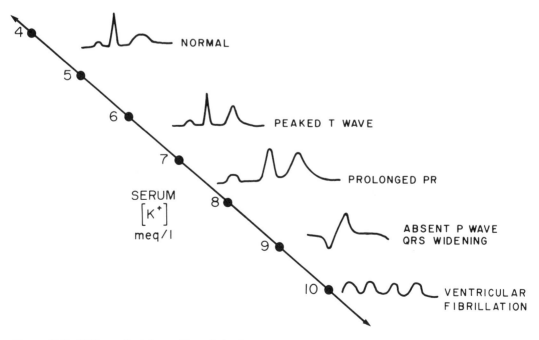

Figure 12.2   ECG manifestations of hyperkalemia.

of 1–3 mEq/l within 1 hour, an effect that may last up to 12 hours.

Calcium stabilizes cardiac conduction by lowering the depolarization threshold. Although Ca^{2+} acts within minutes, its effect usually persists < 2 hours. Precipitates form when HCO_3^- and Ca^{2+} are admixed. Ca^{2+} should be administered with extreme caution in patients receiving digitalis preparations.

Dialysis is most often required in patients with *renal insufficiency*, *severe hyperkalemia*, or *high K^+ loads* that result from multiple trauma or tumor lysis. Hemodialysis may remove up to 40 mEq/hr of K^+, whereas peritoneal dialysis removes only 5–10 mEq/hr. *Loop diuretics* promote K^+ excretion but are only useful in patients with *good urine output and modest hyperkalemia*.

Ion exchange resins lower [K^+] by exchanging Na^+ for K^+ across the bowel wall. More Na^+ is gained than K^+ is lost. Electroneutrality is maintained by loss of Mg^{2+} and Ca^{2+}. Resultant Na^+ retention may produce volume overload in oliguric or anuric patients. Each gram of oral resin binds $\simeq$ 1 mEq of K^+. A typical 50-mg dose of resin decreases serum [K^+] by 0.5–1 mEq/l. When given orally, ion exchange resins require a vehicle to prevent constipation (usually 20% sorbitol solution). Such resins may also be given rectally if oral dosing is not tolerated or advisable. Rectal dosing may prove more efficient than oral dosing at K^+ removal.

Volume expansion with normal saline will rapidly lower [K^+] in dehydrated patients.

CALCIUM DISORDERS

Hypercalcemia

Etiology

The long list of possible causes of hypercalcemia (HC) may be significantly narrowed with a careful *history*, *review of medications*, and a few basic *laboratory tests*. The more common causes of HC are noted below.

Causes of Hypercalcemia

Paget's disease	Hyperparathyroidism
Adrenal insufficiency	Milk-alkali syndrome
Malignancy	Immobilization
Thiazide diuretics	Vitamin D or A
Sarcoidosis	intoxication
	Hyperthyroidism

Signs and Symptoms

The signs and symptoms of HC are *non-specific* but most commonly result from the two major pathophysiologic derangements—*dehydration* and *depressed neuromuscular function*. HC induces an osmotic diuresis resulting in complaints of *polyuria* and *polydypsia*, but if fluid intake is unrestricted, severe Ca^{2+} elevations are unlikely. Unfortunately, the decreased gut motility of HC often produces *nausea, vomiting, abdominal pain*, and *constipation*, negating this potential mode of compensation. The most common manifestations of HC are *neuromuscular disturbances* (lethargy, fatigue, and weakness).

Calcium salts, especially $CaHPO_4$, form when a critical calcium-phosphate product (usually > 60) is reached. These complexes may be deposited in almost any tissue. In the kidney, renal stones and renal insufficiency may result; skin deposits may induce pruritis. Muscle and other soft tissue may also be affected. Pancreatitis or peptic ulcer disease are rare GI presentations. HC may produce hypertension by increasing the peripheral vascular resistance, an effect usually offset by significant volume depletion.

Laboratory Evaluation

Total calcium Ca^{2+} levels must always be evaluated in light of the serum protein concentration because Ca^{2+} is highly protein bound (primarily to albumin). Even ''normal'' levels of total Ca^{2+} may represent *relative HC* in patients with severe hypoproteinemia. Normally, an inverse relationship exists between the PO_4^{3-} and Ca^{2+} in the serum. Vulnerable to changes induced by food intake, the PO_4^{3-} is a highly labile measurement, making it less useful diagnostically.

Alkaline phosphatase may be elevated by any cause of HC. *Urinary Ca^{2+}* is usually very high in hypercalcemic disorders that are not dependent on parathyroid hormone (PTH) activity (sarcoid or vitamin D intoxication). Vitamin D levels are useful in confirming suspected toxicity but are not diagnostic in any other form of HC.

Although frequently assayed, PTH levels are not helpful diagnostically unless markedly elevated in a patient with severe HC and normal renal function. Even mild renal insufficiency severely limits the use of PTH assays, because it decreases the clearance of the commonly assayed carboxy-PTH fragment. For this reason, *mid-molecule* or *amino-terminal* assays are superior. The most common ECG effect of HC is shortening of the QT interval.

Treatment

As with hyperkalemia, the simplest and most rapid method to reduce [Ca^{2+}] in the dehydrated patient is to expand the circulating volume with *isotonic saline*. Following volume expansion, *loop diuretics* are rapidly effective at lowering [Ca^{2+}] if good urine flow is established. Since immobilization worsens HC, *ambulation* is helpful when feasible.

Phosphate therapy is immediately effective but is not generally recommended because of its many side effects, which include soft tissue calcification, "overshoot" hypocalcemia, and acute renal failure. Oral phosphates are safer than intravenous preparations, but GI intolerance (diarrhea) limits their use.

The antimetabolite *mithramycin* inhibits osteoclast function to prevent reabsorption of bone Ca^{2+}. Mithramycin may be helpful in acute severe cases of HC associated with malignancy, but side effects (hepatic, renal, and marrow toxicity) usually prohibit chronic use.

Glucocorticoids are most useful in the HC of malignancy (especially breast carcinoma and lymphoma). By inhibiting gut absorption of Ca^{2+}, steroids are also effective in sarcoidosis and vitamin D intoxication.

Calcitonin inhibits osteoclast function and promotes incorporation of Ca^{2+} into bone but is expensive, unpredictable, and prone to tachyphylaxis. When used, calcitonin is more effective when administered in combination with glucocorticoids.

Diphosphonates prevent osteoclast-mediated bone resorption. They are currently used for the treatment of Paget's disease and have shown promise for use in malignancy-related HC.

Hypocalcemia

Symptomatic hypocalcemia is less common than symptomatic hypercalcemia but is just as life threatening. The urgency of evaluation and treatment depend upon the severity of symptoms.

Clinical Manifestations

Hypocalcemia may be asymptomatic if *ionized* Ca^{2+} remains stable despite low total [Ca^{2+}] or if hypocalcemia develops slowly. Alkalosis lowers *the fraction of ionized Ca^{2+} at any given total Ca^{2+}, aggrevating symptoms.* The threshold at which symptoms develop in hypocalcemia is also highly variable. The majority of symptoms are due to *neuromuscular irritability*. The most common complaints are of paresthesias, cramps, or tetany. Dyspnea or stridor may occur if ventilatory or upper airway muscles are affected. Although usually a consequence of hypocalcemia, tetany may also develop in acute respiratory alkalosis and acute hyperkalemia. More specific signs of neuromus-

cular irritability, including carpopedal spasm (Trousseau's sign) or facial muscle hyperreflexia (Chvostek's sign), may often be elicited in patients with hypocalcemia but are not diagnostic. Other potential CNS effects include seizures, papilledema, hallucinations, confusion, and depression. Hypocalcemia may compromise perfusion by lowering the systemic vascular resistance and decreasing cardiac contractility. The QT prolongation seen with hypocalcemia may result in a variety of arrhythmias (most significantly, torsades de pointes).

Causes

There are four recognized mechanisms of hypocalcemia: (1) *decreased Ca^{2+} intake or absorption*; (2) *binding and sequestration of Ca^{2+}*; (3) *inability to mobilize bone Ca^{2+}*; and (4) *decreases in serum protein concentration*. Because the majority of Ca^{2+} is bound to serum protein, reductions in protein concentration result in hypocalcemia. A reduction in albumin of 1 gm/dl reduces the serum [Ca^{2+}] by $\simeq 0.8$ mg/dl. The globulin fraction of serum protein has less influence.

Ca^{2+} may be removed from the circulation by *binding to other drugs or chemicals* (such as phosphate, chelating agents (ethylenediaminetetraacetic acid (EDTA)), or the citrate of transfused blood). Ca^{2+} may also bind inflamed intra-abdominal fat (in pancreatitis). Hyperphosphatemia may induce hypocalcemia in patients with renal failure or in those who are otherwise unable to excrete PO_4^{3-} normally. Alkalemia (from HCO_3^- administration or massive transfusion) may also induce symptomatic hypocalcemia.

Reductions in Ca^{2+} intake, or impaired absorption resulting from reduced activity of vitamin D may also induce hypocalcemia. Anticonvulsants and glucocorticoids impair Ca^{2+} absorption (probably by inhibiting vitamin D action). Prolonged hospitalization (particularly among patients receiving TPN) may also cause vitamin D deficiency. Renal failure decreases vitamin D production, but hypocalcemia is usually blunted by the development of secondary hyperparathyroidism.

PTH deficiency and resistance to PTH are rare causes of hypocalcemia except in patients undergoing thyroid or parathyroid surgery. In such patients, life-threatening hypocalcemia may develop within hours of operation. Therefore, monitoring postoperative Ca^{2+} assumes added importance following neck surgery. Very rarely, protracted, severe hypotension may result in parathyroid infarction and subsequent hypocalcemia.

Magnesium (Mg^{2+}) levels should be obtained in hypocalcemic patients because Mg^{2+} is necessary, for both PTH secretion and action. Hypocalcemia due to *hypomagnesemia* is particularly common in alcoholics and in patients receiving chronic TPN or diuretics.

Treatment

The first step in the treatment of hypocalcemia is to assure airway patency and adequate ventilation and perfusion. Serum levels of K^+, Mg^{2+}, vitamin D, and PTH should be obtained. *Alkalosis* should be corrected to raise the ionized Ca^{2+} fraction. *Hyperphosphatemia* should be corrected with phosphate buffers (aluminum-containing antacids) and a low phosphate diet.

Ca^{2+} replacement is always empiric because deficits are impossible to calculate accurately. Symptomatic patients should be given intravenous calcium. Slow infusions of 10–20 ml of 10% *calcium gluconate* is the preferred method of supplementation. Such dosing provides 10 mg of elemental Ca^{2+} per milliliter. Maintenance Ca^{2+} administration must be guided by serial determinations of serum $[Ca^{2+}]$. Concomitant *vitamin D* deficiency should be treated. 1,25-OH vitamin D may be required if renal and liver function are compromised, but this drug is very expensive. In patients with preserved hepatic and renal function, nonhydroxylated vitamin D preparations will suffice. *Thiazides* increase renal tubular Ca^{2+} reabsorption, making them potentially useful to increase serum $[Ca^{2+}]$.

MAGNESIUM DISORDERS

Hypermagnesemia

Hypermagnesemia (HM) is uncommon unless magnesium sulfate is infused to control neuromuscular irritability (e.g., during eclampsia) or unless patients with renal insufficiency are given magnesium supplements to dietary intake. However, in patients with severe renal insufficiency or ileus, unintentional gut absorption of Mg^{2+}-containing cathartics may also overload the excretory capacity. Recently, HM has also been described following extravasation of renal "stone dissolving" drugs that contain high concentrations of Mg^{2+} (Ref. 2).

Clinically, HM presents as hyporeflexia when levels exceed 4 mg/dl, somnolence at levels > 7 mg/dl, and paralysis at levels > 10 mg/dl. HM prolongs the PR interval on ECG, impairs conduction, and may produce heart block. Initially,

Ca^{2+} should be administered to reverse the effects of HM. Emergent dialysis should follow.

Hypomagnesemia

Hypomagnesemia almost always results from excessive *renal or GI Mg^{2+} losses*. Because Mg^{2+} is predominately absorbed in the small bowel, inflammatory bowel disease, chronic diarrhea, and malabsorption are common precipitants. Malnutrition (particularly in alcoholics) decreases $[Mg^{2+}]$ by limiting intake. Pancreatitis also causes hypomagnesemia through uncertain mechanisms.

Although any form of renal disease may produce Mg^{2+} wasting, it most commonly results from the use of diuretics (thiazides, loop, and osmotic). "Forced saline diuresis" may also waste Mg^{2+} during chemotherapy or treatment of hypercalcemia. *Aminoglycosides and platinum compounds* aggrevate renal Mg^{2+} losses. Hypomagnesemia itself causes neuromuscular irritability. Perhaps more importantly, it may also induce hypokalemia and hypocalcemia. Hypomagnesemia predisposes patients to almost all types of arrhythmias (particularly those of digitalis toxicity). Hypomagnesemia prolongs the QT and PR intervals and lengthens and flattens the T wave.

Treatment

Magnesium deficits, like Ca^{2+} deficits, are hard to estimate, making the treatment of hypomagnesemia largely empiric. In patients with normal renal function, Mg^{2+} is safe, even in large doses. Oral Mg^{2+} compounds are usually effective at raising the Mg^{2+} but sometimes produce such severe diarrhea that hypomagnesemia actually worsens. Mg^{2+} is usually administered as $MgSO_4$, either intramuscularly or by slow intravenous infusion. Rapid Mg^{2+} infusions produce hypotension and should be avoided.

PHOSPHATE DISORDERS

Hyperphosphatemia

In an intensive care unit setting, high levels of PO_4^{3-} (> 5 mg/dl) usually reflect impaired PO_4 excretion (renal insufficiency with GFR < 20 ml/min) or increased cellular release of PO_4^{3-} (chemotherapy, rhabdomyolysis, sepsis). Symptoms, however, are few, apart from those caused by concurrent hypocalcemia. Attention should first be directed to the primary cause of PO_4^{3-} elevation. When symptomatic hypocalcemia urges treatment, PO_4^{3-} binders (30–45 ml of aluminum hydroxide every 6 hours), saline, acetazolamide, and restricting intake are usually effective. Dialysis may be required in severe or refractory cases.

Hypophosphatemia

As the major intracellular anion, PO_4^{3-} plays a crucial role in phospholipid, phosphoprotein, and phosphosugar metabolism. It is the depletion of the intracellular PO_4^{3-} store that produces clinical symptomatology, imperfectly reflected by depressed serum values. Whereas PO_4^{3-} is easily depleted from skeletal muscle and erythrocytes, levels tend to be well preserved in most other tissues, such as cardiac muscle. Factors predisposing to total body phosphate depletion include: malnutrition, alcoholism, hypomagnesemia, renal tubular dysfunction (diuresis, nonoliguric acute tubular necrosis), and gastrointestinal losses (antacid binding, malabsorption, nasogastric suctioning, emesis, diarrhea).

It is important not to equate hypophosphatemia with intracellular PO_4^{3-} depletion. Extracellular to intracellular transfer of PO_4^{3-} occurs during anabolism, insulin administration, correction of metabolic acidosis, and the acute phase of respiratory alkalosis. Hypophosphatemia is therefore commonly observed in alcohol-dependent patients, during refeeding or caloric loading, during recovery from diabetic ketoacidosis, and during hyperventilation. In many such patients, hypophosphatemia does not reflect pathologic PO_4^{3-} depletion.

Consequences

As a general rule, serum $[PO_4^{3-}]$ must fall below 1.0 mg/dl before symptoms become overt. Dysfunction of the cellular elements of the blood, muscle weakness, GI upset, neural dysfunction, and (rarely) tissue breakdown are the major clinical consequences. Depletion of 2,3-diphosphoglyceric acid (2,3-DPG) diminishes the ability of erythrocytes to unload oxygen to the tissues. Thrombocytopenia, platelet dysfunction, and impaired leukocyte killing have been shown experimentally. Skeletal muscle dysfunction is of major clinical interest in the setting of ventilatory failure, in which PO_4^{3-} depletion contributes to weakness and ventilator dependence. A PO_4^{3-}-related sensorimotor neuropathy is occasionally observed 4–7 days after PO_4^{3-}-poor hyperalimentation is started. Very rarely, severe PO_4^{3-} depletion can produce hemolysis, rhabdomyolysis, or congestive cardiomyopathy.

Treatment

Although PO_4^{3-} should be a component of all nutritional regimens, *urgent* correction should be reserved for situations in which clinical symptoms accompany a serum $PO_4^{3-} < 1.0$ mg/dl. As with K^+ repletion, PO_4^{3-} must traverse the small extracellular compartment to reach its intracellular target, so that *repletion must be cautious.* An intravenous infusion of 2.5–5.0 mg/kg as potassium or sodium phosphate over 6 hours should not cause the calcium-phosphate product to climb to dangerous levels (> 60 mg/dl). Oral PO_4^{3-} supplementation (125 mg twice a day, as potassium phosphate or equivalent) will usually suffice when the serum PO_4^{3-} is only modestly reduced (> 1.0 mg/dl). Concurrent hypomagnesemia must be corrected. Oral PO_4^{3-} supplementation should continue for 5–10 days after re-establishing a normal serum level.

SUGGESTED READINGS

1. Cooke CR, Turin MD, Walker WG: The syndrome of inappropriate antidiuretic hormone secretion (SIADH): pathophysiologic mechanisms in solute and volume regulation. *Medicine* 58:240–251, 1979.
2. Fassler CA, Rodriguez RM, Badesch DB, Stone WJ, Marini JJ: Magnesium toxicity as a cause of hypoventilation in patients with normal renal function. *Arch Intern Med* 145:1604–1606, 1985.
3. Felig P, McCurdy DV: The hypertonic state. *N Engl J Med* 297:1444–1454, 1977.
4. Geheb M, Carlson R (eds): Renal failure and associated disturbances (symposium). *Crit Care Clin* 3(4):699–955, 1987.
5. Knocher JP: The pathophysiology and clinical characteristics of severe hypophosphatemia. *Arch Intern Med* 137:203–220, 1977.
6. Kunau RT, Stein JH: Disorders of hypo and hyperkalemia. *Clin Nephrol* 7:173–190, 1977.
7. Laureno R, Arieff AI: Rapid correction of hyponatremia: cause of pontine myelinolysis? *Am J Med* 71:846–847, 1981.
8. Newman JH, Neff TA, Ziponin P: Acute respiratory failure associated with hypophosphatemia. *N Engl J Med* 296:1101–1102, 1977.
9. Smithline N, Gardner KD: Gaps-anionic and osmolal. *JAMA* 236:1594–1597, 1976.

13 Transfusion and Blood Component Therapy

INDICATIONS FOR BLOOD TRANSFUSION

There are three major reasons for administration of blood products: (1) to increase oxygen carrying capacity; (2) to restore circulating volume; and (3) to reverse deficiencies of clotting proteins or platelets.

Tissue oxygen delivery can remain adequate in the face of anemia if reductions in hemoglobin are offset by proportional increases in tissue perfusion or oxygen extraction. Unfortunately, these compensatory mechanisms are often impaired in critically ill patients. For this reason, hemoglobin (Hgb) concentration is generally maintained above 10 gm/dl (packed cell volume, PCV, > 30%). This is especially important in patients with coronary disease, refractory hypoxemia, or limited cardiac reserve. Conversely, the lower acceptable limit for Hgb can be relaxed somewhat in patients with long-standing anemia, whose tissues and cardiac performance accommodate to chronically reduced O_2 delivery (e.g., chronic renal failure).

THE COMPONENT SYSTEM

Most patients needing transfusion do not require all ten components available in fresh whole blood (Table 13.1). Component therapy "stretches" the blood supply by allowing prolonged storage of non-labile factors and by permitting several patients to receive the specific components they need from a single blood donation. By limiting administered

Table 13.1
Whole Blood Components

Erythrocytes	Factor VIII concentrate
Platelets	Factor IX concentrate
Fresh frozen plasma	Cryoprecipitate
Plasma protein fraction	Globulins
Albumin	Leukocytes

volume, component therapy reduces the risk of fluid overload, the amount of transfused anticoagulant, and the incidence of infection.

Red Blood Cell Components

Whole Blood

Whole blood is used in the emergent restoration of circulating volume and oxygen-carrying capacity, but it is a poor source of clotting factors and platelets if more than 24 hours old. Furthermore, transfusion of whole blood may produce circulatory overload in the euvolemic patient who requires only red blood cells (RBCs). (Whole blood is particularly risky in patients with renal failure or congestive heart failure, CHF.) A 500-ml "unit" of whole blood contains $\simeq$ 60 mEq of sodium and has a PCV averaging 35–40%. The only major indication for whole blood is in support of massively bleeding patients in whom *fresh* whole blood is preferred. Even then, whole blood must usually be supplemented by transfusions of platelets and/or plasma.

"Fresh" Whole Blood

Fresh whole blood is less than 6–8 hours old and is useful in patients needing simultaneous replacement of circulating volume, red cells, platelets, and clotting factors. Platelets become nonfunctional within 24 hours of collection. After 48 hours, essentially all factor VIII is depleted. Within 1 week, even the longer lived factor V is depleted. Furthermore, RBCs lyse as blood ages, reducing the PCV and increasing the plasma potassium concentration. (Thirty percent of RBCs may be lost after 3 weeks of storage.) Reductions in adenosine triphosphate (ATP) and diphosphoglyceric acid (2,3-DPG) produce a leftward shift of the oxyhemoglobin dissociation curve, inhibiting oxygen release to the tissues.

Fresh blood is used to prevent dilutional coagulopathy in massively transfused patients who require 10 or more units of whole blood within a 24-hour period. In actively hemorrhaging patients, repletion of clotting proteins and platelets with fresh whole blood or component therapy should begin after approximately 6–10 units of packed RBCs have been given.

Packed Red Blood Cells

Removing plasma from whole blood leaves a 200–300 ml unit of packed red blood cells (PRBCs) having a PCV of 65–75%. PRBCs are used to restore oxygen-carrying capacity. A unit of transfused PRBCs should raise the PCV of an adult patient by approximately 3%. (Continued bleeding or excessive volume expansion blunts the expected increase.) PRBCs contain few platelets, clotting factors, or leukocytes and are not effective as volume expanders when used alone. PRBCs can be infused as rapidly as whole blood when viscosity is reduced by adding $\simeq$ 75 ml of normal saline per unit.

PRBCs offer several *advantages*: (1) *less volume expansion* than whole blood for a given increase in oxygen-carrying capacity (each unit of PRBCs contains only 8–20 mEq of sodium, a particularly helpful feature in patients with heart or kidney failure; (2) *less anticoagulant* than whole blood, reducing the potential risk of anticoagulant/preservative (citrate) toxicity; and (3) *lower plasma volume*, reducing the risk of viral hepatitis, immunologic reactions from transfused antibodies, and anaphylaxis.

Leukocyte-Poor Components

Leukocyte poor components (LPCs) are indicated for patients who have experienced white cell or leukoagglutinin reactions and are particularly useful in patients with anti-IgA or IgE antibodies. LPCs are produced by removing the leukocyte-rich buffy coat by repeated washing, spin filtering, or freezing. Each method destroys platelets while reducing the white blood cells (WBCs) and plasma by approximately 75–90%. Because of the loss of RBCs in processing, a unit of leukocyte-poor RBCs contains less hemoglobin than a unit of PRBCs. Even LPCs contain limited numbers of viable WBCs; therefore, *all* blood products transfused into immunosuppressed patients must be irradiated to prevent graft-versus-host disease (GVHD).

White Blood Cell Components

Granulocyte Transfusions

Granulocyte transfusions are indicated only in neutropenic patients with overwhelming infections who fail conventional antimicrobial therapy. Because of the risk, expense, and limited benefit of granulocyte transfusions, they are rarely used.

Many problems exist in the transfusion of WBCs. Allergic reactions are nearly universal, and because WBCs have a circulating half-life of only 6 hours, frequent transfusion is required. WBCs must also be ABO compatible. Several types of viral hepatitis are commonly transmitted in WBC components. In patients with severe bone marrow depression, WBC transfusion also carries a nearly certain risk of GVHD. WBCs often aggregate, a tendency that precludes the use of transfusion filters and frequently leads to pulmonary dysfunction. No laboratory measure of effectiveness exists because peripheral WBC counts usually do not rise in most patients receiving WBCs (presumably secondary to sequestration). Concurrent administration of WBCs and amphotericin B may cause acute respiratory failure (ARDS).

Platelet Components

Random Donor Platelets

A unit of pooled random donor platelets (RDPs) contains 40–70 ml of platelet concentrate and large numbers of WBCs that may be removed by spin filtration. Platelet transfusions are indicated for (1) severe thrombocytopenia (platelet counts < 20,000/ mm^3) or (2) active bleeding due to inadequate numbers of circulating platelets (< 100,000/mm^3) or (3) platelet dysfunction. Uremia, liver disease, and aspirin or non-steroidal anti-inflammatory drugs are the most common reasons for platelet dysfunction.

The usefulness of RDPs is limited, however: (1) Repeatedly transfused patients develop antibodies to common platelet surface antigens and eventually require HLA-matched platelets to prevent rapid immune destruction of the transfused platelets. (2) Platelets often produce minor allergic reactions including chills, fever, and rash. (3) WBCs contained in platelet transfusions may produce GVHD in the pancytopenic patient. (4) Platelet transfusions are unlikely to be helpful in the "immune thrombocytopenias" (idiopathic thrombocytopenic purpura, ITP, or thrombotic thrombocytopenic purpura, TTP) because of rapid platelet destruction.

Platelets may be administered as rapidly as they will infuse (5–10 min/unit). The normal life span of circulating platelets is 3–4 days; therefore, platelet transfusions are usually needed every 2–3 days if production is reduced without accelerated destruction. Each unit increases the count by 5–10,000 platelets/mm^3, unless destruction is ongoing. When assessed 1 hour after transfusion, an increment of < 2,000/mm^3 per unit confirms platelet destruction. Platelets are usually administered as "six packs", that raise the platelet count by ≈ 25–50,000 platelets/mm^3. A blunted increment is common in patients with burns, splenic sequestration, fever, infection, and/or platelet antibodies. Because young (large) platelets have enhanced hemostatic function, the presence of many large platelets may indicate a lower risk of bleeding at any given count.

ABO-compatible platelets minimize formation of anti-platelet antibodies and survive longer in the circulation. Because of the very small volume of plasma present in transfused platelets, incompatibility between donor plasma and recipient RBCs is usually insignificant. However, if multiple units of platelets and incompatible plasma are transfused, a positive Coombs' test or overt hemolysis may occur. The small number of RBCs transfused in platelet concentrates makes RBC crossmatching unnecessary. (However, 10% of massively transfused patients will develop ABO sensitization.) Platelets do not contain Rh antigens and therefore Rh sensitization is not a problem. Although platelets should be administered through a filter to prevent aggregation, filtration lengthens infusion time and decreases the number of viable platelets transfused.

HLA-Matched Platelets

In patients refractory to RDPs, HLA-matched donors may undergo pheresis 2 or 3 times weekly to provide large numbers of platelets for transfusion. These pheresed concentrates commonly produce a rise of 30–60,000 platelets/mm^3. Furthermore, HLA-matched platelets from a single donor reduce infection risk.

Clotting Factor Concentrates

Fresh Frozen Plasma

Fresh frozen plasma (FFP) preserves the activity of many clotting proteins (especially factors V and VIII and fibrinogen). A unit of FFP contains 180–300 ml of plasma. Appropriate *indications* for transfusing FFP include: (1) dilutional coagulopathy in the massively transfused patient; (2) excessive anti-coagulation in patients treated with warfarin; (3) congenital or acquired coagulation factor deficiencies; and (4) Von Willebrand's disease.

FFP has several *disadvantages*: (1) Each milli-

liter of transfused plasma contains only 1 unit of each clotting factor; therefore, relatively large volumes of FFP are needed to correct deficiencies compared to factor concentrates. (2) The risk of allergic reactions is high due to residual platelets and leukocytes. (3) Although FFP need not be ABO compatible with recipient plasma, it should be compatible with the recipient's RBCs.

Cryoprecipitate

Cryoprecipitate (CPT) forms when plasma separated from fresh whole blood is rapidly frozen and then allowed to rewarm. The precipitate contains most of the factor VIII (about 80–100 units) and fibrinogen (250 mg) of the original unit of plasma. CPT is indicated for the treatment of: (1) hemophilia A (factor VIII deficiency); (2) Von Willebrand's disease; and (3) hypofibrinogenemic states (e.g., thrombolytic therapy, congenital deficiency, and consumptive coagulopathy).

Factor VIII Concentrate

Factor VIII concentrate, a component used in the treatment of hemophilia A, is prepared from the plasma of many donors (frequently hundreds). In the bleeding hemophiliac, factor VIII activity is negligible and should be increased to > 50% of normal levels to arrest hemorrhage. The dose of factor VIII may be calculated by replacing 1 unit of factor VIII per milliliter of calculated plasma volume per percent of desired factor VIII activity (Table 13.2). Alternatively, the factor VIII requirement may be roughly approximated:

$$\text{dose (units)} = 40 \times (\text{wt in kg})$$
$$\times (\% \text{ factor VIII activity desired})$$

Factor VIII concentrates carry a much higher risk of hepatitis than CPT and have a half-life of only 8–12 hours, necessitating frequent transfusion. (Heat treatment and serologic testing have reduced the risk of acquired immune deficiency syndrome, AIDS.)

Factor VIII doses can be calculated using the equations in Table 13.2.

Table 13.2
Calculation of Factor VIII Doses

Blood volume (ml)	= wt in kg × 70
Plasma volume (ml)	= blood volume × (1 − PCV)
Units of factor VIII	= Plasma volume
	× (desired factor VIII % − current factor VIII %)

PROBLEMS ASSOCIATED WITH MASSIVE TRANSFUSION

Exsanguination

A formal crossmatch procedure requires 45–60 minutes. Therefore, when the patient's condition does not allow completion of a formal crossmatch, O-negative (*universal donor*) or *type specific* (ABO- and Rh-compatible) blood may be given. The ABO determination itself usually takes less than 10 minutes. Therefore, type-specific blood is preferred except in cases in which transfusion must occur even more urgently.

Massive Transfusion

Massive transfusion is usually defined as the administration of > 10 units of blood per 24 hours. Problems resulting from massive transfusion include: (1) dilutional thrombocytopenia and coagulopathy; (2) adult respiratory distress syndrome; (3) hypokalemic alkalosis; (4) hypocalcemia; (5) hypothermia; and (6) transfusion-related infection. The risk of viral hepatitis approximates 1% per unit of transfused blood product.

Dilutional clotting disorders begin to emerge when one blood volume equivalent (5 units of blood) have been replaced. Clotting factor levels then commonly drop below 30% of normal activity and platelet counts fall below 100,000/mm^3. After 5–10 units of blood have been transfused, platelet counts, prothrombin time, and partial thromboplastin time should be monitored. To maintain a normal clotting profile, 2 units of FFP and 6 units of platelets should be transfused per 6–10 units of PRBCs.

ARDS may result from hemorrhage-related hypotension in conjunction with the transfusion of component microaggregates. Although it is not certain that blood filters reduce this risk, they should probably be used during massive transfusion.

COMPLICATIONS OF TRANSFUSION

Immediate Hemolytic Reactions

Hemolytic reactions can be immediate or delayed. If immediate, they are usually due to major ABO incompatibility. The most common cause of major transfusion reaction is misidentification of the patient sample or transfusion of blood into the wrong patient. *These mistakes are essentially always due to clerical errors and usually occur at the bedside.* As a result, stringent rules have been instituted in most hospitals to prevent these occurrences. When notified by the blood bank that an improperly labeled tube has been received, repeat sample collection is indicated.

Most severe reactions occur as the first 50–100 ml of blood product are infused. For this reason, frequent vital signs should be taken in the initial period of transfusion. Major reactions are potentially fatal because they produce intravascular hemolysis, coagulopathy, shock, renal failure, and pulmonary dysfunction. Transfusion reactions may be difficult to recognize in the critically ill patient, particularly if unconscious. New-onset dyspnea, fever, bone pain, or diffuse bleeding are all clues to transfusion reaction. Primary treatment of a major reaction is to stop the transfusion. Using sterile technique, donor blood and blood tubing should be returned to the blood bank. Clotted and anticoagulated samples of the recipient's blood and a urine sample should also be sent to the blood bank with notification of a suspected transfusion reaction. Fluids and vasopressors should be administered as required to maintain perfusion of vital organs. Intravenous sodium bicarbonate may be given to alkalinize the urine, in an effort to prevent precipitation of hemoglobin in the renal tubules and subsequent acute renal failure. Loop and osmotic diuretics may also be useful to preserve urine flow and avert renal failure.

Delayed Hemolytic Reactions

Low titer antibodies (often undetectable by Coombs' test) can cause delayed hemolysis in multiply transfused or multiparous patients. RBC transfusion recalls an immune response that produces IgG antibodies directed against donor cells. Over the subsequent 10–14 days, the direct Coombs' test becomes positive and transfused RBCs are lysed. This problem usually presents as a sudden (but often asymptomatic) drop in the PCV about 2 weeks after transfusion. Although usually benign, a falling hematocrit and rising bilirubin in a postoperative patient often raise concern for hepatic failure or occult bleeding.

Other Causes of Hemolysis

Blood should always be administered through a needle larger than 19 gauge to prevent mechanical shredding of RBCs. Heating above 38°C or freezing will also cause hemolysis. Normal saline is the only suitable solution for the transfusion of RBCs. Solutions containing calcium (e.g., Ringer's lactate) lead to clumping, and iso-osmotic glucose solutions (D5W) may produce cell lysis and aggregation.

Infections

Bacterial infections transmitted through transfused blood are most frequently due to poor sterile technique at the time of the transfusion and prolonged infusion time. *Listeria monocytogenes* is capable of growing at the usual storage temperature of blood and may cause transfusion-related bacteremia.

Because of the large number of donors required for their preparation, the risk of infection is greatest from pooled blood products (e.g., factor VIII concentrate and activated factor complexes). Viral infections occur in up to 10% of all transfused patients and include cytomegalovirus (CMV), hepatitis B, and non-A non-B hepatitis. Because of donor testing, hepatitis B now accounts for < 2% of all transfusion-related hepatitis, whereas non-A, non-B hepatitis accounts for ≃ 90% of cases. Up to 50% of the general population demonstrate serologic evidence of prior CMV infection; therefore, the high rate of transfusion-related CMV infection is not surprising. Other infections transmitted via blood include malaria, syphilis, brucellosis, toxoplasmosis, and Epstein-Barr virus. Since screening tests for HIV were instituted, the risk of transfusion acquired AIDS is < 1/500,000 for each unit of transfused blood component.

Other Risks of Transfusion

Febrile non-hemolytic transfusion reactions may occur due to surface antigens on WBCs or platelets. In patients with previous febrile reactions, the use of leukocyte-poor RBCs and HLA matched components reduce the risk.

Allergic reactions range from urticaria to anaphylaxis. These usually occur in patients with IgG antibodies directed against IgA in the donor blood. Stopping the transfusion and administering antihistamines are usually sufficient to abort the reaction.

RBCs, WBCs, platelets, and CPT should all be administered through standard blood filters to prevent transfusing *aggregates* of these components.

All filters reduce the maximal infusion rate and should be changed after every 2–4 units because of filter plugging.

Hyperkalemia may occur in massively transfused patients given PRBCs stored for long periods of time, especially in patients with renal dysfunction. Potassium concentration in the transfused plasma may rise as high as 20 mEq/l in PRBCs stored more than 3 weeks. Hyperkalemia may be prevented by using *fresh* whole blood or by using RBC products containing little plasma, such as washed or packed RBCs.

Hypothermia is rarely seen outside the setting of *massive* transfusion. Blood warming needs to be performed only with (1) massive transfusion; (2) transfusion rates exceeding 50 ml/min; or (3) cold agglutinin disease. Blood may hemolyze if heated above 38°C.

Hypocalcemia has been touted as a problem in the massively transfused patient, but is a rare event even in this patient group. Prophylactic administration of calcium is not recommended.

Because citrate is used to anticoagulate most blood components, *alkalemia* may develop as the liver converts citrate to bicarbonate. The metabolic alkalosis of citrate infusion is usually clinically insignificant and self-correcting.

SUGGESTED READINGS

1. American Red Cross. Circular of information for the use of human blood and blood components. October 1984 (ARC Publication No. 1751).
2. Boral LI: Platelet transfusion therapy. *Laboratory Med* 16(4):221–227, 1985.
3. Consensus Conference. Fresh-frozen plasma. Indications and risks. *JAMA* 253(4):551–553, 1985.
4. Greenwalt TJ: Pathogenesis and management of hemolytic transfusion reactions. *Sem Hematol* 18(2):84–121, 1981.
5. Insalaco SJ: Massive transfusion. *Laboratory Med* 15(5):325–330, 1984.
6. Solanki D, McCurdy PR: Delayed hemolytic transfusion reactions. An often-missed entity. *JAMA* 239(8):729–731, 1978.
7. Thompson AR, Harker LA: *Manual of Hemostasis and Thrombosis*, ed 3. Philadelphia, FA Davis Co, 1983.

14 Medication Administration

BASIC PHARMACOKINETICS

Four major concepts are key to understanding drug dosing: *bioavailability* (BA), *volume of distribution* (V_d), *clearance*, and *half-life* (t½).

Bioavailability

When a drug is given intravenously, the entire dose is made available to body tissues. All other routes of adminstration reduce BA, i.e., the fraction of unmetabolized drug reaching the circulation, compared with the total dose given. For enterally administered drugs, *hepatic metabolism* is the most important determinant of BA because splanchnic blood flows through the liver en route to the systemic circulation. Severe liver damage increases available concentrations of orally administered medications because of hepatocellular dysfunction and portal-to-systemic shunts (particularly in cirrhosis). Dose, concentration, route of administration, solubility, rate of dissolution, absorptive area, and drug-drug interactions influence BA. Circulation to the site of drug deposition (intramuscular or subcutaneous injections) or to the gut mucosa (enteral route) also affects absorption and BA—a key consideration in states of hypoperfusion.

Volume of Distribution

Drugs distribute unevenly among the intracellular and extracellular compartments, in accordance with serum protein binding, cardiac output, vascular permeability, and tissue solubility. The V_d relates the total amount of drug in the body to its plasma concentration. Knowledge of V_d *is most useful in determining loading doses* of drugs, particularly those that distribute in multiple compartments (such as lidocaine). Distribution effects may account for such phenomena as ultra-rapid buildup and termination of drug effects, and prolongation of drug action with repeated dosing (e.g., narcotics).

Clearance

In simplest terms, *clearance* reflects the rate at which drug is eliminated from the circulation. Drug clearance may occur either through *chemical conversion and subsequent excretion of metabolites* or through *excretion of unchanged drug*. Although other tissues may participate, the liver is the central site of most drug metabolism. Hepatic metabolites are secreted into bile and then either directly eliminated in the stool or, alternatively, reabsorbed across the gut wall, assimilated into the bloodstream, and eliminated by the kidney.

Half-life

After administration, most drugs exhibit a two-phase concentration profile corresponding to distribution and elimination. The serum half-life (t½) is the time required for drug concentration to fall by 50% without further supplementation. The t½ incorporates distribution and clearance effects to give a *useful index for predicting the time required to achieve steady state concentration and determine dosing interval*. With repeated intermittent dosing, most drugs accumulate and wash out exponentially to their final concentrations (first order kinetics).

Under most conditions, 5 half-lives are required before drugs administered in constant dosage achieve a steady state concentration—a delay that may compromise treatment. *Therapeutic drug levels* may be achieved more rapidly by the use of loading doses, but loading doses will not shorten the time to reach the steady state. Drug level monitoring before 5 half-lives have elapsed will *underestimate the eventual steady state peak* and *trough* concentrations (see Fig. 14.1).

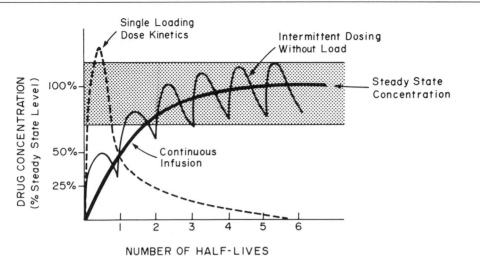

Figure 14.1 Dosing and elimination kinetics. After a single dose, drug concentration falls exponentially to undetectable levels over ≈ 5 half-lives (*dashed line*). During continuous infusion or intermittent administration of smaller maintenance doses (without load), a steady state concentration is not achieved until 5 half-lives have elapsed (*solid line*). The therapeutic range can be achieved and maintained quickly by combining a large initial loading dose with a maintenance schedule of either type.

PHARMACOKINETICS IN DISEASE

Circulatory Failure

In circulatory failure, blood flow is diverted from the skin, splanchnic bed, and muscle to maintain cerebral perfusion. Depressed cardiac output impairs drug absorption from subcutaneous, intramuscular, and gastrointestinal sites. Although intravenous dosing averts the problem of absorption, a smaller V_d often results in high blood levels immediately after injection. (For example, usual doses of lidocaine commonly cause central nervous system (CNS) toxicity after bolus injection.)

Even in the absence of overt liver or kidney failure, circulatory failure compromises the clearance of many drugs by diminishing renal function and hepatic metabolism. Reduced clearance increases the steady state drug level for any given dosage and prolongs the time necessary to reach equilibrium. These two facts help explain why *circulatory failure frequently results in the delayed expression of toxicity of slowly accumulating drugs.* Lidocaine, quinidine, and theophylline are drugs particularly affected by circulatory failure.

Hepatic Failure

As the primary organ of drug metabolism and serum protein formation, the liver plays a key role in pharmacokinetics. Hepatic failure depresses the synthesis of albumin and other serum proteins,

causing the *total serum levels* of highly protein bound drugs to fall. On the other hand, serum *concentrations of free drug* may be normal or increased. (Phenytoin is a classic example.) Reduced liver blood flow impairs hepatic drug clearance. Specifically, porto-systemic shunts (as in cirrhosis) decrease "first pass" metabolism, thereby increasing bioavailability. Unstable patients with vacillating hepatic blood flow or parenchymal function can be difficult to manage with medications subject to extensive first pass metabolism (e.g., diltiazem, morphine, nifedipine, propranolol). To avoid the vagaries of fluctuating liver function, it is often useful to utilize renally metabolized and excreted drugs in patients with impaired hepatic function. (For example, oxacillin, a renally excreted drug, is a logical substitute for hepatically metabolized nafcillin.) Drugs with long half-lives and those with metabolites dependent upon hepatic clearance should be avoided. Biliary obstruction impairs the ability of the liver to concentrate drugs (particularly antibiotics) in the bile. Even drugs that normally enter the bile (e.g., ampicillin) fail to do so in the setting of complete biliary obstruction. Drug therapy may cause artifactual elevations in liver-related laboratory tests; *tetracycline* and *intravenous lipid preparations* may elevate reported values of serum bilirubin, and *Hetastarch* may spuriously elevate serum amylase.

Renal Failure

Many drug dosages must be modified to prevent toxic accumulation during renal failure. Renal failure is frequently accompanied by reduced albumin concentration and diminished protein binding. As in hepatic failure, these changes may result in low total serum drug concentrations but normal *free drug* levels. The clearance of most renally excreted drugs is proportional to the glomerular filtration rate (GFR), which in turn parallels creatinine clearance. *At steady state*, drug dose (as a percentage of normal) can be calculated by estimating creatinine clearance, expressed as a percentage of the normal value (see Chapter 23). *Cefoxitin* produces an artifactual elevation of creatinine if the analysis is performed by colorimetric methods.

Lung Disease

Although lung disease does not directly affect drug metabolism, cor pulmonale and positive pressure ventilation may alter hepatic blood flow and GFR, predisposing to drug toxicity.

Burns

Beginning immediately after the injury, burn patients translocate fluid from the intravascular to the extravascular space, changing V_d and reducing renal and hepatic blood flows. Later (longer than 1 week after injury), the GFR and metabolic rate accelerate, and the concentrations of serum albumin and protein-bound drugs decline. Consequently, larger doses of many drugs (e.g., cimetidine, aminoglycosides) are needed to achieve therapeutic levels.

Acid-Base Disorders

Acid-base status plays a significant role in the absorption, distribution, and elimination of drugs. Ionized drugs traverse cell membranes poorly. Systemic acidosis inhibits the ionization of weak acids (e.g., salicylates, phenobarbital), thereby promoting their translocation to target tissues. For similar reasons, weak bases (amphetamines, quinidine) enter cells more readily under alkalemic conditions. These same acid-base properties can be used to bolster drug excretion. Urinary alkalinization traps weak acids in the urine, increasing the renal excretion of salicylates and phenobarbital, whereas acidosis promotes excretion of amphetamines, quinidine, and phencyclidine (PCP). pH also impacts the binding of certain drugs to serum proteins. Therefore, manipulation of acid-base status can influence drug activity—a principle that should be kept in mind during crisis intervention. (A good example is the use of bicarbonate to sequester free tricyclic antidepressant in protein complexes in the treatment of overdosage.)

GOALS OF DRUG ADMINISTRATION

The aim of drug therapy is to rapidly achieve and maintain effective and nontoxic tissue drug concentrations. In critically ill patients, these goals are met by combining appropriate loading and maintenance regimens. During intermittent dosing, drug levels may demonstrate peaks and troughs that potentially expose patients to toxicity and subtherapeutic levels (Fig. 14.1).

In an attempt to avoid these fluctuations, many drugs used in the intensive care unit are infused at a constant rate. Unfortunately, even constant infusions do not guarantee constant drug levels. Drugs with long half-lives or those with a large V_d may accumulate for long periods of time before toxic side effects emerge. Deterioration of renal or hepatic function may impair drug excretion. The addition of new drugs to an established regimen may also alter metabolism, compete for protein binding, or alter absorption.

ROUTES OF ADMINISTRATION

Inhalation (Aerosols)

Endobronchial administration normally achieves high local drug concentrations without adverse systemic effects. However, certain inhaled solutions reaching the pulmonary parenchyma are rapidly absorbed across the massive surface area of the capillary bed (e.g., isoproterenol).

Intratracheal Instillation

The intratracheal route may be used to produce therapeutic drug levels rapidly in settings where intravenous access is limited or denied (e.g., cardiopulmonary resuscitation). Drugs given via the intratracheal route must be delivered in at least 10 ml of liquid to permit the majority of the dose to access the alveolar compartment where absorption occurs.

The intratracheal route has been demonstrated effective for emergent use of lidocaine, epinephrine, naloxone, and atropine (Table 14.1). Interestingly, intratracheal administration may prolong the duration of action of certain drugs (lidocaine, atropine).

It is unwise to mix drugs when dosing via the intratracheal route. Furthermore, some commonly used drugs should never be given intratracheally (norepinephrine and calcium chloride, for example, may cause pulmonary necrosis). Because so-

Table 14.1
Intratracheal Drugs

Drug	Dose (mg)
Lidocaine	50–100
Epinephrine	1 (1:10,000 dilution)
Atropine	1–2
Naloxone	2–5

dium bicarbonate depletes surfactant, massive atelectasis may result from intratracheal use.

Intravenous Injection

Intravenous injection is the most reliable route of drug administration. Intravenous infusions avoid problems of bioavailability and eliminate delays associated with absorption. Therapeutic levels can be immediately obtained. Intravenous injection also allows the administration of drugs that otherwise would be too caustic, unstable, or poorly absorbed to dose via other routes. At steady state, uninterrupted, continuous intravenous infusion sustains drug levels, limits peaks and troughs, and avoids the associated problems of subtherapeutic levels and toxicity. It should be noted, however, that fluctuating drug clearance may cause important changes in drug concentrations—even at an unchanging rate of infusion.

Intramuscular Injections

Because uptake of drug from muscle into the intravascular compartment is a gradual process, the duration of action of an intramuscular injection is usually longer than that of an equivalent intravenous bolus. Under normal circumstances, *aqueous solutions* are more promptly absorbed than *oily or viscous preparations*. Drug absorption may be erratic if local perfusion is impaired, as during shock or cardiopulmonary arrest.

Problems occurring with intramuscular injections include pain or abscess formation at the injection site and hematoma formation in patients with clotting disorders. Intramuscular injections also raise the serum creatinine phosphokinase and may interfere with the diagnosis of myocardial infarction and rhabdomyolysis.

Subcutaneous Injections

Subcutaneous injections (particularly of insulin, epinephrine, or heparin) may be appropriate if the drug is non-irritating and administered in a small volume (< 1 ml). Rates of absorption vary widely, depending on the drug given and local blood flow. For example, subcutaneous epinephrine is absorbed with sufficient speed to be a mainstay of emergent asthma therapy. Conversely, insulin must not be given subcutaneously to the hypotensive diabetic. Delayed absorption of some drugs (e.g., heparin) may be useful to allow *prolonged* low-level drug effects.

Intra-arterial Injections

Direct injection into peripheral arteries delivers massive concentrations of drug to a local region and may produce serious complications (tissue ischemia and necrosis), particularly if vasoactive drugs are infused. Consequently, the only common use of intra-arterial therapy is the deliberate, selective, and closely metered administration of vasoconstrictors by catheterization of mesenteric vessels in the treatment of gastrointestinal bleeding. Rarely, selective infusions of anti-neoplastic agents into visceral arteries may be performed.

Intrathecal Therapy

Intrathecal therapy is rarely employed, except when high CNS concentrations of drugs that cross the blood-brain barrier poorly must be obtained. Refractory CNS infection (i.e., fungal meningitis, gram-negative meningitis, or abscess) constitutes one such indication. Intraventricular or spinal access to the cerebrospinal fluid may be appropriate, depending on the organism and clinical condition of the patient. Rarely, intrathecal anti-neoplastic drugs may be used for leukemic meningitis.

Intraperitoneal Therapy

Intraperitoneal antibiotics are often used to treat peritonitis developing in patients undergoing peritoneal dialysis. (Gram-positive coverage is usually provided by a cephalosporin or vancomycin, and gram-negative coverage is provided by an aminoglycoside.) Intravenous loading doses are given initially, but serum levels are sustained by absorption of drug given via the intraperitoneal route. Because intraperitoneal concentrations of drug equilibrate with those in the serum, the concentration of drug in the dialysate should equal that desired in the serum. For example, if a serum level of 7 mg/dl is desired, the dialysate concentration of drug should be kept at 7 mg/dl.

Transcutaneous Administration

Cutaneous drug absorption depends upon skin permeability, blood flow, moisture content, and the presence of skin disorders. The highest penetration of transcutaneously administered drugs is for lipid-soluble preparations applied to moist skin. At the current time, nitroglycerin, clonidine, and scopolamine are the only systemic drugs commonly administered *transcutaneously*.

Systemic Absorption of Dermatologic Preparations

High concentrations of topical *corticosteroids* applied over large areas may occasionally result in significant systemic absorption. Chronic use of long-acting (fluorinated) topical corticosteroids can suppress the pituitary-adrenal axis, particularly if applied to inflamed skin under occlusive dressings. Certain *topical antibiotics* used in burn therapy may also produce metabolic acidosis (mafenide) or salt-wasting (sodium nitrate) (see p. 293).

Intraocular Drugs

Even eye drops may be absorbed systemically in significant concentrations if given *frequently*, in *high doses*, or if there is significant *corneal inflammation or trauma*. Corticosteroids and beta blockers (e.g., timolol) both have the potential for producing systemic effects when administered intraocularly. (Intraocular beta blockers are contraindicated in asthma or congestive heart failure.)

Oral Drug Administration

Bioavailability of orally administered drugs is limited by acid digestion, poor absorption across the gut wall, and first pass metabolism by the liver. Effective oral therapy requires gut motility, adequate mucosal perfusion, and epithelial integrity. Patients with ileus, gut hypoperfusion, or atrophic or injured gut epithelium are poor candidates for oral dosing. Drugs given in aqueous solutions are more rapidly absorbed than those given in oily solutions, and non-ionized drugs are more readily absorbed than ionized drugs. Drugs destroyed by an acidic pH may be partially protected by enteric coating. Conversely, some drugs *require* acid for activation or absorption (e.g, sucralfate, ketoconazole, and iron), a point that deserves consideration in patients receiving antacid therapy.

Although not often considered, significant fluid overload may result from giving such fluid intensive oral preparations as sodium-potassium exchange resin (Kayexalate) or bowel preparations, e.g., saline or polyethylene glycol.

Sublingual Administration

Because only minute quantities of drug are absorbed across intact oral epithelium, an effective sublingual drug must be potent and lipid-soluble. Nitroglycerin is one of the few drugs that fits this description. If swallowed and absorbed enterally, nitroglycerin is rapidly eliminated by first pass liver metabolism. However, because drugs absorbed from the sublingual space drain directly to the superior vena cava, such first pass clearance is bypassed, increasing bioavailability.

Rectal Administration

Rectal administration of certain drugs can occasionally be useful in *children*, *combative patients*, and patients with *problematic venous access or refractory vomiting and/or ileus*. Hepatic first pass metabolism is less extensive with rectally administered drugs than with orally administered drugs, but it is still significant. Unfortunately, rectal administration results in *erratic and incomplete absorption* and therefore is less desirable than either oral or parenteral dosing. Rectal dosing is best confined to sedatives, antiemetics, antipyretics, laxatives, and theophylline compounds.

Intravesicular Administration

Amphotericin bladder lavage is commonly employed when yeast is found in the urine, but it is of limited usefulness. Intravenous amphotericin should be employed if *invasive Candida* or *Aspergillus* infection of the bladder is suggested by evidence of *hyphal forms* or *clumps* of fungus, urine, or histologic evidence of *bladder wall invasion*. *Yeast* in the urine of an asymptomatic patient rarely requires treatment (particularly in patients with indwelling Foley catheters). Intravesicular therapy may result in hyponatremia if aqueous solutions are used, and fluid overload may result from isotonic saline. Bladder lavage with glycine-containing solutions is often used to control bleeding after urinary tract surgery.

SUGGESTED READINGS

1. Bennett WM, et al: Drug prescribing in renal failure: dosing guidelines for adults. *Am J Kidney Dis* 3:155–193, 1983.
2. Friedman H, Greenblatt DJ: Rational therapeutic drug monitoring. *JAMA* 256:2227–2233, 1986.
3. Greenblatt DJ, Koch-Weser J: Drug therapy: intramuscular injection of drugs. *N Engl J Med* 295:542–546, 1976.
4. Pentel P, Benowitz N: Pharmacokinetic and pharmacodynamic considerations in drug therapy of cardiac emergencies. *Clin Pharmacokinet* 9:273–308, 1984.
5. Pond SM, et al: First-pass elimination. Basic concepts and clinical consequences. *Clin Pharmacokinet* 9:1–25, 1984.
6. Richard C, et al: The effect of mechanical ventilation on hepatic drug pharmacokinetics. *Chest* 90:837–841, 1986.
7. Sellers EM, et al: Drug metabolism in the elderly. *Drug Metab Rev* 14:225–250, 1983.
8. Williams RL: Drug administration in hepatic disease. *N Engl J Med* 309:1616–1622, 1983.

15 Nutrition and Alimentation

NUTRITIONAL REQUIREMENTS

In the intensive care unit (ICU), more pressing concerns often divert attention away from nutritional support. Yet, by impairing immune function, prolonging weaning from the ventilator, and delaying wound healing, malnutrition may prove decisive. It should be noted, however, that despite the inherent appeal of providing nutritional supplementation, there is surprisingly little documentation that nutritional support improves outcome. Furthermore, it is likely that certain catabolic patients (e.g., those with sepsis) ineffectively utilize nutrients in any form.

Calories

Formulas for calculating calorie requirements, (basal energy expenditure, BEE) are often complicated, as exemplified by the Harris-Benedict equation:

BEE (men) $= 66 + (13.7 \times wt) + (5 \times ht) - (6.8 \times age)$

BEE (women) $= 655 + (9.6 \times wt) + (1.8 \times ht) - (4.7 \times age)$

where weight (wt) and height (ht) are expressed in kilograms and centimeters, respectively. Despite their apparent complexity, the Harris-Benedict formulas still require adjustment for additional stress. A well-nourished, minimally active patient should receive 1.25 times the basal energy expenditure. The severely anabolic patient may require up to 1.75 times the BEE. Although detailed calculations may occasionally prove helpful, adequate caloric requirements can usually be estimated by simple assessment of the patient's general condition and lean body weight. In most hospitalized patients, 35 kcal/kg/day are needed. In the severely stressed patient, 45 kcal/kg/day or more may be required (see Fig. 15.1).

About 80% of all calories should derive from non-protein sources. Typically, glucose provides $\frac{1}{2}$–$\frac{3}{4}$ of this, with the remainder coming from lipids. The exact proportions of glucose and lipid are not of crucial importance. However, at least 100–150 non-protein calories per gram of nitrogen must be provided to avoid using amino acids as an energy source. Some glucose is required for protein sparing effects. However, when given in excess of 7 mg/kg/min, glucose is largely converted to fat, leading to potential complications of overfeeding (volume overload, hyperglycemia, increased CO_2 production, and fatty liver).

Protein

Normal adults require $\simeq 0.8$ gm/kg/day of protein; however, the average ICU patient requires 1–2.5 gm/kg/day (see Fig. 15.2). The amount of nitrogen supplied may be calculated by dividing grams of protein by 6.25. In addition to the normal routes of catabolism, important protein losses may also occur through the urine (nephrotic syndrome), surgical drains, or chest tubes.

CHOOSING CANDIDATES FORSUPPLEMENTAL NUTRITION

Most patients are able to withstand calorie deprivation for 1 week or more before supplementation is mandatory. However, nutritional support should not be delayed in patients who clearly will be deprived of food for long periods or in those who have massive nutritional requirements. Likely candidates for nutritional supplementation include: (1) those *unable to eat for long periods* because of endotracheal intubation or gastrointestinal (GI) tract interruption; (2) patients with *high caloric requirements* (e.g., burns, sepsis, major surgery, or trauma; and (3) patients who sustain *high protein losses* (e.g., corticosteroid or tetracycline usage, nephrotic syndrome, or draining fistulas).

Complex scales for nutritional assessment have

CALORIC REQUIREMENTS IN STRESS

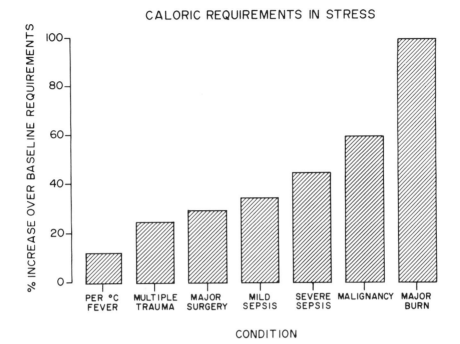

Figure 15.1   Caloric requirements in stress.

PROTEIN REQUIREMENTS IN STRESS

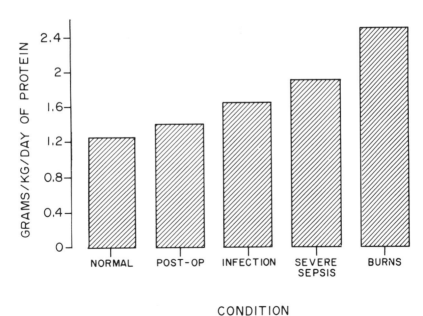

Figure 15.2   Protein requirements in stress.

been developed that include anthropomorphic measurements, clinical nutrition history, and analytical laboratory criteria. Whereas such precise indices of nutritional status may occasionally be helpful, simple clinical evaluation—*history of weight loss*, *dietary history*, and knowledge of *underlying disease*—provides a good working assessment. Of the widely available clinical measures of nutritional status, clinical history, absolute lymphocyte count, serum cholesterol, and serum protein levels are perhaps the most useful data.

Malnutrition is almost certain in patients losing 5% of their body weight in a month or more than 10% in 6 months. Absolute *lymphocyte counts* < 1200 cells/mm^3 and < 800/mm^3 signify moderate and severe malnutrition, respectively. Because *albumin* normally has a half life of $\simeq 18$ days, weeks of nutritional deficiency are usually needed to produce severe hypoalbuminemia. Faster losses of serum proteins may occur during intense catabolic stress. *Transferrin* and *thyroid-binding globulin (TBG)-prealbumin* are more sensitive acute indicators of response to nutritional depletion or therapy because they have shorter half-lives. *Complement levels* and skin fold thickness, however, are not reliable indices of nutritional status. In the absence of hypothyroidism or nephrotic syndrome, severe depressions of serum cholesterol reliably indicate calorie deprivation. Fever, sepsis, steroids, tumors, and immunosuppressant drugs reduce the value of the *antigenic skin test response*.

THE ADVERSE EFFECTS OF MALNUTRITION

Malnutrition depresses the immune system by reducing immunoglobin levels and by decreasing T-cell function. Poor nutrition may impair wound healing and increase rates of infection in burns, trauma, and postoperative states. Starvation impairs ventilatory capacity by decreasing drive and diaphragm bulk. Severe nutritional deficiencies may be fatal, even in otherwise healthy patients. (Even under optimal conditions, otherwise healthy adults succumb to subacute losses $> 40\%$ of lean body mass.)

INDICES OF ADEQUATE NUTRITION

The same indices used to detect malnutrition may also be used to determine the effectiveness of nutritional supplementation. Because *albumin* turns over slowly, it is not a useful index of *acute* improvement or deterioration in nutritional status. With much shorter half-lives, both *pre-albumin*

and *transferrin* are more helpful. *Weight gain* is not always a dependable sign; edema may produce rapid weight increases without any improvement in nutritional status.

Nitrogen balance is possibly the best indicator of nutritional homeostasis. Because non-urinary (skin and stool) losses of nitrogen are usually small ($\simeq 2$ gm/day), the 24–hour urine collection effectively quantitates nitrogen losses. Urine urea nitrogen (UUN) accounts for 80% of total urinary N$_2$ losses. Hence, unless excessive non-urinary nitrogen losses occur (e.g., through fistulas or open surgical wounds), the balance between nitrogen intake and loss can be approximated using this formula:

$$N_2 \text{ balance} = \underbrace{\text{Protein}/6.25}_{\text{INTAKE}} - \underbrace{[(\text{UUN} + 20\%) + \text{non-urinary losses}]}_{\text{EXCRETION}}$$

ROUTES OF NUTRITIONAL SUPPLEMENTATION

Enteral Therapy

The enteral feeding route should be used whenever possible. It is less expensive, impedes ulceration, and preserves mucosal integrity and small bowel function better than intravenous nutrition. Because enteral feeding stimulates insulin secretion, hyperglycemia is a less likely complication than during TPN. Enteral feeding also provides iron and trace elements more effectively than TPN. Oral feeding poses the risk of aspiration, however, even in patients with an intact gag reflex and normal peristalsis. Oral tolerance for clear liquids is probably the best clinical indicator that a patient is able to swallow safely.

When the upper GI tract must be bypassed, soft small bore (6–8 French) feeding tubes are preferable to the larger Levin or Salem tubes. In most patients with ileus, peristalsis of the small bowel returns before gastric motility; therefore it may be advantageous to deliver nutrients directly to the small bowel. Feeding tubes should migrate to a final position in or beyond the duodenum for optimal function, a process that may require 12 hours or longer to complete. Before instituting nasogastric (NG) feeding it is important to assure proper tube placement by x-ray. Neither the aspiration of what appears to be stomach contents nor characteristic gurgling with air insufflation indicates satisfactory positioning. (Feeding tubes malpositioned in the airway may produce similar sounds.) Initiating feeding before confirming that the tube is in the GI tract invites disaster.

Continuous feedings are preferable to bolus

feedings because they *reduce the aspiration risk*, *produce less bloating*, and *generate smaller residual volumes*. Gastric residuals should be checked to assure that the stomach is not overfilling, thereby predisposing to regurgitation and aspiration. As a general rule, gastric residuals should approximate the hourly infusion rate of continuous tube feeding and should always be < 200 ml. Even when delivered to the duodenum, tube feeding stimulates gastric secretion (sometimes up to 3–4 l/day). Under normal circumstances the stomach should empty its contents within 2–3 hours of loading. Therefore, gastric motility may be assessed by serial aspirations of gastric contents or alternatively by following the progress of contrast dye radiographically. In patients with depressed gastric motility, metaclopromide may promote peristalsis. This same drug is also helpful in moving small bore feeding tubes into the duodenum.

Selection of Feeding Formulas

Certain products are available to supplement oral diets and enteral feedings. A *calorie boost* can be provided by complex carbohydrates (Polycose) or oils (MCT oil, Microlipid). Certain *protein supplements* may be particularly helpful for patients on liquid or fat restriction diets (Citrotein, Pro Med). Puddings made from complete formulas are ideal for fluid restricted patients.

Nutritionally balanced feedings may be obtained either in *polymeric* form, in which protein, fat, and carbohydrates are all present as complex molecules, or as *elemental diets*, wherein amino acids provide nitrogen and oligosaccharides serve as the carbohydrate source. Polymeric tube feedings are useful when the gut digestion of fat and protein is normal. The most commonly used formulations (Isocal, Ensure, Osmolite, Precision LR) can provide adequate protein, fat, and 1–2 kcal/ml. The high fat content of polymeric feedings enhances palatability. The potential for diarrhea from polymeric feedings is low because they have a small lactose content, a low residual, and low osmolarity. Certain formulations containing fiber (e.g., Complete B) may help to regularize bowel evacuation. Elemental diets (Vivonex, Vital HN, and Travasorb) contain virtually no fat, no lactose, and have little residual material. Therefore, they require minimal digestion, making them ideal for patients with short bowel syndrome, inflammatory bowel disease, and pancreatic insufficiency. Their low viscosity renders them useful for catheter-needle jejunostomy feeding. Unfortunately, they are quite expensive, and their high osmolarity predisposes to diarrhea, despite their low residual.

When initiating hypertonic tube feedings, a half strength solution is begun at 25–50 ml/hr. At this rate, discomfort, bloating, and diarrhea are seldom encountered. However, prolonged continuation of such a protocol delays full calorie and protein supplementation. Isotonic formulas may usually be started at full strength, but the patient's overall condition and the period of abstinence must be considered. After 24 hours it is reasonable to advance feeding solutions to full strength, then to increase the infusion rate to 100–150 ml/hr over a 2–3 day period, as tolerated. For feedings delivered to the duodenum or jejunum, feeding rate should be increased before increasing concentration of the formula.

Tube Types

Gastrostomy tubes offer the advantages of stable position and large caliber. The large bore gastrostomy tube allows administration of pulverized medications, an advantage over jejunostomy or NG tubes, which frequently obstruct. Although gastrostomy tubes enter the stomach directly through the abdominal wall, they do not prevent regurgitation and aspiration. Endoscopic placement of *percutaneous gastrostomy* tubes, the "PEG" tube, has recently gained popularity, avoiding expense and risks of open surgery. Jejunostomy feeding requires direct surgical placement of a small-bore catheter. *Jejunostomy* prevents regurgitation and may later be withdrawn (without re-operation) to leave a self-closing fistula.

Problems and Complications of Enteral Nutrition

Aspiration, the most important and life-threatening complication of enteral alimentation, may be reduced by feeding continuously at a well-tolerated infusion rate, checking gastric residuals, and elevating the head of the bed to 30° from horizontal. Reductions in feeding volume, solution osmolarity, and carbohydrate content reduce the incidence of *diarrhea*. The addition of pectin to the feeding solution may be a useful countermeasure. (Diarrhea in patients receiving tube feedings commonly results from bacterial overgrowth and from the use of antibiotics and drugs with cholinergic properties.) Nasogastric tubes often *obstruct* and require replacement. Obstruction may be avoided if pill fragments are not administered through the tube and if the lumen is flushed several times daily with water. Placement of small-bore feeding tubes using a metallic stylet is dangerous and should be avoided. *Esophageal perforation* and *translaryngeal introduction* of the catheter into the lung or pleural space are possible complications. The pH-neutralizing effect of enteral feedings encourages overgrowth of pathogenic bacteria, predisposing to gastrointestinal and pulmonary infections.

Parenteral Feeding

The cost of intravenous nutrition (TPN) often reaches $150/day for hospitalized patients. TPN solutions may be delivered into peripheral or central veins, with each route having specific advantages and disadvantages.

Peripheral TPN

Peripheral TPN alone may be an ideal supplement for the well-nourished patient with minimal requirements; however, it is *not* acceptable for catabolic patients requiring protracted support. Similar protein solutions are used in both central and peripheral TPN mixtures. However, to avoid osmolality-related phlebitis, the glucose concentration of peripheral TPN is lower than that of central TPN. Consequently, fewer calories are available in a given infused volume. If lipid is not used as a major calorie source, up to 7 liters/day of peripheral TPN may be needed to fully satisfy calorie and protein requirements. Even when $\simeq 60\%$ of calories are derived from intravenous lipid, 3–3.5 liters of fluid are still needed to deliver 2100 calories (3 liters of glucose plus amino acids and 500 ml of 20% lipid solution). Consequently, *underfeeding* is common when peripheral TPN is used, because of volume limitations alone.

The corrosive nature of the TPN solution presents another major problem of peripheral administration. Venous inflammation results from the high osmolarity and potassium content of TPN solutions. Used alone, glucose and amino acid mixtures are highly irritating. Up to 50% of patients receiving 600 mOsm (standard) TPN solutions develop phlebitis within 2 days. Therefore, peripheral intravenous sites should be changed at least every other day. However, the concurrent infusion of lipid through a Y connector reduces the risk of chemical phlebitis.

Central TPN

Central administration of TPN incurs all of the risks of large vessel cannulation. Catheter tip position must be checked before starting feeding to prevent inadvertent infusion of fluids into the pericardium or pleural space. To minimize the infection risk, central catheters should be changed at 10 day intervals (unless a skin-tunneled catheter is placed). For similar reasons, feeding catheters should not be used for medication delivery or non-TPN solutions. (Multi-use triple lumen catheters are less than ideal, because multiple catheter entries increase the risk of infection.) After a central catheter is properly positioned, a highly concentrated (usually 1400–1800 mOsm/l) solution of 5–10% amino acids mixed with 40–50% glucose is administered. An 8.5% amino acid solution is usually mixed with an equal volume of D50 or D25 glucose to yield a solution containing 150–200 kcal/gmN$_2$. The specific vitamins and trace metals added to standard TPN solutions vary on a hospital-to-hospital basis. To prevent bacterial growth in TPN solutions, individual bottles should not hang longer than 24 hours.

Normal electrolyte composition of TPN solution includes sodium (40–50 mEq/l), potassium (30–45 mEq/l), chloride (40–220 mEq/l), phosphate (14–30 mEq/l), magnesium (25 mEq/l), calcium (20 mEq/l), plus an anion (usually acetate) needed to electrically balance the solution.

Soy bean (Intralipid) or safflower (Liposyn) oil mixtures provide extra calories and prevent essential fatty acid deficiency. Iso-osmolar lipid solutions normally provide all essential fatty acids (linoleic, linolenic, and oleic acid). As little as 500 ml of 10% lipid solution given weekly will prevent essential fatty acid deficiency. Lipid solutions also serve as a concentrated source of calories, providing 1.1 Kcal/ml for 10% solutions. No more than 60% of total daily calories should be provided as fat. Lipids are contraindicated in patients with hyperlipidemia. Rapidly administered large-volume infusions of lipid may produce pulmonary dysfunction or thrombocytopenia. Adding heparin to lipid solutions (up to 1000 U/l) may accelerate triglyceride clearance by activating lipoprotein lipase.

Intravenous Nutrition for Special Patients

Malignancy

TPN improves the weight and nutritional parameters of many patients with cancer. However, catabolic mediators (e.g., tumor necrosis factor) released in response to many neoplasms blunt the beneficial effects of TPN. TPN may also improve the tolerance to chemotherapy, but there is no evidence to demonstrate that survival is improved. Protein gain is not as rapid in cancer patients as in other TPN candidates, but fat gain is similar.

Renal Failure

Carefully provided nutritional support improves the outcome of *acute* renal failure. (In contrast, the benefits are not well documented in chronic renal failure.) TPN does not hasten recovery of renal function but may improve uremic symptoms by *limiting catabolism.* Goals of TPN in acute renal failure are to provide daily 2000–3000 calories and 0.25 gm/kg of protein with high biologic value. High glucose concentrations are used to minimize administered volume, and only essential amino acids are given if high serum levels of urea nitrogen are present. Solutions low in sodium and potassium are used unless volume depletion or sodium wasting is a problem. Determinations of urine sodium may help guide the TPN sodium concentration.

In *chronic* renal failure, an appropriate goal is to provide 0.5–1.0 gm/kg/day of high-grade protein; intake should seldom be restricted to < 20 gm/day. Because losses can be massive in the *nephrotic syndrome*, protein intake should not be limited in this group. Patients with end-stage renal disease should be dialyzed at a rate sufficient to allow nearly normal protein ingestion. Vitamin depletion is a potential problem of patients with renal failure since almost all low protein diets are vitamin deficient, and water soluable vitamins are lost during dialysis.

Hepatic Failure

The TPN prescription must be radically altered in hepatic failure. Because fat metabolism is impaired, hyperlipidemia may result when a large fraction of non-protein calories are provided as lipid. Carbohydrate intolerance is also common, and high carbohydrate loads may lead to fatty liver. Heightened aldosterone secretion and depressed free water clearance require low sodium and low volume when TPN is used. Encephalopathy may be precipitated by large protein loads, particularly when aromatic amino acids are the major nitrogen source. The substitution of intravenous branched chain amino acids for their aromatic counterparts reduces ammonia formation and improves mental status in the setting of hepatic encephalopathy.

Monitoring TPN

Careful monitoring is required to prevent complications and to assure that TPN accomplishes its goal. *Daily weights* should be obtained to monitor fluid status. (Weight gains in excess of 1 pound/day are likely to result from accumulating fluid.) Frequent sampling of *glucose* during the initiation of TPN therapy is necessary to avoid hyperglycemia and hyperosmolarity. Gross *examination of the serum for lipemia* 3 hours after fat infusion or ingestion may confirm hyperlipidemia induced by lipid supplements. *Electrolytes* (including magnesium, calcium, phosphorus), *liver function tests, creatinine, protein, and albumin* should be monitored at least twice weekly. Each week a 24-hour determination of *urine urea* helps to assess nitrogen balance.

Complications of TPN

Complications of parenteral nutrition are reduced by an experienced team versed in all aspects of TPN, including the local care of infusion catheters. Metabolic complications are more likely to occur in starved and severely malnourished patients and those with diabetes or impaired hepatic or renal function. *Catheter-related sepsis* occurs in < 3% of patients when proper precautions are taken.

Hyperosmolarity is common when glucose is infused at rates > 0.5 mg/kg/hr, particularly in dehydrated patients. Certain free fatty acids (linoleic, linolenic, and arachidonic acid) are considered essential because they cannot be synthesized by the body. *Essential fatty acid* requirements are met easily by 500 ml lipid emulsion (10%) given once or twice weekly. Deficiency of essential fatty acids may also be avoided by giving 15–30 ml of corn oil orally each week. *Vitamin deficiencies* are common during TPN use. Many hospitals do not include vitamins K, B_{12}, or folic acid in TPN solutions. B_{12} injections are not required more than monthly, and weekly injections are usually adequate to prevent vitamin K deficiency. Folate requirements do not exceed 1 mg/day, except in patients undergoing dialysis. During prolonged use, *deficiencies of trace elements* (including zinc, iron, cobalt, iodine, copper, selenium, and chromium) may produce skin disorders, immunologic defects, and other metabolic problems.

Bone pain and *increased alkaline phosphatase* may occur with the chronic use of TPN, but the mechanism is unknown. (Both are usually associated with normal vitamin D levels and decreased serum phosphorus.) *Hypophosphatemia* occurs in $\simeq 1/3$ of patients started on TPN and is particularly likely when markedly elevated serum glucose levels induce an osmotic diuresis. Hypophosphatemia shifts the oxyhemoglobin dissociation curve leftward and decreases glycolysis but does not produce obvious weakness until levels fall below 1 mg/dl. Hemolysis, impaired phagocytosis, and rhabdomyolysis may all be seen with severe phosphate depletion. *Hypomagnesemia* may present as refractory hypocalcemia, hypokalemia, or both. Hypomagnesemia is particularly common in patients with pancreatitis and underlying alcoholism.

Mild increases in serum glucose (< 250 mg/dl) are desirable because they produce protein-sparing effects. However, problematic *hyperglycemia* occurs commonly in infants, diabetics, cirrhotics, the elderly, and patients receiving corticosteroids. Insulin should be added to TPN if the serum glucose remains > 250 mg/dl for more than 1 day. It is best to add insulin directly to the TPN bottle to match insulin dosing to the rate of TPN infusion. (Hypoglycemia is particularly common when insulin is continued, as TPN is tapered or discontinued.) To prevent *hypoglycemia* as TPN is stopped, the infusion rate may first be slowly tapered to ≃ 1 1/24 hr. D10W can then be substituted for an additional 24 hours. (The need for tapering TPN, however, is debated.)

Acalculous cholecystitis and *cholelithiasis* are seen with increased frequency in patients receiving TPN, probably secondary to diminished gall bladder secretion and emptying. The incidence of symptomatic gallbladder disease may reach 1 in 4 patients receiving TPN for more than 12 weeks. It is especially high in patients with impaired small bowel absorption (e.g., Crohn's disease).

Lipid administration encourages *cholestasis* by inhibiting hepatic bilirubin excretion. Restricting lipid intake to < 2 gm/kg/day and keeping a 200:1 ratio of calories to protein may help to prevent this problem.

Rapid infusion of amino acids (particularly histidine, alanine, and glycine) may cause *hyperchloremic acidosis*. The addition of acetate to TPN solution can prevent these changes. Amino acid infusions also promote gastric and pancreatic secretion and stimulate ventilatory drive.

Mild, selective *increases in liver function tests* (LFTs) are almost universal in patients receiving TPN for > 10 days. About ½ of all patients experience a 50% rise in alkaline phosphatase and serum glutamic oxaloacetic transaminase (SGOT) levels. Serum glutamic pyruvic transaminase (SGPT) is less commonly affected. Fatty infiltration is the presumed cause. High insulin levels produced by continuous glucose infusion may inhibit lipolysis and favor triglyceride synthesis. Decreases in the glucose infusion rate usually correct the problem. LFT abnormalities may be decreased or prevented by giving < 60% of non-protein calories as glucose. Patients who remain normoglycemic rarely develop hepatic function test abnormalities. Even when TPN solutions are continued, LFT abnormalities usually revert to normal in 3 weeks.

SUGGESTED READINGS

1. Apelgren KN, Wilmore DW: Nutritional care of the critically ill patient. *Surg Clin N Am* 63(2):497–507, 1983.
2. Askanazi J, Weissman C, Rosenbaum SH, et al: Nutrition and the respiratory system. *Crit Care Med* 10(3):163–172, 1982.
3. Barrocas A, Tretola R, Alonso A: Nutrition and the critically ill pulmonary patient. *Resp Care* 28(1):50–61, 1983.
4. Ormes JF, Clemmer TP: Nutrition in the critical care unit. *Med Clin N Am* 67(6);1295–1304, 1983.
5. Pingleton SK: Nutritional support in the mechanically ventilated patient. *Clin Chest Med* 9(1):101–112, 1988.
6. Pingleton SK, Harmon GS: Nutritional management in acute respiratory failure. *JAMA* 257(22):3094–3099, 1987.
7. Rochester DF, Esau SA: Malnutrition and the respiratory system. *Chest* 85(3):411–415, 1984.
8. Wilson DO, Rogers RM, Hoffman RM: Nutrition and chronic lung disease. *Am Rev Respir Dis* 132:1347–1365, 1985.

Section **2**

Medical Crises

16 Cardiopulmonary Arrest

Cardiopulmonary resuscitation (CPR) is applied to unresponsive patients found without effective pulse and/or ventilatory efforts. In the community, most such events are *cardiac* in origin and occur in patients with underlying heart disease. In contrast, primary *respiratory* events (respiratory failure, pulmonary embolism) are more common in hospitalized patients—a principle that must be kept in mind during resuscitative efforts and prophylaxis.

PRIMARY PULMONARY EVENTS (RESPIRATORY AND PULMO-CARDIAC ARREST)

Patients are often found unresponsive without respirations but with an effective pulse. These conditions define a respiratory arrest. Failure to achieve effective ventilation results in progressive acidosis and hypoxemia that may culminate in cardiovascular dysfunction, hypotension, and eventual circulatory collapse. Although the etiology of many respiratory arrests remains uncertain even after detailed investigation, the cause can often be traced to *respiratory center depression* (due to iatrogenic sedation or electrolyte disturbance) or to failure of the respiratory muscle pump (due to *excessive workload*, *impaired mechanical efficiency*, or *muscle weakness*). Although tachypnea is usually the first response to stress, the respiratory rhythm disorganizes, slows, and eventually ceases as overloading continues.

The partial pressure of arterial oxygen (PaO_2) plummets dramatically shortly after ventilation ceases. Furthermore, body stores of oxygen are restricted and rapidly consumed, in contrast to carbon dioxide, which has a huge storage pool and an efficient buffering system. On the other hand, if effective circulation is maintained, $PaCO_2$ builds rather slowly, at a rate of 6–9 mmHg in the first apneic minute and 3–6 mmHg/min thereafter. (Once the apneic patient develops metabolic acidosis, however, H^+ combines with HCO_3^- to generate CO_2 and water, increasing the rate of CO_2 production dramatically.) *Thus, life-threatening hypoxemia will occur long before significant respiratory acidosis.*

Initially, hypoxemia enhances the peripheral chemical drive to breathe and stimulates heart rate. Profound hypoxemia, however, depresses neural function and produces bradycardia refractory to atropine. At this point, cardiovascular function is usually severely disturbed, not only because cardiac and vascular smooth muscle function poorly under conditions of hypoxia and acidosis but also because cardiac output is the product of stroke volume and heart rate. The end result of this process is a pulmo-cardiac arrest.

PRIMARY CARDIOVASCULAR EVENTS (CARDIO-PULMONARY ARREST)

The heart may abruptly fail to achieve an effective output because of a new *dysrhythmia* or suddenly *impaired pump function* resulting from diminished preload, excessive afterload, or decreased contractility. The normal heart compensates for changes in heart rate over a wide range through the Starling mechanism. (Thus, cardiac output is normally maintained despite slowing of rate by chamber dilation and increasing stroke volume.) Patients with dilated or stiff hearts lose this reserve and are highly sensitive to rate changes. Thus, bradycardia is tolerated poorly by patients with congestive heart failure.

Common Causes of Inappropriate Bradycardia

Hypoxemia	Pharmacologic effects
Intense vagal stimulation	Beta blockade
Sinus/AV node ischemia	Verapamil
Drug overdosage	Digitalis

Decreases in preload sufficient to result in cardiovascular collapse are usually the result of reflex venodilation, massive hemorrhage, pericardial tamponade, or tension pneumothorax. The right ventricle is unable to adjust quickly to increased afterload. Therefore, abrupt increases in afterload sufficient to cause catastrophic cardiovascular collapse usually affect the right (rather than left) ventricle. These often result from embolism to the pulmonary circuit by clot or air. Acute dysfunction of the cardiac muscle fiber itself can result from hypoxemia, acidosis, electrolyte disturbance, or myocardial infarction. Regardless of the precipitating event, patients with diseased coronary arteries are particularly susceptible to the adverse effects of a reduced perfusion pressure.

Neural tissue is disproportionately susceptible to reductions in blood flow. A circulatory arrest *always produces profound coma* within seconds, and respiratory rhythm ceases very rapidly thereafter. Thus, ongoing respiratory efforts indicate *very* recent cardiovascular collapse or the continuation of effective blood flow below the palpable pulse threshold. (In a person of normal body habitus, a systolic pressure of $\simeq$ 80 mmHg, 70 mmHg, or 60 mmHg must be present to be felt at radial, femoral, or carotid sites, respectively.)

The outcome from a full-blown arrest (cessation of pulse and respiratory efforts) depends critically on the speed with which appropriate interventions are made to re-establish the native circulation and oxygenate the blood. The multiplicity of potential causes for arrest mandates a methodical, nearly reflex approach to analysis and management.

BASIC PRINCIPLES OF RESUSCITATION

Chaos often surrounds initial attempts at CPR. A prompt, well-directed resuscitative effort is critical to restore cardiopulmonary and neurological function. The primary activities of resuscitation include: (1) chest compression; (2) airway management and ventilation; (3) preparation and administration of drugs; (4) establishing and maintaining intravenous access; and (5) specialized procedures (defibrillation, pacemaker placement, chest tube placement).

Thus, managing the complete cardiopulmonary arrest routinely requires four persons in addition to the team leader. Additional personnel may be needed for specialized tasks such as chart review and communicating with the laboratory, pharmacy, or other physician specialists. Once all equipment is at the bedside, limiting the number of people involved in CPR avoids excessive confusion.

Principle 1: Define the Team Leader

A single person must be in charge of the resuscitation team. This person should integrate all pertinent information and establish priorities for response. The team leader should monitor the electrocardiogram (ECG), order medications, and direct the action of the other team members but should not be distracted from the leadership role by performing procedures.

Principle 2: Maintain Ventilation and Chest Compression

Establishing Effective Ventilation

Basic support of the airway and circulation should not be interrupted for long periods to perform adjunctive procedures. In the pulseless apneic patient, establishing an airway and achieving effective ventilation (with pure oxygen, if available) is the initial priority. Except in unusual circumstances, this can be accomplished with mouth-to-airway or bag-mask ventilation. Because position, body habitus, and limitations of available equipment often compromise either upper airway patency or the seal between the mask and face, bag-mask ventilation often requires two people for effective use. Although cricoid pressure may help seal the esophagus, gastric distention and vomiting may still occur if inflation pressures are excessive. Furthermore, inflation pressures generated by bag-mask ventilation may cause barotrauma.

When the airway is patent, the chest should rise smoothly with each attempted inflation. Once effective chest compression and ventilation have been achieved, the most experienced person should intubate the airway to achieve definitive control. Intubation attempts should not interrupt ventilation or chest compression for more than 15 seconds. Therefore, all materials including laryngoscope, endotracheal tube, and suction equipment should be *assembled and tested before any attempt* at intubation. Inability to establish effective bag-mask ventilation should prompt an immediate intubation attempt. When neither intubation nor effective bag-mask ventilation can be accomplished because of abnormalities of the upper airway, restricted cervical motion, or patient agitation, sedation/paralysis or fiberoptic guidance may be helpful, depending on cause. Very rarely, all such attempts fail and an emergent temporizing measure must be undertaken. Insufflation of oxygen via a large bore (14–16 gauge) needle puncture of the cricothyroid membrane or emergent cricothyroidotomy can accomplish adequate oxygenation until a more definitive airway is established.

Esophageal obturator airways have no role in the resuscitation of hospitalized patients because they are less effective than endotracheal intubation at providing ventilation or preventing aspiration. Complications include: (1) tracheal intubation (quickly fatal); (2) esophageal and gastric rupture; (3) hypoventilation; and (4) vomiting and aspiration.

During CPR, ventilation should normalize arterial pH and provide adequate oxygenation. *The cornerstone of pH correction is adequate ventilation—not bicarbonate administration.* Reductions in pulmonary blood flow limit the capacity for CO_2 excretion. Consequently, hypocapnia is seldom produced *at the tissue level* during ongoing CPR. Conversely, excessive HCO_3^- can produce hyperosmolality and paradoxical cellular acidosis (see Ref. 11). Adequacy of ventilation and oxygenation should be guided by serial arterial blood gas determinations. However, newer evidence suggests that perfusion adequacy might be better judged from central venous pH and/or the end-tidal CO_2 concentration of exhaled gas.

Establishing Effective Circulation

Blood flow during (closed-chest) CPR has been theorized to occur by two basic mechanisms: cardiac compression, and thoracic pumping. Both mechanisms probably contribute to circulatory output during CPR.

The *cardiac compression* theory proposes that chest compression generates positive intraventricular pressure, simulating cardiac muscle contraction. According to this schema, the heart valves function normally to achieve a forward blood flow with each compression.

The *thoracic pump* theory proposes that the heart serves only as a passive conduit for blood flow. This mechanism is currently thought to predominate in adults. Chest compression creates a positive pressure relative to extrathoracic structures, and flow is valved at the thoracic inlet. Retrograde vena caval flow is prevented by jugular venous valves and functional compression of the inferior vena cava at the diaphragmatic hiatus. This theory may account for augmented flow with phasically increased intrathoracic pressure and for improved flow observed during simultaneous chest compression and positive pressure inflation (the *"new"* CPR).

At best, *closed chest compression* of the arrested circulation provides about ⅓ of the usual output of the beating heart. Improperly performed, CPR is not only ineffective but also potentially injurious. Several points of technique deserve emphasis. Short-duration chest compressions simulate the low stroke volume of heart failure, whereas failure to fully relax chest compression simulates pericardial tamponade or excessive levels of positive end-expiratory pressure. Maximal blood flows occur when $\simeq 60\%$ of the cycle is in the compression phase. (Unfortunately, higher outputs do not necessarily guarantee increased cerebral perfusion; some blood appears to flow into the external carotid circulation.) When a 60% compression ratio is used, the compression *rate* becomes much less critical. In most patients a compression rate of 70 beats per minute is about right. *Open cardiac compression* may provide double the cardiac output of closed chest technique, but it has obvious practical logistical problems and has not improved survival.

Although experimental data suggest that phasic increases in intrathoracic pressure improve blood flow during CPR, there is as yet no evidence that simultaneous ventilation and chest compression improves outcome. Similarly, although theoretically attractive, abdominal binding, military antishock ("MAST") trousers, and volume loading are unproven interventions. During CPR it is difficult to determine whether blood flow is adequate, because pulse amplitude does not directly parallel blood flow (i.e., pressure does not equal flow).

Principle 3: Correct Systemic Acidosis

Adequate ventilation is key to pH correction. When used, bicarbonate should be administered cautiously, guided by blood gas analysis. HCO_3^- is rarely necessary if circulation and ventilation are promptly restored. An arterial pH above 7.15 is usually adequate for cardiovascular function when the heart is actively beating. However, what the appropriate guideline is for the arrested circulation is highly controversial. Previously recommended doses of sodium bicarbonate (1 mg/kg) may produce unwanted side effects including: (1) arrhythmogenic alkalemia; (2) increased CO_2 production; (3) hyperosmolarity; (4) hypokalemia; (5) paradoxical central nervous system (CNS) and intracellular acidosis; and (6) a leftward shift in the oxyhemoglobin dissociation curve, limiting delivery of O_2 to tissues.

Principle 4: Create an Effective Cardiac Rhythm

Asystole

Any rhythm is better than asystole, the complete absence of electrical activity (a flat ECG). Therefore, another key aim is to stimulate electrical activity and then to modify the rhythm to one with a pulse. Asystole usually indicates extended interruption of perfusion and carries a grave prognosis. It makes little sense to countershock the truly asystolic patient because there is no "rhythm" to modify. However, *low-amplitude ventricular fibrillation* may go unrecognized unless detected by a full 12-lead ECG. Ventricular fibrillation may be best distinguished from "asystole" in leads II and III. *Epinephrine* (in 1-mg doses) and *atropine* (in 1-mg increments to a total dose of 2–4 mg) are useful in restoring a vestage of electrical activity, even if disorganized. Manipulation of electrolyte balance (Ca^{2+}, K^+) may also be useful in refractory cases.

Ventricular Fibrillation

Blind direct current countershock should be administered to all pulseless unresponsive adult patients as soon as possible; ventricular fibrillation (VF) is the most common rhythm in victims of sudden death, and the success of defibrillation declines with each passing minute. The goal of cardioversion is to abolish all chaotic ventricular activity, allowing an intrinsic pacemaker to emerge. Many defibrillators allow a "quick look" at the cardiac rhythm before countershock is attempted, but careful inspection of the rhythm is not mandatory before proceeding. Blind cardioversion will not harm patients with bradyarrhythmias or asystole and usually benefits those with pulseless tachycardias or VF. Conversely, because *respiratory arrest* is much more common than VF as a cause of sudden death in *children*, blind countershock without examining the rhythm is not recommended.

The success of defibrillation is influenced by the amplitude of VF, which correlates inversely with the duration of fibrillation. If two initial attempts at defibrillation prove unsuccessful, "coarsening" the rhythm and increasing vascular tone with epinephrine may be helpful. (Once an organized rhythm has been re-established, epinephrine increases vascular tone, improving brain and heart perfusion.) On the other hand, inappropriately high doses of epinephrine may be deleterious because of increased myocardial oxygen consumption.

Defibrillation Technique

Defibrillators are calibrated to discharge through a 50-ohm impedance, a value less than the electrical impedance of the adult chest (70–80 ohms). Therefore, the *delivered energy is usually lower than is indicated by the nominal machine settings.* There is no consistent relationship between body weight and the energy required for defibrillation, but most optimally prepared patients have a defibrillation threshold of 100–150 joules. Although higher energy levels are often needed, defibrillation with the least effective energy level reduces cardiac damage and the risk of high-grade atrioventricular (AV) block. Thoracic impedance declines with repeated shock. Therefore, if defibrillation initially fails, patients should be *rapidly* reshocked at the same electrical dosage.

Improper paddle positioning dissipates energy and reduces the rate of successful defibrillation. In the anterolateral technique, paddles are placed at the cardiac apex and just below the clavicle to the right of the sternum. In some patients, anterior-posterior paddle placement delivers energy to the heart more efficiently than does the anterior-lateral approach. Defibrillator paddles should not be placed over ECG monitor leads or transcutaneous drug patches because of the possibility of electrical arcing, equipment damage, and explosion. Contact between defibrillator and chest wall should be maximized by use of conducting gels or gauze pads soaked in saline, but conducting fluids must not bridge the chest paddles. The standard-size paddles on adult defibrillators provide optimal electrical impedance matching between machine and chest wall. Once cardioversion has been accomplished, ventricular irritability should routinely be suppressed with intravenous lidocaine (or procainamide) unless contraindicated by high grade conduction disturbances or medication allergy (see Arrhythmias, Chapter 4). Attention is then turned toward normalizing blood pressure, arterial blood gases, and electrolytes.

Refractory Ventricular Fibrillation

In patients resistant to defibrillation, check the following: (1) Confirm effective *oxygenation and ventilation* by chest auscultation or preferably by arterial blood gas analysis if immediately available; (2) *Ensure that the defibrillator is working.* One of the most common reasons for failure of the defibrillator to discharge in the setting of VF is for the machine to be set in the *synchronized* cardioversion mode. (If there is no QRS complex, there is no signal to trigger a "synchronized" discharge of the defibrillator.) (3) Correct serious acidemia (pH < 7.2), but be cautious—overcorrection (to pH > 7.5) may render the heart resistant to defibrillation.

If defibrillation consistently produces a *brady-cardic rhythm* that degenerates to VF, try to increase heart rate with epinephrine, isoproterenol, atropine, or pacing, to prevent recurrence due to underperfusion. If counter-shock returns *any tachycardia* that repeatedly degenerates, consider the possibility of excessive catecholamine stimulation and decrease infusion rate or try appropriate antiarrhythmics (lidocaine, procainamide, bretylium).

Hypokalemia, a frequent cause of *refractory* VF, is found in ≃ ⅓ of all patients suffering sudden death. In this desperate setting, up to 40 mEq of potassium may be cautiously administered over 30 minutes. *Hypomagnesemia* may also result in refractory VF, but magnesium levels are unlikely to be measured during the time span of a resuscitative effort. Magnesium (1–2 gm over 15 minutes) may be given empirically in patients without renal dysfunction. Hypomagnesia, a cause of both hypokalemia and hypocalcemia, should be considered in patients who exhibit these electrolyte abnormalities.

Ventricular Tachycardia

The primary therapy of hemodynamically compromising ventricular tachycardia (VT) is immediate electrical shock. A precordial "thump" creates a small electrical discharge that may occasionally cardiovert *witnessed* VT or VF but is rarely effective in other settings. In pulseless patients, wide complex tachycardia of unproven origin *should be treated as VT* with countershock or drug therapy, depending upon the hemodynamic status of the patient.

Intravenous *lidocaine* is generally considered the drug of choice in patients with VT and a stable blood pressure (see Arrhythmias, Chapter 4). VT unresponsive to lidocaine may respond to *procainamide* or *bretylium*. The latter drug has a biphasic action that initially produces adrenergic discharge, followed by adrenergic blockade. Bretylium has a long delay between administration and peak action (15–45 minutes) and can produce severe postural hypotension once effective circulation is restored. Advantages of bretylium include its ability to lower the defibrillation threshold, making cardioversion easier and occasionally producing "chemical defibrillation." Verapamil may cause asystole in patients with VT; therefore in

cases in which the supraventricular origin of tachycardia is uncertain, it should probably be withheld.

Electromechanical Dissociation

Electromechanical dissociation (EMD) is characterized by the inability to detect pulsatile activity in response to coordinated ECG complexes. When cardiac in origin, EMD carries a dismal prognosis because it is usually a sign of massive pump destruction or free wall rupture. Additionally, mechanical obstructions to the normal transit of blood through the heart may cause EMD. Hence, atrial myxoma, mitral stenosis, and aortic stenosis may cause refractory EMD. However, other reversible conditions can produce this syndrome. These include: (1) *hypovolemia*, particularly from acute blood loss. (Vasopressors are relatively ineffective in the setting of hypovolemia; hence, adequate circulating volume must be assured.) (2) *pericardial tamponade* suspected on the basis of venous engorgement, a history of cardiac trauma, or preexisting pericardial disease, for which pericardiocentesis should be attempted; (3) *tension pneumothorax*; and (4) *massive pulmonary embolism* by clot or air. Thrombo-embolism may fragment and migrate during CPR, opening the central pulmonary artery and re-establishing effective output. Air embolism can be treated by positioning the patient (left side down, Trendelenburg) and/or transvenously aspirating air from the right heart.

Recent controversy has arisen about the use of calcium in EMD. Calcium benefits only a few patients (particularly those with hypocalcemia) and has the potential for serious complications. Nonetheless, it is probably worth trying when other measures (e.g., HCO_3^-, epinephrine) have failed.

Bradyarrhythmias

Bradyarrhythmias that cause sudden death have a particularly bad prognosis. In the adult, these are often a manifestation of hypoxemic, hypercarbic respiratory failure. Indeed, the most important measure in treating the hypotensive bradycardic patient is *assuring adequate ventilation and oxygenation*—not giving vagolytic drugs. In general, the slower the rate and wider the complex, the less effective the myocardial contraction. The vagolytic action of atropine is most useful in narrow complex bradycardias resulting from sinoatrial node failure or AV blockade. Doses of at least 1 mg should be administered. (Lower doses of atropine may paradoxically increase AV block.) Isoproterenol or epinephrine may also be helpful for their chronotropic action. While useful for symptomatic bradycardia, transvenous or transthoracic ventricular pacing is difficult to achieve during CPR and rarely proves effective in asystole due to massive myocardial infarction.

POST-RESUSCITATION ARRHYTHMIAS

A low threshold for the treatment of dysrhythmias (particularly premature ventricular contractions) should be maintained in recently resuscitated patients. Chapter 4 provides a discussion of arrhythmias, but two specific types of rhythm disturbances deserve emphasis here.

Digitalis-related Arrhythmias

In the setting of digitalis toxicity the cardiac rhythm should be stabilized by stopping the drug and by correcting hyperkalemia and hypomagnesemia. Digitoxic arrhythmias may be exacerbated by the administration of calcium. Cardioversion (with the lowest effective wattage) is indicated if ventricular arrhythmias cause symptomatic hypotension. Phenytoin, lidocaine, and procainamide are especially useful drugs for the treatment of digitalis-induced arrhythmias. Pacing is usually required for high-grade AV block.

Torsades de Pointes

Torsades de Pointes is a form of polymorphic VT frequently associated with prolongation of the QT interval. Torsades de Pointes is characterized by a constantly changing QRS axis that produces an apparent "twisting of points" about the isoelectric axis (Fig. 16.1). A host of reversible precipitating factors has been identified, including hypokalemia, hypomagnesemia, tricyclic antidepressants, and type 1a antiarrhythmics (quinidine, procainamide, and diisopyramide). Cardioversion is almost always effective in pulseless patients, but torsades de pointes frequently returns within a short time. Lidocaine may also be transiently beneficial, but the most effective measures include those that correct the underlying stimulus and shorten the QT

interval, usually by increasing the heart rate with atropine, isoproterenol, or pacing. Type 1a antiarrhythmics are contraindicated.

Intracardiac Injections

Although intracardiac (IC) injection has traditionally been used to administer drugs during resuscitation, it is not the route of choice. Many such attempts fail to puncture the heart. Complications include *coronary laceration*, *pneumothorax*, and *cardiac tamponade*. IC injection may expose the myocardium to massive concentrations of vasoactive drugs, destabilizing its electrical properties. Inadvertent injection of medication into the myocardial wall may result in intractable ventricular arrhythmias. There is little if any indication for IC injection because most drugs used for resuscitation may be given as effectively and in more appropriate concentrations via the intravenous or endotracheal routes (see Medication Administration, p. 133).

Use of Calcium in Cardiac Resuscitation

Until recently, calcium was widely recommended in cardiac resuscitation. Although contractility may improve in patients with low circulating levels of *ionized* Ca^{2+}, excessive Ca^{2+} exacerbates the arrhythmic tendency of unstable ischemic myocardium, impairs cardiac relaxation, and may hasten cellular death. Furthermore, extremely high Ca^{2+} levels may occur with indiscriminate dosing. One gram is usually sufficient for maximal therapeutic effect. (However, even at these doses, potentially toxic levels of Ca^{2+} may result.) Ca^{2+} exacerbates digitoxicity, enhances coronary artery spasm, and forms insoluble precipitates when administered with sodium bicarbonate. Ca^{2+} administration appears warranted when there has been a prolonged period of arrest and absent or ineffective pump activity. Outside the setting of CPR, the use of intravenous Ca^{2+}

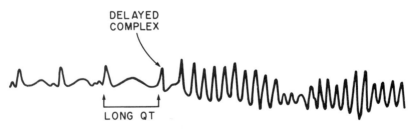

DELAYED
COMPLEX

LONG QT

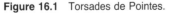

Figure 16.1   Torsades de Pointes.

should be restricted to symptomatic patients with *hypocalcemia, calcium channel blocker overdose*, and *hyperkalemia*.

DECIDING WHEN TO FOREGO OR TERMINATE RESUSCITATION

Certain clinical disorders are associated with a virtually hopeless long-term prognosis (e.g., refractory metastatic carcinoma, acquired immune deficiency syndrome, AIDS). However, each case must be considered individually with regard for the wishes of the patient and family. The importance of clarifying the "code status" of all seriously ill patients should be emphasized. When doubt exists as to the propriety of resuscitative efforts, CPR should generally be initiated unless specifically countermanded by the attending physician.

A single set of guidelines regarding termination of effort cannot be applied to all clinical situations. During ongoing CPR, neurological signs are unreliable predictors of outcome and should not be used in the decision to terminate resuscitative efforts. Resuscitation is seldom successful when more than 20 minutes are required to establish coordinated ventricular activity. Several studies have reported that, with rare exception, failure to respond to 30 minutes of advanced life support predictably results in death. Best results occur when sudden electrical events are promptly corrected with cardioversion. Prolonged resuscitation with a good neurological outcome may occur when *hypothermia* or profound pharmacologic central nervous system (CNS) depression (e.g., barbiturates) precipitates the arrest.

SEQUELAE OF RESUSCITATION

Immediate Post-Resuscitative Period

Although a prompt response improves the chance for cardiac and neurological recovery, antecedent sepsis, renal failure, and pneumonia are predictors of poor outcome. Long-term survival of severe anoxia is unusual in patients with underlying vital organ dysfunction, perhaps because further organ injury occurs or because neural centers critical to autonomic control and maintenance of protective reflexes are damaged by the event.

Iatrogenic *alkalosis, hypokalemia*, and other *electrolyte abnormalities* are extremely common following resuscitation. Hepatic and aortic lacerations, pneumothorax, flail chest, and flail sternum may occur as a result of CPR but are especially common when improper chest compression technique is used. *Aspiration pneumonitis* is frequent, and seizures from cerebral ischemia or lidocaine

toxicity often emerge. *Gastrointestinal (GI) bleeding* from stress ulceration affects as many as ½ of all resuscitated patients. After resuscitation, impressive elevation of hepatic (and/or skeletal muscle) enzymes are frequently seen, although frank ischemic necrosis and failure of the liver rarely occur. Creatine phosphokinase (CPK) is routinely elevated in patients receiving high-dose countershock. However, noteworthy elevation of the myocardial band (MB) isoenzyme of CPK is unusual unless repeated high-energy electrical shocks have been delivered.

Long-Term Prognosis

The primary goal of CPR is full cerebral resuscitation. The best current strategy is to provide early CPR and defibrillation. For uncertain reasons, glucose levels > 300 mg/dl in the immediate post-CPR period appear to correlate inversely with meaningful neurological recovery. The effect of glucose may relate to excessive production of lactate during cerebral ischemia. After "successful" CPR, $\simeq ⅓$ of patients do not awaken. Of the patients who recover consciousness, $\simeq 1$ in 3 suffers a serious permanent neurological deficit. *The probability of awakening following cardiac arrest is greatest in the first day following resuscitation and declines exponentially thereafter* to a very low stable level. (Almost all awakening occurs within 96 hours of resuscitation. Nonetheless, recovery from comatose or vegetative states has been reported after 100 days.)

Pupillary response to light, cephalic reflexes, and patterns of motor response to stimulation are valuable clues to eventual outcome. In the initial post-CPR period, abnormal pupillary and oculomotor responses are the best single predictors of an adverse outcome, whereas defective motor responses predict nonfunctional recovery best after 24 hours of observation (see Ref. 5). "Brain resuscitation" with calcium antagonists, steroids, or barbiturates is experimental and cannot be advocated on the basis of the evidence currently available. The diagnosis of irreversible brain damage or brain death is made by using the specific clinical and electroencephalographic criteria outlined in Chapter 28.

SUGGESTED READINGS

1. Auerbach PS, Geehr EC: Inadequate oxygenation and ventilation using the esophageal gastric tube airway in the prehospital setting. *JAMA* 250:3067–3071, 1983.
2. Lo B, Strull W: Survival after cardiopulmonary resuscitation. *N Engl J Med* 310:463, 1984.
3. Clark MB, Dwyer EM, Greenberg H: Sudden death

during ambulatory monitoring. *Am J Med* 75:801–806, 1983.

4. Eisenberg MS, Hallstrom A, Bergner L: Long-term survival after out-of-hospital cardiac arrest. *N Engl J Med* 306:1340–1343, 1982.

5. Levy DE, Caronna JJ, Singer BH, et al: Predicting outcome from hypoxic-ischemic coma. *JAMA* 253:1420–1426, 1985.

6. Longstreth WT, Jr, Inue TS: High blood glucose level on hospital admission and poor neurological recovery after cardiac arrest. *Ann Neurol* 15:59–63, 1984.

7. Luce JM, Cary JM, Ross BK, et al: New developments in cardiopulmonary arrest. *JAMA* 244:1366–1370, 1980.

8. Ornato JP, et al: Hypokalemia and cardiac arrest. *Pract Cardiol* 12(2):31–32, 1986.

9. Randomized clinical study of thiopental loading in comatose survivors of cardiac arrest. *N Engl J Med* 314:397–403, 1986.

10. Ruskin JN, McGovern B, Garan H, et al: Antiarrhythmic drugs: a possible cause of out-of-hospital cardiac arrest. *N Engl J Med* 309:1302–1306, 1983.

11. Stacpoole PW: Lactic acidosis. The case against bicarbonate therapy. *Ann Intern Med* 105:276–278, 1986.

12. Urban P, Scheidegger D, Buchmann B, et al: Cardiac arrest and blood ionized calcium levels. *Ann Intern Med* 109:110–113, 1988.

13. Weaver WD, Cobb LA, Dennis D: Amplitude of ventricular fibrillation waveform and outcome after cardiac arrest. *Ann Intern Med* 102:53–55, 1985.

14. Weil MH, Rackow EC, Trevino R, et al: Difference in acid-base state between venous and arterial blood during cardiopulmonary resuscitation. *N Engl J Med* 315:153–156, 1986.

15. Weisfeldt ML, Halperin HR: Cardiopulmonary resuscitation: beyond cardiac massage. *Circulation* 74:443–448, 1986.

17 Angina and Myocardial Infarction

UNSTABLE ANGINA

Pathophysiology

Myocardial ischemia results from an imbalance between oxygen supply and demand. Anginal chest pain is the clinical expression of this imbalance. Because the left ventricle (LV) comprises the majority of cardiac muscle mass and has the greatest afterload, it is most commonly affected by ischemia. Myocardial oxygen delivery may be limited by: (1) atherosclerosis; (2) plaque rupture with thrombosis; (3) coronary artery spasm; (4) anemia; (5) hypoxemia; and (6) limited diastolic filling time (tachycardia). In addition to a limited oxygen supply, three major factors increase cardiac oxygen demand: (1) tachycardia/exercise; (2) heightened LV afterload causing increased transmural wall tension (hypertension, heart failure, aortic stenosis); and (3) increases in LV mass (hypertrophy). Rarely, increases in right ventricular (RV) afterload (pulmonary embolism) may precipitate RV ischemia—a phenomenon most common in patients with underlying coronary narrowing. *Unstable angina* (UA) is synonymous with preinfarction angina, crescendo angina, intermediate coronary syndrome, or acute coronary insufficiency. UA is a disorder that represents a *transition period* during which most patients undergo accelerated myocardial ischemia over a period of up to 3 months. If unchecked this transition often culminates in acute myocardial infarction (MI).

Diagnosis

History and Physical

The term "unstable angina" denotes new pain or a departure from a previous anginal pattern. UA occurs *at rest*, *more frequently*, or *with less exercise* than stable angina. Pain *lasting longer than 15 minutes* is also suggestive. UA may *awaken* patients from sleep or present as *pain at a new site*

such as the jaw or arm. *Autonomic manifestations* (nausea, vomiting, or sweating) also favor "instability". Blood pressure frequently rises *before* the onset of pain, even in resting patients. Rising blood pressure boosts afterload, increasing the wall tension and myocardial O_2 consumption ($M\dot{V}O_2$).

Laboratory

During episodes of ischemic chest pain *electrocardiogram (ECG) features* may include: (1) ST segment elevation *or* depression; (2) T wave inversion; (3) premature ventricular contractions (PVCs); or (4) conduction disturbances, including bundle branch block. It is important to recognize that ECG findings are absent in up to 15% of symptomatic patients with UA. Therefore, a normal ECG does not exclude a diagnosis of UA or MI. (Furthermore, up to 70% of all ECG documented episodes of ischemia are clinically silent.) *Holter monitoring* is useful in diagnosing such silent episodes.

In UA the *total creatine phosphokinase (CPK) and myocardial band (MB) fraction* may be elevated to the upper limits of normal, but it is unclear if these elevations reflect true myocardial necrosis.

Therapy of Unstable Angina

Patients with UA should be admitted to an electrocardiographically monitored bed and receive aggressive anti-anginal treatment. Unstable angina can *usually* be stabilized medically and does not require immediate coronary angiography or other invasive procedures. A small percentage of patients presenting with UA will progress to subendocardial or transmural MI. The two basic approaches to the treatment of UA are to reduce myocardial O_2 demand or to improve O_2 supply.

Reducing Myocardial Oxygen Consumption

The principal measure to decrease myocardial oxygen consumption is to *limit physical activity*.

(Exercise studies are contraindicated because frank infarction may ensue). *Arrhythmias* (particularly tachycardias) *should be controlled* to optimize diastolic filling time, maximizing cardiac output and coronary perfusion.

Controlling hypertension and congestive heart failure decreases wall tension and hence facilitates myocardial perfusion (see Hypertensive Emergencies, Chapter 18). *Beta blockers* are particularly useful in UA with hypertension but are contraindicated in heart failure or coronary artery spasm.

Increasing Myocardial Oyxgen Supply

Often myocardial oxygen supply can be increased by boosting *oxygen* saturation or correcting *hemoglobin* to levels > 10 gm/dl. *Coronary vasodilators* may also increase myocardial perfusion. Nitroglycerin (TNG) is most commonly used and may be administered sublingually, orally, transcutaneously, or intravenously. (In unstable patients the intravenous route is most reliable.) Apart from dilating coronary vessels, TNG also decreases wall tension of the LV by reducing preload and, to a lesser extent, afterload. Acting through these mechanisms TNG also reduces the risks of life- threatening arrhythmias in acute ischemia. Nitrates are effective both for *classical and variant angina* because of their direct coronary vasodilating properties.

TNG is titrated to relieve the chest pain or to reduce the blood pressure by 10–20% (usually intravenous doses of 0.7 to 2 mcg/kg/min suffice). Intravenous TNG is usually begun at 5–15 mcg/min and titrated upward as necessary in 5 mcg/min increments every 5 minutes. Headache is a common side effect but usually responds to mild oral analgesics. Occasionally, hypotension accompanies TNG-induced vasodilation. This adverse effect can usually be offset by volume expanders or alpha agonists. Since alcohol is used as a vehicle in TNG infusions, violent adverse reactions may occur in patients taking antabuse. High doses for prolonged periods may also produce intoxication.

Coronary spasm, a primary contributor to ischemia in certain settings, may be ameliorated by nitrates or calcium channel blockers. Blockers of the slow Ca^{2+} channel (e.g., nifedipine) are usually rapidly effective in reversing coronary spasm and should be tried in most patients with angina refractory to sublingual TNG.

Most patients with UA have an ulcerated athrosclerotic plaque covered by an accumulation of platelets and red blood cells. Hence, *anticoagulants and antiplatelet drugs* represent an attractive

therapeutic option. Aspirin may halve the mortality in UA by irreversibly inhibiting intracoronary platelet aggregation. (There is little evidence that dipyrimadole is required for this effect.) Inhibition of platelet aggregation may complicate subsequent coronary artery surgery, but aspirin-related clotting defects are reversible with platelet transfusions.

Full anticoagulation with heparin immediately terminates the accumulation of platelets and red cells on plaque fissures. Conversely, warfarin takes days to achieve full anticoagulation and it should not be used in the acute treatment of UA.

Mechanical opening of coronary arteries with angioplasty, surgery, or thrombolytic agents may also be helpful (see below).

The *intra-aortic balloon pump* (IABP) may prove useful for hemodynamic stabilization while awaiting coronary artery surgery, particularly in patients with proximal coronary occlusion, hypotension, or acute mechanical defects (mitral regurgitation or ventricular septal defect). Balloon inflation during diastole augments coronary perfusion, and deflation during systole decreases LV afterload. Unless a rapidly correctable mechanical defect is present, use of IABP does not improve outcome.

MYOCARDIAL INFARCTION

Mechanisms

Myocardial infarction most commonly results from the same processes responsible for UA—structural narrowing, thrombosis, or spasm of the coronary arteries. If angiography is promptly performed, a fresh coronary thrombus may be demonstrated in the vast majority of cases ($\simeq 85\%$). Rarely, coronary flow may be interrupted by *embolism* in patients with endocarditis, prosthetic valves, or rheumatic valvular disease. Only 5–10% of patients sustaining an MI have *normal coronary arteries* (the mechanism of infarction remains unknown in these patients).

Diagnosis

History

A classical history of UA preceeds myocardial infarction in only 1 of 4 patients. More typically, myocardial infarction is characterized by the abrupt onset of *squeezing* or *heavy substernal chest pain* radiating to the neck and/or medial aspect of the left arm. It must be emphasized that the pain description may be highly atypical—"burning", "stabbing", "sharp", or may be localized only to the arm or neck. Autonomic symptoms (nausea, vomiting, and sweating) are more common than in UA. Up to 20% of myocardial infarctions are painless (particularly true in diabetics and the elderly). A history of palpitations is not helpful.

Physical Examination

Blood pressure and *pulse rate* are usually mildly increased. (Tachycardia is more common in anterior or lateral myocardial infarctions than in inferior or posterior MIs, in which bradycardia is more likely.) *Fever* may accompany uncomplicated MI but rarely exceeds 102°F or persists beyond 1 week.

An *S4* gallop is very common, whereas an *S3* suggests congestive failure, especially if accompanied by pulmonary rales. A paradoxically split S2 indicates increased LV ejection time. A systolic *murmur* at presentation should raise the suspicion of acute papillary muscle dysfunction. A pericardial *friction rub* commonly appears in the first 48 hours following MI and may be easily confused with a murmur.

Laboratory

Cardiac Enzymes.   Although the creatine kinase (CPK) is the most sensitive test for MI in patients presenting within 24 hours of the onset of symptoms, total CPK may be elevated by skeletal muscle injury (e.g., severe exercise or intramuscular injection). Electrical cardioversion may increase total CPK levels, but unless multiple high wattage shocks are given the myocardial or MB fraction of CPK (CPK-MB) should not rise significantly. CPK-MB is *relatively* specific for cardiac muscle but may also be released during *massive* skeletal or smooth muscle damage (e.g., rhabdomyolysis, polymyositis, and small bowel surgery). The CPK begins to rise within 6 hours of the onset of coronary occlusion and peaks at 24–36 hours. CPK peaks earlier in non-Q wave infarctions and in patients who have received thrombolytic therapy to abort an acute infarction. The rapid washout of CPK associated with thrombolysis may produce peak enzyme levels as early as 30 minutes after reperfusion. Typically, CPK returns to normal within 3–4 days. The MB fraction peaks earlier and resolves more quickly than total CPK. An elevated total CPK with an MB fraction > 5% is diagnostic, although an MB fraction exceeding 5% may occur with a normal CPK. Peak CPK activity correlates with the degree of muscle loss.

Although sensitive, the serum glutamic oxaloacetic transaminase (SGOT) is not sufficiently specific for unequivocal diagnosis. Similarly, total lactic dehydrogenase (LDH) rises in most cases of MI but has a *low specificity*. Levels of the LDH-2 isoenzyme normally exceed those of the LDH 1 isoenzyme. Reversal of the ratio suggests MI. LDH begins to rise 12–24 hours following coronary occlusion, peaking at 2–4 days and resolving in 7–10 days. Because LDH rises later than CPK, it may be used to diagnose infarction in patients presenting > 24 hours after onset of symptoms.

Electrocardiogram.   A single ECG cannot be used to exclude a diagnosis of angina or MI. Often the ECG remains normal early in infarction and damage to certain portions of the heart (particularly the high lateral wall) may be electrocardiographically silent. Furthermore, in patients with an abnormal baseline ECG (particularly left bundle branch block), the tracing may be uninterpretable for infarction. As an MI evolves, injury proceeds from the endocardial to the epicardial surface. When damage does not extend to the epicardial surface, a ''subendocardial infarction'' pattern, characterized by ST segment depression and T wave inversion, is the rule. Conversely, *transmural* MIs reflect the epicardial damage pattern of ST segment elevation and delayed Q wave development in leads overlying the infarcted region (Table 17.1). While Q wave formation is highly specific for transmural MI, it is not a sensitive marker.

The *T waves invert* within hours following coronary occlusion and usually remain so for 24–48 hours. (Occasionally T wave inversion fails to reverse). The ST segment in MI is usually *flattened and elevated* above the isoelectric baseline. The typical ECG evolution of transmural MI is illustrated in Figure 17.1.

For anatomic reasons, the posterior epicardium cannot be directly monitored by leads placed on the anterior surface of the chest. Therefore, true posterior transmural infarctions differ in their ECG presentation, producing ST depression (rather than elevation) and R waves (rather than Q waves) in leads V1 and V2. ST segment elevation of peri-

Table 17.1
Anatomic Patterns of Myocardial Injury

Location of Injury	Affected Leads
Inferior	II, III, F
Anterior/septal	V2–V4
Anterolateral	V3–V6
Lateral	I, AVL, occasionally V6
Apical	II, III, F, V5–V6
Posterior*	V1 and V2

*ST segment depression with R waves; T wave is inverted initially and then becomes upright

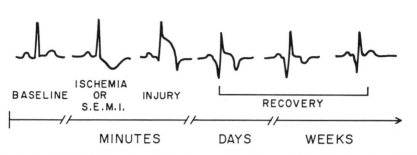

Figure 17.1 Electrocardiographic evolution of acute myocardial infarction. S.E.M.I., subendocardial (non-transmural) myocardial infarction.

carditis or cardiac contusion may usually be distinguished from acute MI by a "non-stereotyped" ECG pattern failing to correspond to distributions typical for the coronary circulation. Elevated leukocyte counts, glucose levels, and erythrocyte sedimentation rates are suggestive but not diagnostic of acute MI.

Echocardiography. Although echocardiography (ECHO) cannot be considered a definitive test for ischemia, it is a helpful adjunctive technique. ECHO offers suggestive evidence for ischemia or infarction when dyskinesis is demonstrated, helps to rule out competing diagnoses to explain hypotension or congestive symptoms (e.g., valvular disease, aortic dissection), and proves instrumental in diagnosing complications (chordal disruption, papillary muscle dysfunction, septal perforation, ventricular aneurysm, mural thrombus, etc.).

Nuclear Scans. Infarct-avid scanning (technetium) is most useful in detecting infarction in patients with *abnormal baseline ECGs*, or those with *"non-Q wave"* infarcts, *chest pain following cardiac surgery*, and patients with *previous infarcts*.

Technetium pyrophosphate concentrates in areas of myocardial damage, producing scintigraphic "hot spots" over recently infarcted regions. This test may be positive as early as 10–12 hours following MI but reaches peak sensitivity at ≃ 72 hours. Pyrophosphate scanning is highly sensitive in *transmural* MI, but ≃ 50% of all patients with *subendocardial* injury fail to demonstrate localized uptake. Technetium scans rapidly become positive (hours) if thrombolytic therapy re-establishes perfusion to an infarcted area. Four days after infarction, > ½ of positive pyrophosphate scans revert to normal.

Thallium (Th) scanning demonstrates scintigraphic "cold spots" in non-perfused areas of myocardium. Th has a lower specificity than technetium because "cold" spots occur in patients with *reversible* areas of impaired perfusion or *infarcts of any age*. Thallium scans are most useful in demonstrating areas of reversible ischemia. (Injection of the radionuclide during peak exercise will demonstrate a cold spot in ischemic areas that becomes perfused at rest.) Thallium is difficult to obtain and delivers a relatively high radiation dose—both disadvantages to its use. Other potentially useful diagnostic tests (e.g., radionuclide ventriculogram, echocardiography) are reviewed elsewhere (see "Hemodynamic Monitoring", Chapter 2).

Complications of Myocardial Infarction

Half of all patients sustaining MI have no significant complications. Of those with a complicated course most serious events occur within the first 5 days. Complications generally fall into one of two categories—electrical or mechanical.

Electrical Complications

Premature Ventricular Contractions

Premature ventricular contractions (PVCs) occur in almost all patients sustaining MI but their incidence rapidly declines with time. (Baseline levels are usually restored within 24–48 hours). Isolated unifocal PVCs are of little importance. However, in the setting of acute ischemia PVCs should be suppressed if *frequent*, *multifocal*, or *coupled*. As a practical matter most patients receive lidocaine prophylaxis over the initial 12–24 hours post-infarction, independent of rhythm.

Ventricular Tachycardia

In patients with acute ischemia, ventricular tachycardia (VT) occurs commonly and should almost always be suppressed. One particular form of VT, idioventricular rhythm (IVR), deserves special mention. Usually self-limited, IVR is a series of wide QRS complexes of ventricular origin. When IVR occurs at a rate of 60–100 beats per minute it is termed "accelerated". This rhythm most commonly occurs following reperfusion of ischemic myocardium or as an escape mechanism in patients with high grade atrioventricular (AV) block. If perfusion is adequate, no treatment is indicated. Indeed suppression may cause asystole.

Ventricular Fibrillation

Ventricular fibrillation (VF) as a primary event is seen in 2–10% of all MIs. Because "warning arrhythmias" do not invariably occur, most physicians favor prophylactic lidocaine. VF carries little prognostic import if defibrillation is successful and if the disturbance occurs as an isolated electrical event early in the course of a small MI. Reversible factors increasing the risk of VF (particularly *electrolyte imbalances*, *anemia*, and *hypoxemia*) should be addressed.

Bradycardia

Bradyarrhythmias occur more commonly in inferior and posterior MIs because of intense vagal stimulation and a higher incidence of sinoatrial (SA) and AV nodal ischemia (see Arrhythmias/Cardioversion, Chapter 4).

Mechanical Complications

Pericarditis

The pain of pericarditis may be distinguished from continued or recurrent myocardial ischemia by its *sharp*, *pleuritic* or *positional* nature, its *failure to radiate*, its *poor response to antianginal therapy*, and the presence of a *friction rub*. Histological pericarditis occurs in almost all *transmural* MIs but is usually mild and clinically insignificant. Symptoms typical for pericarditis occur in only a small proportion of such cases. In affected patients symptoms usually emerge 2–4 days following the MI. Non-steroidal anti-inflammatory drugs (e.g., indomethacin) are helpful in controlling the inflammation. Although effective, corticosteroids increase the risk of free ventricular wall rupture. Large pericardial fluid accumulations occur in < 10%. Rarely, in anticoagulated patients, pericardial fluid may become hemorrhagic and accumulate sufficiently to cause tamponade. Delayed episodes of immunologically-mediated febrile pleuro-pericarditis (Dressler's syndrome) may complicate either MI or pericardiotomy anytime within 3 months.

Pump Failure

Most in-hospital deaths from MI occur within 96 hours of admission secondary to shock and LV failure. Clinical evidence of *heart failure* develops when ≥ 20% of the LV sustains damage. (Persistent sinus tachycardia may be a hint to incipient heart failure if present ≥ 48 hours after infarction.) Fatal pump failure usually ensues when > 40% of the LV mass is infarcted or dysfunctional. The muscle mass lost is a much more powerful predictor of outcome than the anatomical location of the infarction. Contractility of ischemic but salvagable muscle may return after a period of hours to days ("stunned myocardium"). Ischemia-induced decreases in LV compliance usually require increased filling pressures to maintain stable cardiac output. Under most circumstances, a pulmonary capillary wedge pressure of 18 mmHg is optimal. Pulmonary edema should be treated with diuretics, vasodilators, and inotropic drugs as dictated by hemodynamics and ventilatory parameters. In most patients with pump failure secondary to LV infarction, reduction of afterload represents a preferred alternative—relieving pulmonary congestion while usually increasing CO. Because a substantial portion of the limited cardiac output must be diverted to the respiratory pump, mechanical ventilation can boost oxygen delivery to deprived vital organs and should be considered whenever respiratory distress becomes evident. Treatment of severe heart failure and cardiogenic shock are detailed in Chapter 3, Support of the Circulation. Unfortunately, the prognosis of cardiogenic shock remains dismal.

Right Ventricular Infarction

Right ventricular (RV) infarction is seen in up to 40% of all *inferior* MIs. Hypotension, jugular venous distention, and clear lung fields are key diagnostic features. The diagnosis may be confirmed electrocardiographically by ST segment elevation in right precordial leads (V3R and V4R). Pulmonary artery catheterization may also be confirmatory when right atrial pressures are disproportionately elevated in relation to a wedge pressure. (Hemodynamic monitoring is also useful to exclude the presence of pericardial tamponade, a condition with similar clinical appearance.) RV infarction, the result of right coronary artery occlusion, rarely occurs as an isolated event. Inferior LV infarction almost always accompanies RV infarct because LV wall thickness and afterload exceed those of the RV and because both the RV and inferior LV wall share a common blood supply.

The presenting symptom of RV infarction is hypotension, not pulmonary edema. Therefore, the treatment of the RV infarct differs in several important respects from symptomatic LV infarction. As a first priority, *the filling pressure of the right ventricle must be optimized*. This may require mean right atrial pressures > 20 mmHg to maintain an acceptably high wedge pressure and cardiac output. Once adequate RV filling has been assured cautious trials of afterload reduction and/or ionotropic drugs may also prove helpful.

Atrial infarction occurs rarely, usually in combination with infarction of the inferior wall of the left ventricle. Fed by branches of the right coronary artery, the right atrium is the most commonly affected chamber. Ischemia of the SA node and conduction pathways accounts for its *most common manifestations: bradycardia, atrial arrhythmias, and heart block*. Thrombi formed within the infarcted right atrium may embolize to the pulmonary artery.

Mitral Regurgitation

Papillary muscle dysfunction or rupture is the most common mechanical complication of MI. Mitral regurgitation (MR) has a wide range of presentations from minimal malfunction to frank rupture. *MR most commonly results from malfunction of the posterior papillary muscle* because it is fed by the single posterior descending artery while the anterior papillary muscle is supplied by branches of both the left anterior descending and circumflex arteries. Frank papillary muscle *rupture is a rare but highly lethal event* that carries a 24–hour mortality of 70%.

MR typically occurs 2–10 days following posterior or inferior MI and should be suspected in any MI patient developing a new murmur (often at the cardiac apex). The rapid onset of shock, heart failure, or pulmonary edema also suggests MR. Regurgitant flow is greatest after papillary muscle rupture and less intense when dysfunction is caused by ischemia without structural damage.

The diagnosis may be confirmed by echocardiography or pulmonary artery catheterization. Echocardiography may reveal a hyperdynamic (unloaded) LV and often visualizes a flail mitral leaflet. Doppler studies may demonstrate the regurgitant left atrial jet. Invasive monitoring is indicated in almost all MI patients who develop a new murmur, particularly if pulmonary congestion is present. Although pulmonary artery pressure

tracings usually reveal large V waves produced by retrograde flow of blood across an incompetent mitral valve, V waves are much more sensitive than specific. Ventricular septal defect, mitral stenosis, or severe heart failure occasionally mimic MR by producing large V waves.

The *primary objective in treating acute MR is to reduce left ventricular impedance* (afterload). In stable patients with mild MR, LV afterload reduction may be sufficient. However when florid pulmonary edema follows papillary muscle rupture, vasodilators (nitroprusside or nitroglycerine) and intra-aortic balloon pumping should be followed by immediate surgery.

Ventriculoseptal Defect

The ventricular septum ruptures in ≃ 1% of all MIs. Ventriculoseptal defect (VSD)-related left to right shunting reduces effective output and causes pulmonary edema. The anterior portion of the interventricular septum is predominately supplied by a single vessel (the left anterior descending) whereas the posterior portion is fed collaterally from several sources. Therefore, *post-infarction VSD is usually a consequence of an anterior MI* that involves the left anterior descending artery (LAD). Conversely, VSD developing after a (true) posterior MI is a marker of diffuse multi-vessel disease and carries a worse prognosis. Predisposing factors for post-infarct VSD include an anterior-septal MI, hypertension, female gender, advanced age, and first infarction.

In the vast majority of patients, physical examination reveals biventricular heart failure and a new murmur. The new murmur is usually loud, harsh, holosystolic, and of maximal intensity at the left lower sternal border. An accompanying thrill is common.

Pulmonary artery catheterization demonstrates an unexpected step-up in hemoglobin saturation between the right atrium and pulmonary artery (usually > 10%). Hemodynamic compromise and magnitude of the left-to-right shunt parallel the size of the defect. Echocardiography may demonstrate a VSD, particularly if Doppler techniques are used. A "bubble" echocardiogram occasionally shows bidirectional ventricular flow.

Therapy for a VSD depends upon systemic and pulmonary capillary wedge pressures. Hypotensive patients with a low wedge pressure should receive fluids initially. If the blood pressure is adequately maintained and the wedge pressure is < 18 mmHg, observation with delayed surgery minimizes operative risk. If blood pressure is adequate with a low cardiac output and an elevated wedge pressure, vasodilators are useful. If the patient is hypotensive with a high wedge pressure, temporary support by balloon pumping, ionotropes, and vasodilators should precede immediate surgical correction.

The eventual outcome of post-MI VSD is very poor, with mortality mounting to ≈ 90% at 2 months. The strategy of delaying surgical intervention (for 6 weeks) is highly questionable. Surgery probably offers less to those surviving 6 weeks than to those who die early in the course.

Free Wall Rupture

Almost invariably, rupture of the ventricular free wall is rapidly fatal. Although unusual, ventricular rupture occurs more commonly than either papillary muscle rupture or VSD; 20% of deaths due to MI result from free wall rupture. Unfortunately, therapeutic options are so limited that little attention has been accorded it. Most frequently, the anterior or lateral wall ruptures 3–6 days following the MI. Hypertension accentuates wall stress and contributes to muscle disruption at the border of the normal and infarcted tissue. Ventricular rupture is most likely in elderly patients with extensive transmural damage and little collateral flow.

The clinical presentation of wall rupture is usually one of *recurrent chest pain without ECG changes*, rapidly followed by shock and death. Differential diagnosis includes pericardial tamponade, tension pneumothorax, and massive muscle damage. Immediate thoracotomy must follow temporary stabilization with volume expansion, transfusion, and pericardiocentesis. If immediately available, echocardiography may visualize a defect of the LV wall.

Systemic Embolism

The incidence of mural thrombi and arterial embolism may reach 30% in selected subsets of patients with MI. *Large infarctions*, particularly those involving the *anterior and apical segments* of the left ventricle, predispose to systemic embolism. Patients with large infarctions, mural thrombi, or overtly dyskinetic segments on echocardiography should be anticoagulated unless contraindications are present.

Treatment

Traditionally, the therapy of MI has been primarily supportive, with close monitoring and treatment of the electrical and mechanical complications outlined above. A second therapeutic goal is to limit infarct size. This can be accomplished by mechanical or pharmacologic coronary vasodilation in conjunction with adjunctive measures to improve oxygen delivery and minimize oxygen demand. Unfortunately, therapy aimed at reducing myocardial oxygen demand (e.g., beta blockers), the inflammatory response (e.g., steroids, nonsteroidal anti-inflammatory agents), or at boosting diastolic perfusion pressure achieves little success—particularly when coronary occlusion is complete and the collateral circulation is poor.

Until recently vasodilators (e.g., nitroprusside, nitrates) and spasmolytics (Ca^{2+} channel blockers) were the only commonly employed means to improve myocardial blood flow. However, these methods are relatively poor at increasing perfusion except in small subsets of patients. Additionally, such drugs may be detrimental if they redistribute blood flow away from ischemic areas or significantly lower coronary perfusion pressure. Therefore, in recent years thrombolysis, angioplasty, and coronary surgery have assumed increased importance. Although the specific approach varies with the expertise of the cardiology and surgical services, it is generally agreed that any effort to reperfuse jeopardized myocardium must be undertaken urgently. Myocardial reperfusion is the preferred method of alleviating chest pain, but direct analgesia (e.g., morphine) may be necessary. Anemia and hypoxemia should not be overlooked as methods of correcting ischemia.

The oxygen required by the heart muscle can be reduced by lowering total body oxygen consumption and by decreasing myocardial wall stress, a parameter influenced by the "triple product" of heart rate, contractility, and blood pressure.

General Support

In the supportive phase of management measures are taken to minimize stress. A liquid diet is usually provided for 24 hours following infarction. Temperature extremes of foods are avoided to minimize the risk of arrhythmias. Sedation and stool softeners to prevent anxiety and straining may also decrease the risk of arrhythmias. Subcutaneous heparin is indicated for the prevention of deep venous thrombosis in patients with MI at strict bed rest.

Thrombolytic Therapy

If angiography is promptly performed (< 4 hr), the vast majority (≈ 85%) of patients sustaining acute MI have acute coronary thrombosis. This finding has prompted the development of thrombolytic agents aimed at clot dissolution. Three agents, streptokinase (SK), urokinase (UK), and tissue plasminogen activator (TPA), are currently approved for use. All three agents accelerate conversion of plasminogen to plasmin, an enzyme that attacks fibin. In addition, accelerated thrombolysis usually produces a hypocoagulable state by reducing circulating levels of most clotting proteins (especially fibrinogen). TPA differs from UK or SK in that it binds to fibrin in preformed clots and produces only a *local* fibrinolytic effect. Its very short circulating half-life and a local mechanism of action probably result in less marked reductions in serum fibrinogen and fewer hemorrhagic complications. To prevent ischemic myocardium from becoming necrotic, thrombolysis must occur promptly ($< 4–6$ hr). Reperfusion within 2–4 hours improves survival and limits infarct size, thereby maximizing post-infarct ventricular performance. Because thrombosis usually involves portions of the coronary circulation previously narrowed by atherosclerosis, surgical measures (e.g., angioplasty, coronary artery bypass) are often required to assure long-term patency, even when thrombolysis is initially successful.

Although thombolysis transiently reperfuses the occluded coronary in $\simeq 75\%$ of patients, the therapy suffers from many limitations. SK is a foreign protein that predisposes to allergic and anaphylactic reactions. This risk is minimized by using TPA or UK, but all three agents suffer from the tendency to induce bleeding. Contraindications to use include: (1) active bleeding; (2) history of central nervous system (CNS) disease (stroke, arteriovenous malformation, surgery, tumor, or head trauma) especially if recent; (3) underlying coagulopathy; (4) severe uncontrolled hypertension; (5) recent (< 14 days) invasive procedure or operation (producing a site at which potential bleeding could not be tamponaded); (6) recent cardiopulmonary resuscitation; (7) left heart thrombus. SK is also contraindicated in patients with a known history of recent streptococcal infection.

Although bleeding may occur with any of these drugs, it is most common in patients given high doses for prolonged periods and in those with impaired platelet function or breached vascular integrity. Intracoronary (IC) injection is probably associated with fewer bleeding complications than intravenous therapy but does not appear to be substantially more effective. Furthermore, IC injection may cause an unacceptable delay in the initiation of therapy if a catheterization team must be assembled. Administration via the IC route offers the option of subsequent angioplasty if lytic therapy is unsuccessful or residual high-grade coronary obstruction remains. Obviously, IC therapy carries the same risks as any coronary catheterization.

Percutaneous Coronary Angioplasty

Percutaneous coronary angioplasty (PTCA) is the most rapid method of restoring coronary flow through amenable (proximal) coronary occlusions. Unfortunately, few patients present promptly enough to benefit from acute PTCA. Furthermore, only a small number of tertiary care hospitals have the resources to rapidly assemble an experienced team and perform PTCA within the 4–6 hour window required to assure reasonable myocardial salvage. Such limitations make intravenous thrombolytic therapy the preferred option for reperfusion in most patients. Present data suggest that PTCA of residual stenosis can be safely deferred for $\simeq 24$ hours following thrombolysis. Elective PTCA following thrombolysis is also associated with lower rates of acute reocclusion and chronic restenosis. Despite its limitations, emergency PTCA retains a role in patients who cannot receive or who have failed to improve with thrombolytic therapy. Additionally, in some centers, coronary reocclusion following thrombolysis due to high-grade residual stenosis is approached with PTCA. Recurrent unstable angina or MI following initially successful reperfusion with maximal anticoagulation and antianginal therapy is often treated with PTCA.

Coronary Artery Bypass Grafting

As with other forms of reperfusion, surgery must re-establish blood flow within 6 hours of the onset of symptoms if it is to be successful. Because coronary artery bypass grafting (CABG) requires preoperative coronary angiography, many patients may be reperfused with PTCA, alleviating the need for acute surgery. However, in some patients demonstrating *multivessel high-grade* stenosis, CABG is often the better option. Patients with cardiogenic shock as a result of proximal coronary occlusion (usually left main or LAD) who require intra-aortic balloon assistance are also candidates for CABG. Thus, in patients with single-vessel occlusions, acute CABG is usually reserved for patients failing both thrombolysis and PTCA and in whom adequate time remains to revascularize the ischemic area. CABG in such a setting may be complicated by thrombolytic drug-induced coagulopathy. CABG after 4–6 hours is unlikely to salvage myocardium and is associated with higher morbidity and mortality.

Beta Blockade

Beta blockers reduce infarct size and improve survival rates by lowering myocardial oxygen consumption through reductions in both heart rate and blood pressure.

Beta-blockers also exert independent antiarrhythmic effects. A large number of studies suggest that intravenous beta blockade given early in the course of MI reduces *early* (first week) mortality. Mortality statistics are improved because of lower rates of reinfarction, cardiac rupture, and life-threatening arrhythmias. Long-term (1–2 yr) beta blocker therapy also improves the risk of death from cardiac events. Such reductions are mostly the result of a lower rate of *sudden* cardiac death. If feasible, the early administration of 5–10 mg of propranolol, atenolol, or metoprolol by *slow* intravenous infusion followed by chronic oral therapy provides the maximal survival advantage. Despite the apparent benefits of beta blockers, many patients with MI are unable to tolerate their most common side effects—bronchospasm, heart failure, and conduction system disturbances. Intravenous dosing of beta blockers must be closely monitored and the drug discontinued if marked bradycardia, hypotension, or increased AV block develop.

Calcium Channel Blockers

Although highly effective for reversing coronary spasm and beneficial in relieving pain in many patients with coronary thrombosis, Ca^{2+} blockers (nifedipine, verapamil) have not improved survival in multiple clinical trials. Therefore, their routine use in MI cannot be advocated.

Outcome of Myocardial Infarction

Overall, MI carries a mortality of 10–20%. Most deaths due to myocardial infarction are the result of prehospital arrhythmias, which to a large degree cannot be prevented. Conversely, most deaths in patients reaching the hospital result from refractory pump failure. Therefore, survival is improved by limiting infarct size and by promptly treating mechanical and electrical complications. Survival is best predicted by the patient's *age* and degree of *left ventricular impairment* (a reflection of the volume of lost myocardium).

SUGGESTED READINGS

1. Cintron GB, Hernandez E, Linares E: Bedside recognition, incidence and clinical course of right ventricular infarction. *Am J Cardiol* 47:224–227, 1981.
2. Cohn JN, et al: Right ventricular infarction. Clinical and hemodynamic features. *Am J Cardiol* 33:209–214, 1974.
3. Epstein SE, Palmeri ST, Patterson RE: Evaluation of patients with acute myocardial infarction. Indications for cardiac catheterization and surgical intervention. *N Engl J Med* 307:1487–1492, 1982.
4. Forrester JS, Diamond GA, Swan HJC: Correlative classification of clinical and hemodynamic function after myocardial infarction. *Am J Cardiol* 39:137–145, 1977.
5. Meister SG, Helfant RH: Rapid bedside differentiation of ruptured interventricular septum from acute mitral insufficiency. *N Engl J Med* 287:1024–1025, 1972.
6. Mueller HS, Roberts R, Teichman SL, et al: Thrombolytic therapy in acute myocardial infarction: Part 1. *Med Clin No Am* 72:197–226, 1988.
7. Roberts R (ed): Early intervention after acute myocardial infarction -an ACCP concensus conference. *Chest* 93(Suppl):1S-32S, 1988.
8. Yusuf S, Collins R: IV nitroglycerin and nitroprusside therapy in acute myocardial infarction reduces mortality. Evidence from randomized controlled trials (abstr). *Circulation* 72:Suppl III 224, 1985.
9. Yusuf S, Peto R, Lewis J, et al: Beta blockade during and after myocardial infarction: an overview of the randomized trials. *Prog Cardiovas Dis* 27:335–71, 1985.

18 Hypertensive Emergencies

DEFINITIONS

Diastolic blood pressures > 120 mmHg without evidence of end-organ injury define *accelerated hypertension* (AH). The diagnosis of *malignant hypertension* (MH) is made in patients with comparable elevations of blood pressure who exhibit overt organ damage. Organ damage in MH is due to a necrotizing vasculitis that produces ischemia by small-vessel occlusion. MH is most common in smokers, younger patients, black males, and patients with secondary hypertension (e.g., renovascular). Ninety percent of *untreated* patients with MH are dead within 1 year of the diagnosis, most commonly from uremia, heart failure, or stroke.

In MH, the systemic blood pressure (BP) frequently exceeds 200/130 mmHg; however, similar elevations can be observed in other clinical situations. *Retinopathy*, a sensitive monitor of organ injury, is the sine qua non distinguishing MH from AH. *Papilledema*, *exudates*, *flame hemorrhages*, and *arteriolar constriction* characterize the retinopathy of MH and correlate well with renal involvement. After control of BP, retinal hemorrhages and papilledema resolve or heal over weeks to months.

Patients with MH are usually symptomatic but have nonspecific complaints. Headache occurs in $\simeq 85\%$ of patients and blurred vision in $> 50\%$. Cardiac symptoms (angina, congestive heart failure) are a common presentation, whereas nausea, vomiting, and focal neurological deficits are distinctly uncommon.

Objective evidence of ventricular enlargement or renal insufficiency (serum creatinine > 3.5 mg/dl) is present in about ¼ of cases. The urinalysis commonly shows albuminuria, hematuria, and cast formation. The peripheral blood smear may demonstrate microangiopathic hemolysis. Hypokalemic alkalosis frequently occurs as a result of

secondary hyperaldosteronism consequent to diuretic usage.

TREATMENT PRINCIPLES OF SEVERE HYPERTENSION

Malignant Hypertension

The aggressiveness of antihypertensive therapy should be guided by symptomatology and evidence for organ damage, not by the absolute values of recorded BP. Patients requiring immediate treatment should be admitted to an intensive care unit for closely monitored therapy. An arterial catheter should be inserted for accurate BP measurement in most patients receiving parenteral antihypertensives (see p. 166). Whenever possible, *oral therapy* should be initiated concurrently to minimize the duration of intravenous drug administration.

When myocardial infarction, aortic dissection, pulmonary edema, cerebral hemorrhage, or hypertensive encephalopathy complicate MH, steps should be taken to lower the mean BP to $\simeq 120$ mmHg within minutes.

Rapidly progressive renal failure, borderline left ventricular failure, or recent myocardial infarction present a less threatening problem and mandate less urgent treatment, with the aim of reducing BP more gradually over 6–12 hours.

Accelerated Hypertension

Although important to reverse quickly, AH does not present the same therapeutic crisis as MH. In contrast to MH, AH does not always require parenteral treatment; many oral regimens are successful. Most recently, oral nifedipine has been used effectively for this purpose. The BP usually starts to fall quickly, with peak action occurring at $\simeq 30$ minutes. The effects of oral or sublingual nifedipine are due primarily to gastric absorption; therefore, ''squirt and swallow'' or ''chew and swallow'' techniques that accelerate gastric absorption result in the most rapid onset of action. Patients with the highest BP show the largest declines in response to nifedipine. As a side benefit, coronary dilating properties may help to prevent myocardial ischemia.

SPECIFIC PROBLEMS IN HYPERTENSION

Hypertensive Encephalopathy

Hypertensive encephalopathy (HE) is a central nervous system (CNS) vasculopathy that usually occurs in patients with chronic hypertension whose diastolic BP suddenly exceeds 130 mmHg. This serious problem may complicate either MH or AH. In pregnancy or glomerulonephritis, this syndrome may occur with BP as low as 160/100 mmHg. The rapidity of increase in BP is as important as the absolute level. HE must be distinguished from other treatable disorders including ischemic or hemorrhagic stroke, hypoglycemia, subarachnoid hemorrhage, meningitis, encephalitis, brain tumors, and seizures. The distinction may be difficult because many of these conditions may be accompanied by secondary elevations of BP.

Headache is the most common complaint in HE, followed by nausea, vomiting, blurred vision, and confusion. Focal neurological deficits, including hemiparesis and cranial nerve palsies (particularly of the facial nerve) may also be seen. Arteritis of the vessels nourishing the optic nerve (not increased intracranial pressure) produces the papilledema seen in most cases of HE. The sine qua non of HE is rapid mental clearing in response to BP control.

There are no specific laboratory findings in HE. For example, the electroencephalographic features are nondiagnostic, and although the opening pressure recorded during a lumbar tap may be elevated, the fluid analysis is usually unremarkable.

The goal of therapy in HE is to lower the BP to "safe" levels as quickly as possible with nitroprusside (NP), diazoxide, or trimethaphan (TMP). A diastolic blood pressure of 100 mmHg (mean 120 mmHg) is an appropriate target that must not be undershot.

Normally, cerebral blood flow (CBF) is auto-regulated to maintain constant perfusion over a wide range of mean arterial pressures (Fig. 18.1). Failure of cerebral auto-regulation may allow excessive perfusion (resulting in cerebral edema) or transient periods of hypoperfusion and ischemia. Normal auto-regulatory mechanisms are modified by the presence of chronic hypertension, making

mean arterial pressures of 100–120 mmHg necessary for adequate cerebral perfusion. Therefore, it is important not to lower perfusion pressure excessively.

Aortic Dissection

Aortic dissection should be suspected in MH when there are characteristic symptoms (e.g., tearing chest or back pain) and an arm/leg BP difference, absent pulses in the lower extremities, or asymmetry in BP between arms. *Artifactual hypotension* may result if blood flow to the left subclavian artery is compromised by dissection. The goal of BP reduction is to immediately *decrease both mean BP and the rate of increase in systolic pressure (dP/dt)* while preserving vital organ perfusion. Reducing dP/dt decreases the shear force on the aortic wall, helping to limit dissection. Reduction in dP/dt can be achieved by beta-adrenergic or ganglionic blockade. Unfortunately beta blockade alone does not usually provide a sufficiently rapid reduction in BP. Therefore, a beta-blocker used in conjunction with NP or TMP alone are appropriate regimens.

Renal Failure

Perfusion-related and reversible increases in creatinine (Cr) and blood urea nitrogen (BUN) frequently follow BP reduction in AH or MH. In this setting, re-establishing a safe BP is the main priority. Although other reversible causes (dehydration, renal artery occlusion, lower tract obstruction) should be sought, an increasing BUN or Cr should not dissuade the clinician from continuing antihypertensive therapy. In patients presenting with Cr > 3.5 mg/dl, progressive *renal failure* is a likely and often unavoidable consequence of therapy.

Pulmonary Edema

In most cases of MH, pulmonary edema is primarily the result of excessive LV afterload and usually responds rapidly when systemic vascular resistance is lowered. Heightened afterload is most likely to cause pulmonary edema in patients with pre-existing left ventricular dysfunction or aortic insufficiency. In general, therapy should focus on reduction of afterload, not on reduction of preload.

Cerebral Ischemia and Hemorrhage

Sudden onset of focal neurological deficits, obtundation, headache, and vomiting are the most frequent symptoms of cerebral hemorrhage. Auto-regulation is lost in areas of acute bleeding or ischemic infarction. The role for BP reduction in

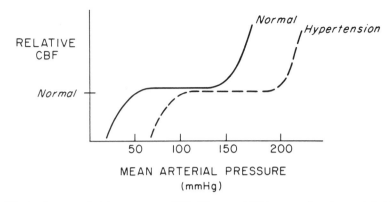

Figure 18.1   Effects of mean arterial pressure on CBF. Whereas CBF is normally auto-regulated in the range of 50–150 mmHg, chronic hypertension shifts this curve rightward and necessitates a higher minimal pressure for adequate flow.

patients with *bland cerebral infarction* is unknown, but in the absence of effective auto-regulation, limiting hypertension may salvage areas bordering the infarct. Excessive reductions in BP may worsen CNS deficits.

Without a predisposing anatomic abnormality, hypertension alone rarely results in *subarachnoid hemorrhage*. However, blood may enter the subarachnoid space of patients with *intracerebral hemorrhage* by dissecting via the internal capsule or putamen into the lateral ventricles. The sedative effects of clonidine, methyldopa, and reserpine impair monitoring of mental status and should be avoided in patients with cerebral complications of hypertension. Diazoxide is also a poor choice, because it decreases CBF disproportionately. Indeed, except for hypertensive encephalopathy, diazoxide is contraindicated in cerebral disorders complicating hypertension.

Angina and Myocardial Infarction

In acute myocardial ischemia, reductions in BP preserve endangered myocardium by decreasing wall stress and increasing myocardial perfusion. In MH and myocardial ischemia, unopposed use of drugs that produce tachycardia and increase myocardial oxygen consumption (arterial vasodilators) should be avoided. Caution should also be used with nitroprusside, a drug that tends to divert blood away from the most ischemic areas of myocardium. Calcium channel blockers and beta blockers are attractive options because they improve the ratio of oxygen supply to demand. Nitroglycerin, primarily a venodilator, affects both peripheral and coronary circulations, thereby reducing preload and decreasing BP. The specific conditions for use of antihypertensives are listed in Table 18.1.

Catecholamine Excesses

Conditions resulting in catecholamine-induced hypertension include: (1) pheochromocytoma; (2) cocaine overdose; (3) monoamine oxidase (MAO) inhibitor crisis; and (4) antihypertensive withdrawal syndrome. Patients with these disorders commonly present with tachycardia, pallor, pounding headache, and vomiting.

Rebound hypertension is especially common in intensive care unit patients following abrupt discontinuation of antihypertensive drugs. Although this syndrome is most frequently associated with the centrally acting alpha agents (clonidine, methyldopa, and guanabenz), withdrawal of beta blockers may also produce rebound hypertension. Such drugs probably should not be given to noncompliant patients and, when discontinued, should be tapered over several days.

Used alone, beta-blockers are contraindicated in catecholamine excess because unopposed alpha effects may paradoxically worsen hypertension. Alpha adrenergic blockers (e.g., phentolamine) or direct vasodilators (e.g., NP) are the mainstays of therapy.

PARENTERAL THERAPY FOR HYPERTENSIVE EMERGENCIES

Diuretics

Because *most patients with severe hypertension have normal or reduced circulating blood volume*, diuretics should be avoided in the emergency setting unless overt signs of heart failure, pulmonary edema, or fluid overload are present. (In more chronic usage, however, most antihypertensive agents tend to cause sodium retention and should be used in conjunction with a diuretic.)

Table 18.1
Antihypertensives in Specific Conditions

Condition	Preferred Drugs	Drugs to Avoid

Dissecting aneurysm	Trimethaphan
	Nitroprusside + beta blocker
		Direct vasodilators alone
		  (Nitroprusside, Diazoxide,
		  Hydralazine)

Pulmonary edema	Nitroprusside Nitrates	Beta blockers Trimethaphan Labetalol
Angina/MI (without CHF)	Beta blockers* Nitrates Calcium blockers	Direct vasodilators Phentolamine
Cerebral hemorrhage	Nitroprusside Trimethaphan	Methyldopa Clonidine Diazoxide
Hypertensive encephalopathy	Nitroprusside Diazoxide	Methyldopa Clonidine
Catecholamine excess states	Phentolamine Trimethaphan Nitroprusside + beta blocker*	Beta blockers alone Diazoxide Labetalol

*Contraindicated in patients with CHF.

Nitroprusside

NP is a direct-acting arteriovenous dilator with an immediate onset of action (usually < 1 minute) and the potential for rapid termination of action (1–3 minutes). The photoinstability of NP mandates frequent changes of solutions and use of light-protected containers. Infusion is started at a dose of 0.5 μg/kg/min and titrated upward to produce the desired BP. Doses required for hypertension are generally higher than those required for the treatment of congestive heart failure but should not exceed 10 μg/kg/min. Because of its potency, controlled administration by pump infusion is mandatory. At low dosage rates, reductions in systemic resistance are compensated by increases in cardiac output. Thus, BP may initially remain stable despite a beneficial action; actual reduction of BP often requires dosing in the higher range. The effects of NP are most pronounced in patients taking multiple antihypertensive drugs and those who are volume depleted.

NP is hepatically metabolized to thiocyanate, which is then cleared renally. Thus, renal failure may result in thiocyanate toxicity. Levels > 10mg/dl may cause hepatic failure, metabolic acidosis, dyspnea, and vomiting. Cyanide may accumulate in hepatic failure, but toxicity is very rare when NP is administered at doses < 3 μg/kg/min for < 72 hours. Nitrates, cyanocobalamin, and thiosulfate are useful in the treatment of thiocyanate toxicity.

Diazoxide

Diazoxide, a direct arteriolar vasodilator, frequently induces hypotension when given suddenly in !arge (5 mg/kg) doses. Recent studies have shown that a "mini-bolus" technique is equally effective and rarely produces hypotension. Intravenous boluses of 1–2 mg/kg (given at 10-minute intervals) and constant infusion (at rates of up to 15 mg/min) are alternative methods of administration. With an onset of action of 1–2 minutes and a mean duration of action of 8 hours, diazoxide is useful in patients who cannot be monitored on a minute-to-minute basis.

Nausea and vomiting are common side effects of diazoxide, limiting its usefulness in patients with altered levels of consciousness. Furthermore, cerebral perfusion may be reduced disproportionately to BP. Reflex increases in heart rate make diazoxide alone a poor choice in patients with ischemic heart disease or aortic aneurysm. The potent fluid-retaining properties of diazoxide almost always require the concurrent use of diuretics after BP has been controlled. Hyperglycemia and hyperuricemia are other common side effects.

Labetalol

Labetalol is a combined alpha and beta blocker with rapid onset but variable duration of action

(1–8 hours). A significant advantage is the rarity of ''overshoot hypotension''. An initial bolus of 20 mg is almost always effective in lowering BP, whereas doses of 20–80 mg at 20–40-minute intervals provide continued BP control. Labetalol is available in tablet form, facilitating conversion from intravenous to oral therapy. The primary disadvantage of labetalol lies in its potential to exacerbate heart failure or bronchospasm.

Trimethaphan

TMP, a ganglionic blocker, exerts direct peripheral vasodilating effects. Although its rapid onset (1–2 minutes) is desirable, the sustained (10-minute) duration of action may be problematic in patients who develop hypotension in response to an excessive dose. Like NP, TMP must be administered by an infusion pump because of its potency. Severe orthostatic hypotension is seen in almost all patients receiving the drug, and positional sensitivity should be kept in mind when difficulty is encountered in obtaining precise BP control. Tachyphylaxis limits its efficacy to 3–4 days. TMP routinely reduces cardiac output and renal blood flow. Furthermore, parasympathetic blockade may result in such distressing symptoms

as dry mouth, blurred vision, constipation, and abdominal distention.

Hydralazine

The action of hydralazine, a direct vasodilator, begins within 10 minutes if given intravenously and within 30 minutes if given intramuscularly. Unfortunately, its prolonged duration of action (3–6 hours) may cause persistent overshoot hypotension. *Because hydralazine is not consistently effective at lowering BP*, it is a poor choice for acute treatment of life-threatening hypertension. Unless counteracted by a beta-blocker, the arteriolar dilating effects of hydralazine often result in reflex tachycardia and contractility, thereby worsening coronary ischemia and aortic dissection.

Methyldopa

Methyldopa is a long-acting central sympatholytic with a delayed onset of action (2–4 hours). Its delayed action and tendency to cause sedation make it undesirable for use in hypertensive emergencies. However, in patients with non-life-threatening AH, methyldopa has the advantage of lowering blood pressure gradually (over several hours). Overshoot hypotension is uncommon.

Table 18.2
Parenteral Drug Therapy in Severe Hypertension*

Drug	Site of Vasodilation	Advantages	Side Effects/Problems
Nitroprusside	Direct dilator (balanced)	Immediate action Easy to titrate No CNS effects	Hypotension Reflex tachycardia Cyanide toxicity Methemoglobinemia
Nitroglycerin	Direct dilator (venous > arterial)	Coronary dilator	Headache Absorbed into some intravenous tubing ETOH vehicle
Hydralazine	Direct dilator (arterial >> venous)	No CNS effects	Reflex tachycardia Lupus syndrome
Diazoxide	Direct dilator (arterial >> venous)	Rapid action Not sedating	Imprecise dosing Reflex tachycardia Hyperglycemia Hyperuricemia
Trimethaphan	Ganglionic blocker (balanced)	Aortic aneurysm Subarachnoid	Anticholinergic effects ↓ cardiac output
Phentolamine	Alpha blocker + direct vasodilator (balanced)	Pheochromocytoma MAO crisis	Reflex tachycardia Tachyphylaxis
Labetalol	Alpha and beta blockers	No "overshoot" hypotension Maintained cardiac output, heart rate	Exacerbation of CHF, asthma, AV block

*Abbreviations: ETOH, alcohol; MAO, monoamine oxidase; AV, atrioventricular.

Phentolamine

Phentolamine is an alpha blocking drug with an abrupt onset of action (1–2 minutes). Its twin effects of alpha blockade and non-alpha-mediated vasodilation precipitate hypotension, tachycardia, nausea, and vomiting in a large percentage of patients who receive it. Associated reflex tachycardia may worsen coronary ischemia.

Parenteral Drug Therapy in Severe Hypertension

The advantages and disadvantages of parenteral drug therapy for severe hypertension are listed in Table 18.2.

SUGGESTED READINGS

1. Huysmans FTM, et al: Acute treatment of hypertensive crisis with nifedipine. *Br J Clin Pharmacol* 16:725–727, 1983.
2. Huysmans FTM, Thien TA, Koene RAP: Combined intravenous administration of diazoxide and beta-blocking agent in acute treatment of severe hypertension or hypertensive crisis. *Am Heart J* 103:395–400, 1982.
3. Lavin P: Management of hypertension in patients with acute stroke. *Arch Intern Med* 146:66–68, 1986.
4. Ram CVS: Hypertensive encephalopathy—recognition and management. *Arch Intern Med* 138:1851–1853, 1978.

19 Venous Thrombosis and Pulmonary Embolism

DEFINITIONS AND MECHANISMS

Pulmonary embolism (PE) may result when any insoluble substance gains access to the systemic veins. Because blood filtering is a natural function of the lung, asymptomatic embolism may occur periodically, even in healthy persons. Distinctive syndromes have been described for embolism of air, oil, fat, tumor cells, amniotic fluid, foreign objects, and injected particulates, as well as for bland and infected fibrin clots. In critical care, *fat embolism*, *septic embolism*, and *bland thrombotic embolism* are the major syndromes of interest.

Oil or fat embolism (during lymphangiography or trauma to long bones) does not impede blood flow. Rather, symptoms develop because the fatty acid products of lipid digestion produce vascular injury, capillary leak, and edema (adult respiratory distress syndrome, ARDS) (see p. 179).

Similarly, the major threat to life in *septic embolism* is not vascular obstruction. Small friable fragments of infected material embolize to cause fever, toxicity, and a characteristic radiograph: multiple ill-defined infiltrates or nodules of varied sizes that frequently cavitate and usually display soft, irregular outlines. Perfusion defects on lung scan are unimpressive compared to the radiograph. Pelvic inflammation, venous catheters or right heart valves, phlebitis, and nonsterile injections (related to drug abuse) are common sources of infected material. After identification, the source must be surgically isolated or removed and the infection treated vigorously with antibiotics directed at the offending organism.

Among the most frequent preventable causes of sudden death in hospitalized patients, *bland pulmonary embolism* is a disease that requires skillful integration of clinical and laboratory data. Its subtlety requires considerable judgment regarding the need for invasive pursuit of the diagnosis.

DEEP VENOUS THROMBOSIS

Diagnosis

Predisposing Factors

Stasis of venous blood, *injury to the vascular intima*, and *hypercoagulability* characterize high-risk patients. Thus, bed rest, immobilization, chronic venous disease, trauma, sepsis, and heart failure are common predisposing factors. Hypercoagulability associated with systemic lupus, or deficiencies of antithrombin III, and proteins C or S should be suspected in patients without other recognized risk factors and in those with a personal or family history of recurrent thrombosis. The vast majority of pulmonary emboli result from deep venous thrombosis (DVT) *above* the knee. Clot confined to the calf is of little physiologic importance. Approximately $1/3$ of *calf* thrombi propogate above the knee. Of thrombi in the thigh veins, again $\approx$ $1/3$ produce symptomatic PE.

Indwelling central venous catheters provide an iatrogenic source of emboli in critically ill patients. Embolization is particularly likely to occur upon catheter withdrawal. Heparin treated catheters may be temporarily exempt from thrombosis until the heparin is leached out (24–36 hours).

Physical Examination

Superficial thrombophlebitis manifested by erythema, tenderness, and a palpable "venous cord" poses little embolic risk unless it extends to the deep system. Such extension is strongly suggested by generalized and asymmetric leg swelling, a highly unusual feature of uncomplicated superficial inflammation.

The signs of DVT relate to inflammation and obstruction. Unilateral lower extremity erythema, heat, swelling, and pain are suggestive, as are unilateral ankle and leg edema. Unfortunately, neither inflammation nor obstruction may be present or

168

obvious, and other processes unrelated to thrombosis may cause the same findings. At least half of large vessel clots go unsuspected on physical examination. The Homans' sign is a non-specific indicator of calf inflammation, seldom present in DVT.

Several common conditions mimic DVT. A ruptured *Baker's cyst* presents as a mass in the calf with pain and erythema, usually in patients with rheumatoid arthritis. *Rupture of the plantaris tendon* may also mimic DVT on examination but history reveals recent exertion with the *acute onset* of excruciating pain. *Crystalline arthritis* (gout or pseudogout) may produce intense joint space inflammation that extends into the calf. *Cellulitis* seen in the setting of direct trauma, chronic fungal infection of the feet, or coronary bypass surgery is the condition most commonly confused with DVT. *Pulmonary osteoarthropathy* presents with pain, tenderness, and swelling over the *anterior* tibia, with or without clubbing. Diagnosis is confirmed radiographically. In patients with hemophilia or those taking anticoagulants, *hematoma* formation in the muscles of the calf may also produce a syndrome clinically similar to DVT. *Post-phlebitic syndrome* usually presents with recurrent *painless calf swelling* following an episode of DVT.

Diagnostic Methods

Iodine-131 fibrinogen scanning is a sensitive technique for detecting active fibrinogen turnover in the calf veins of nonheparinized patients. Unfortunately, it is expensive, time consuming, and carries the potential for hepatitis. *Doppler ultrasound* is a flow-probing method that, when positive, accurately predicts large vein obstruction, unless compromised by low cardiac output or central venous congestion. It is not as sensitive as iodine-131 fibrinogen scanning in detecting nonobstructive clots. *Impedance plethysmography* (IPG) has the same low rate of false-positive results as the Doppler technique and somewhat better sensitivity. It depends upon changes in the electrical conductance of the leg that occur as the venous circulation is obstructed, then released. In current practice, IPG is perhaps the screening test with the highest yield/morbidity ratio. Unfortunately, IPG cannot diagnose pelvic disease and is insensitive to calf vein thrombosis.

Occasionally diagnostic, the *radionuclide venogram* is well worth doing in patients undergoing lung scan, since both studies can be obtained with the same isotope injection. Sensitivity and specificity, however, are not comparable to a contrast study, especially at or below mid-thigh level. The *contrast phlebogram* is simultaneously the most sensitive, definitive, time-consuming, and potentially injurious method for defining clots of the deep veins. Unfortunately, vein patency neither assures that emboli will not recur nor guarantees that an intraluminal clot did not break free or recanalize before the study. Furthermore, contrast may precipitate renal insufficiency, allergic reactions, and local phlebitis. It is most useful in separating large vessel occlusion from cellulitis or other causes of swelling and inflammation in the extremities.

Prevention of Deep Venous Thrombosis

Subcutaneous ("*minidose*") *heparin* is of proven benefit in general surgery patients. Those recovering from hip or prostatic surgery do not appear to benefit, however. Other patients at high risk for embolism may be helped, but the data are less convincing. Subcutaneous heparin causes symptomatic thrombocytopenia in a small fraction of patients but does not routinely prolong clotting tests. Other agents such as aspirin and dipyridamole have not been shown to be effective.

Prevention is the most important treatment of DVT. A major step toward this goal is *early postoperative ambulation* and *minimizing* the period of *bed rest*. Venous stockings or pneumatic compression devices promote venous flow and may decrease stasis in surgical patients who must avoid anticoagulation. Before a compressive device is applied for prophylaxis, an active clotting process must be ruled out. Prophylactic fixed dose subcutaneous heparin (5000 units every 8–12 hours) is a highly effective method of preventing DVT but is inadequate treatment for pre-formed clot. Such low dose therapy does not predictably prolong the partial thromboplastin time (PTT) or cause hemorrhagic complications. In some surgical procedures (e.g., hip or knee replacement), preoperative warfarin (Coumadin) effectively reduces the risk of DVT without increasing bleeding complications. Dextran infusions also reduce the risk of DVT but frequent side effects (e.g., aggravation of bleeding tendency) limit their use.

Treatment of DVT

The goals of treatment in DVT are to prevent clot extension and subsequent pulmonary embolism, preserve the venous architecture and relieve pain. Continuous heparin infusions maintaining the PTT at 1.5 to 2.5 times the control value are indicated for established DVT, unless the contraindications to anticoagulation are compelling. The "clot burden" of DVT is usually less than that in PE. Therefore, patients with DVT usually require less daily heparin than patients with PE. Because the treatment of DVT and pulmonary embolism is essentially the same, the diagnosis of either usually obviates the need to search for the other condition. There is no certain advantage in maintaining the PTT > 2 times control value, and doing so *may* increase the risk of bleeding. (Spontaneous hemorrhage is rare unless there is breeched vascular integrity, impaired platelet function, or massive heparin overdose.) PTT values < 1.5 times the control value are associated with an increased likelihood of recurring DVT or PE. Heparin should be continued for a full 7–10 days to allow thrombus organization and endothelialization. Warfarin is begun several days before stopping heparin to maintain effective anticoagulation without a therapeutic break. A prothrombin time (PT) kept 1.5–2.5 times control will prevent clot recurrence. Warfarin is usually recommended for 6–12 weeks following an uncomplicated episode of DVT.

PULMONARY EMBOLISM

Many critically ill patients die *with* PEs, if not *from* them. Perhaps as many as 1/3 of patients with untreated, symptomatic PE succumb to a fatal recurrence. The diagnosis of PE is often elusive because of the non-specificity of symptoms, physiologic disturbances, physical findings, and radiographic features.

Symptoms and Physical Findings

Signs and symptoms are modified in severity and duration by underlying cardiopulmonary status. No symptom or physical finding is either universal or specific. Therefore, when PE is suspected, the patient must be treated empirically or the diagnosis confirmed by specialized diagnostic testing. The symptoms of embolism resolve rapidly, usually in the first few hours or days after the event. Signs disappear more slowly. In the Urokinase Cooperative Trial of patients with massive and submassive emboli, the following were observed: dyspnea and tachypnea (90%); pleuritic pain (70%); apprehension, rales, and cough (50%); and hemoptysis (30%). Tachycardia (> 100/min) and fever occurred in a significant minority of cases (Ref. 7).

Pleural pain (and infarction) is most likely to be caused by emboli of moderate size occurring in patients with pre-existant heart or lung disease. Syncope usually results from massive embolism.

Pulmonary artery pressures do not rise markedly unless the embolism obstructs > 50% of the capillary bed or the capillary bed was previously compromised. Hence, a right-sided gallop and increased pulmonic component of the second heart sound (P_2) correlate with massive acute obstruction, or moderate obstruction in a patient with underlying vascular disease.

Pleural Effusion

Effusions occur in approximately half of all cases; most (but not all) are exudative. A bloody effusion before anticoagulation suggests infarction, or an alternative diagnosis (tuberculosis, malignancy, trauma). Embolic effusions tend to appear *early* and tend to be *unilateral*. Most are small or moderate in volume.

Routine Diagnostic Tests

Routine diagnostic tests (chest x-ray, electrocardiogram, blood gases, leukocyte count) are most useful to exclude alternative diagnoses (e.g., pneumonia, pneumothorax, myocardial infarction, and pulmonary edema).

Electrocardiogram

The electrocardiogram (ECG) is sensitive but nonspecific. Even in patients without prior cardiopulmonary disease, the ECG is normal in only a small proportion. Nonspecific ST and/or T wave changes occur in the majority of patients. Except for moderate sinus tachycardia, rhythm disturbances are unusual. Atrial fibrillation and flutter seldom occur in patients without preexisting cardiovascular compromise. Similarly, bundle branch block is highly unusual. Left and right bundles are affected equally often. ECG evidence of acute cor pulmonale (S-I, Q-III, T-III pattern, or acute right bundle branch block) appears only in patients with severe vascular obstruction.

Blood Studies

Although hypoxemia is the rule, partial pressure of arterial oxygen (PaO_2) (corrected for the effect of hyperventilation by the alveolar gas equation) exceeds 80 mmHg in 10% or more of patients with submassive or massive embolism.

Biochemical tests, fibrinogen, and fibrin-split-product assays rarely assist in diagnosis. Although lactic dehydrogenase (LDH), serum glutamic oxaloacetic transaminase (SGOT), and bilirubin are each occasionally elevated, this "classical" triad is both unusual and not entirely specific.

Chest X-ray

Nonspecific findings, including consolidation, elevated hemidiaphragm, small pleural effusion, and atelectasis, are frequent. Indeed, the chest x-ray (CXR) remains unchanged from the pre-event film in less than half of all patients. More specific features, including segmental oligemia (Westermark's sign) and Hampton's hump (a wedge shaped peripheral density resulting from pulmonary infarction), are unusual.

Infiltrate may represent parenchymal hemorrhage (resolving rapidly without effusion) or infarction (resolving slowly, often accompanied by a bloody effusion). Fresh infarcts are always pleural based and cavitate frequently. Because the dual parenchymal blood supply usually protects against tissue ischemia, infarction occurs most commonly in patients with prior cardiopulmonary disease. When resolving, the infiltrate often rounds up to form a spheroid "nodule". Multiple, widely scattered, cavitating infiltrates that develop acutely suggest septic emboli.

Special Studies

Perfusion Scan

A perfusion scan is performed by injecting radioactive macroaggregated albumin, a compound with a particle size exceeding that of the alveolar capillary. The radioactive albumin then becomes trapped in the small capillaries of perfused lung.

Because infiltrates change rapidly in hospitalized patients, a comparison CXR must be taken within hours before the scan. A perfectly *normal perfusion lung* scan effectively *rules out* a clinically significant *embolism*. The single rare exception to this rule may be submassive PE confined to the pulmonary outflow tract, producing symmetrical reduction in flow. However, a "low-probabililty" scan is *not* a normal scan; a substantial fraction of low-probability scans occur with proven disease. Therefore a "low-probability" scan should not preclude further diagnostic testing if the clinical suspicion remains high. Conversely, perfusion defects highly suggestive for pulmonary emboli are reported in a substantial proportion of angiogram-negative patients.

Criteria for high probability (positive) or low probability (negative) vary with the interpreter but generally depend on the size, number, and distribution of perfusion defects, as well as their relationship to CXR and ventilation scan abnormalities. Experts often disagree among themselves. Consequently, the false-positive rate may be very high in some centers. The problem of false-positive scans is most prominent in the intensive care unit (ICU) where the prevalence of cardiopulmonary disease is high. Emboli isolated to the upper lobes are unusual in ambulatory patients, whose blood flow when upright distributes preferentially to the bases. *(Bedridden patients often violate this rule.)* Likewise, solitary embolic defects occur infrequently. A perfusion defect much larger than a density on chest film in the same area suggests embolism; a defect the same size or smaller than the radiographic abnormality suggests that embolism is unlikely. A similar rule applies even more strongly to areas of ventilation-perfusion mismatching.

Ventilation Scan

The addition of a ventilation scan improves specificity for embolism; gross ventilation/perfusion ($\dot{V}/\dot{Q}$) mismatching often allows a diagnosis to be made with confidence. However, $\dot{V}/\dot{Q}$ matching sometimes occurs even in embolic disease due to bronchoconstriction, atelectasis, or secretion retention. Conversely, apparent mismatching can result when no embolus is present.

Angiography

Angiography is the definitive test. With appropriate care it can be performed safely in the great majority of hemodynamically stable patients and often remains positive long after the initial event. Although best performed quickly, it is still worth considering as long as 1 week after clinical presentation. Criteria for a positive diagnosis must include an *intraluminal filling defect* or an *abrupt "cut-off"*. (Oligemia and tortuosity are nondiagnostic.) In the absence of overt lower extremity thrombosis, a negative angiogram, carefully done within 48 hours of the onset of symptoms, indicates a negligible risk of clinically significant embolization for weeks afterward. Even when not diagnostic alone, the lung scan may guide subsequent selective angiographic injections. Angiograms done without selective injections, multiple views, and magnification miss a substantial fraction of small emboli. The clinical significance of such small emboli, however, is unclear.

Risks of arteriography have been greatly overstated. There is a low risk of allergic dye reaction and vascular damage (right ventricular or pulmonary artery perforation). Catheter-induced arrhythmias are usually self-limited or easily treated. The greatest risk occurs during contrast injection in patients with pulmonary hypertension. Avoiding contrast injections in such patients or use of special precautions is prudent. If subsequent thrombolytic therapy is contemplated, catheters should be introduced via peripheral cut down to minimize bleeding complications.

Bedside arteriography using a balloon flotation catheter may be helpful in critically ill patients unable to leave the ICU. Unfortunately, bedside injections are much less sensitive and specific than studies done in the angiography suite. Therefore, this test is helpful if positive but cannot confidently exclude emboli. Digital subtraction angiography is gaining in popularity, but current technique does not appreciably lower the risk over conventional arteriography and produces inferior quality images.

Workup of a Suspected PE

Because of the complexity of making the diagnosis, no universally applicable diagnostic protocol can be recommended. It is generally agreed that a negative angiogram rules out embolic disease and documents a low risk of future embolization. It is also clear that a normal perfusion scan rules out the need for angiography. Between these limits, the decision to perform or withhold angiography is based in large part upon the need for diagnostic certainty and the reliability of lung scan in detecting perfusion defects. Many clinicians use the perfusion lung scan only for its value in excluding embolism or as a map for selective angiography. Others rely heavily on patterns of scan defects for guidance. Based upon currently available information, the following strategy seems defensible:

Angiogram Definitely Needed

High risk for anticoagulation (central nervous system trauma, active peptic ulcer, etc.)

Thrombolytic therapy or surgical intervention contemplated

Parenchymal disease renders nuclear scans uninterpretable

Paradoxical embolism suspected (to document right to left shunt or PE)

Angiogram Probably Not Needed

Embolism Unlikely

Normal perfusion scan

Perfusion defect much smaller than radiographic abnormality

Ventilation defect much larger than perfusion defect

Embolism Likely

Multiple or large defects on perfusion scan and suggestive history

$\dot{V}/\dot{Q}$ scan shows $\geq$ 1 lobar or $\geq$ 2 segmental mismatched defects, with a suggestive history and CXR without acute changes in involved areas

With less convincing data, the decision to perform angiography should be based on the height of clinical suspicion, the consequences of an undiagnosed embolic syndrome in patients with limited cardiopulmonary reserve, and the ability of the patient to safely undergo the procedure.

Prognosis and Rate of Resolution

A small percentage of patients die of massive PE before the diagnosis is made, usually within the first hour. A patient adequately anticoagulated with heparin who survives two hours or more has an excellent prognosis. If heparin is not begun, further clinically significant embolization occurs in at least $\frac{1}{3}$ of cases. This risk falls to < 5% with adequate therapy. Whether or not embolism is treated, most recurrent episodes occur within the first several days of presentation. In well-anticoagulated patients, such early episodes represent embolization of pre-formed thrombus, not further thrombus proliferation. Hemodynamic abnormalities usually reverse rapidly in patients who survive long enough to begin treatment, due to distal migration or fragmentation of clot. Angiographic findings can resolve within 12 hours, but usually require 2–3 weeks or longer for complete resolution. Scan defects may also disappear quickly (over days), but most resolve over weeks to months. Perfusion defects persisting 3 months or longer are likely to be permanent.

Chronic pulmonary hypertension and cor pulmonale due to multiple "silent" emboli rarely occur; however, repetition of *symptomatic* embolic episodes can cause this problem. Furthermore, in a small percentage of cases, clot organizes within central vessels to produce a surgically treatable form of pulmonary hypertension.

Management

Anticoagulation

Acute Phase

Heparin is the drug of choice, given initially by a large loading bolus ($\simeq$ 20,000 units) and subsequently by a continuous infusion begun 1–2 hours afterward ($\simeq$ 1,000 units/hour). Effective heparin therapy can also be given subcutaneously if necessary ($\simeq$ 7,500 units every 6 hours), but dosage must be guided by PTT measurements. In the acute period it is better to err on the side of over anticoagulation than undertreatment. Therefore, it is important to ensure that full anticoagulation has been achieved within a few (4–6) hours of starting the maintenance infusion. Heparin should not be withheld pending the results of other studies, unless the risk of anticoagulation outweighs clinical suspicion. Because heparin catabolism varies considerably among patients and over time in any given individual, the rate of heparin administration should be readjusted to maintain the partial thromboplastin time (PTT) $\simeq$ 1.5 $\times$ normal.

As a general rule the half-life of heparin is $\simeq$ 90 minutes in patients with active thrombosis. Therefore, interruption of heparin infusions for $>$ 2 hours exposes patients to recurrent thrombotic risk. Rarely, "therapeutic" PTT values are difficult to achieve. In such patients preformed antiheparin antibody and deficiencies of antithrombin III or proteins C or S should be suspected. The great majority of heparin failures (re-embolization) occur in patients who have not been kept well anticoagulated. Heparin infusion should be continued $\simeq$ 10 days—sufficient time to allow fresh clot to dissolve or organize. The patient should be prevented from ambulating for the first 5–7 days of therapy to avoid dislodging nonadherent clots.

Chronic Phase

After the completion of heparin therapy, antithrombotic prophylaxis is usually maintained with warfarin. However, the prothrombin time should be "in range" 1–3 days before heparin is stopped. Large "loading" doses of warfarin do not prolong the PT more rapidly and may paradoxically increase the thrombotic tendency by rapidly depleting vitamin K-dependent anti-clotting proteins. Patients not believed to have an ongoing risk factor should receive minidose heparin until fully ambulatory. *Duration* of anticoagulation must reflect not only the risk for recurrence but its potential physiologic consequences. Because the rate of recurrence falls hyperbolically with time from discharge, an arbitrary duration of 3–6 months appears reasonable in patients recovering from trauma or surgery. Patients at continued high risk of recurrence, including those who have had two or more episodes, should be anticoagulated indefinitely or until the risk abates. Although a bit more effective than fixed low doses of subcutaneous heparin, outpatient warfarin requires surveillance of the PT and is associated with a higher incidence of bleeding complications.

Thrombolytic Therapy

There is no question that streptokinase, urokinase, and tissue plasminogen activator accelerate the rate of clot resolution. However, these drugs have not been convincingly shown to decrease morbidity or mortality from PE, and the incidence of adverse bleeding is considerably increased. For these reasons many physicians question whether there is any valid indication for these agents in DVT. Although thrombolytics accelerate the resolution of venous clots, it seems reasonable to reserve these drugs for use in patients with angiographically proven massive PE and unstable hemodynamics.

Many problems are associated with thrombolytic agents (for a full discussion see Chapter 17, Angina and Myocardial Infarction). Contraindications include any condition that predisposes to serious bleeding. Puncture of noncompressible venous sites (e.g., subclavian) must not be performed while thrombolytics are administered. These drugs are begun as soon as possible after the thrombotic event has been proven, using a loading dose and continuous volumetric (pump) infusion over a 12–72-hour period, depending upon the condition treated and its clinical response. Ideally, the infusion rate is altered to keep thrombin time or euglobulin lysis time between 2 and 5 times the control value. Protime and PTT are also variably prolonged. At the conclusion of therapy, heparin is begun as thrombin time and PTT fall to twice normal. Aminocaproic acid can be used topically to stop local oozing or systemically to counteract thrombolysis if serious bleeding occurs. Reversal of the coagulation disorder can also be accomplished with fresh frozen plasma or cryoprecipitate.

Surgery: Caval Interruption and Embolectomy

Surgical interruption of the vena cava should be considered for those patients who: (1) sustain recurrent life-threatening emboli from the lower extremities or pelvis despite adequate anticoagulation; (2) cannot receive heparin safely; (3) suffer massive embolism and paradoxical systemic emboli; (4) develop septic embolism from the lower extremities; (5) clearly cannot withstand the hemodynamic effects of another embolism.

Recurrent emboli during the first few days of heparin infusion may be due to the original clot and do not necessarily indicate that heparin is ineffective. To be called a *heparin failure*, embolism must recur after the PTT has been held continuously in the therapeutic range over several days. Options for interruption of the inferior vena cava (IVC) include *ligation*, narrowing the caval lumen by *clipping*, and percutaneous placement of an umbrella or Greenfield *filter*. The clipped or umbrella-filtered vena cava clots off eventually in ⅓ or more of cases within the first 2 years. Ligation of the IVC forces the collateralizing process earlier and usually results in pedal edema (less of a problem with the other techniques). In experienced hands the Greenfield filter may have a significant advantage over open procedures and other inserted appliances. Reported rates of clotting are lower and efficacy greater than with alternative techniques. Rarely such IVC filters perforate the cava or migrate to the heart or pulmonary outflow tract—potentially lethal events.

Each surgical method effectively stops life-threatening embolism for at least several months if the source of embolism is the deep veins of the pelvis or thigh. Large collaterals may develop, but most published surgical reports suggest that the risk of clinically important embolization through these vessels is low. Because venous return is impeded for a few days after caval ligation, the procedure itself can be dangerous in patients with impaired cardiac function. Caval clipping and filter insertion are better tolerated than ligation and are just as effective, except in treating septic embolism.

Emergent pulmonary embolectomy is a highly morbid procedure that has few valid indications. Most patients surviving long enough for the diagnosis to be made angiographically respond to thrombolytic or anticoagulant therapy alone. It is only in those patients who are gravely ill and deteriorating under treatment that this heroic form of therapy should be considered. On the other hand, a surgical approach to a persistent central embolus may offer the only chance of relieving disability and potentially lethal pulmonary hypertension in carefully selected individuals. Magnetic resonance imaging (MRI) may be diagnostically helpful in these cases. Although less risky than acute embolectomy, the procedure itself remains hazardous.

SUGGESTED READINGS

1. Bell WR, Simon TL, DeMets DL: The clinical features of submassive and massive pulmonary emboli. *Am J Med* 1977;62:355–60.
2. Hull R, et al: Pulmonary angiography, ventilation lung scanning and venography for clinically suspected pulmonary embolism in the abnormal perfusion scan. *Ann Intern Med* 1983;98:891–99.
3. Hull RD, Hirsh J, Carter CJ, et al: Diagnostic efficacy of impedance plethysmography for clinically suspected deep-vein thrombosis. A randomized trial. *Ann Intern Med* 1985;102:21–28.
4. MacMillan JC, Milstein SH, Samson PC: Clinical spectrum of septic pulmonary embolism and infarction. *J Thorac Cardiovasc Surg* 1978;75:670–79.
5. Moser KM, Fedullo PF: Venous thromboembolism. Three simple decisions. *Chest* 1983;83:117–21, 256–60.
6. Sharma GV, et al. Thrombolytic therapy. *N Engl J Med* 1982;306:1268–76.
7. Urokinase-streptokinase pulmonary embolism trial: A national cooperative study. *JAMA* 1984;229:1606–13.
8. Wheeler AP, Jaquiss RDB, Newman JH: Physician practices in the treatment of pulmonary embolism and deep venous thrombosis. *Arch Intern Med* 1988;148:1321–1325.

20 Respiratory Failure

This chapter outlines the basic principles that underpin scientific management of oxygenation and ventilation failure. Much of the background needed to understand these disorders is provided in the applied physiology section of *Respiratory Medicine for the House Officer* (Ref. 4). Other crucial information is provided in chapters on "Hemodynamics", "Mechanical Ventilation", "Positive End-Expiratory Pressure", and "Support of the Circulation" in this volume.

DEFINITIONS

Respiratory failure may be thought of as a problem in one or more of the steps necessary to sustain energy production at the mitochondrial level. Dysfunction may occur in *ventilation* (the movement of gases between the environment and the lungs); in *intrapulmonary gas exchange* (the process in which mixed venous blood releases CO_2 and becomes oxygenated); in *gas transport* (the delivery of adequate quantities of oxygenated blood to the metabolizing tissue), or in *tissue gas exchange* (the ability of peripheral tissues to extract or utilize O_2 and release CO_2).

The latter two steps in this process may fail independently of the performance of the lung or ventilatory pump. Tissue O_2 delivery depends not only on the partial pressure of arterial oxygen (PaO_2), but also on non-pulmonary factors—cardiac output, hemoglobin (Hgb) concentration, and the ability of Hgb to release O_2. Cardiogenic shock, anemia, and carbon monoxide poisoning provide clinical examples of O_2 transport failure. Laboratory abnormalities characteristic of such conditions are lactic acidosis and reduced O_2 content and/or saturation of mixed venous blood (even in the face of adequate arterial oxygen tension).

Failure of O_2 uptake refers to the inability of tissue to extract and utilize O_2 for aerobic metabolism. The clearest clinical examples of derangement in this terminal phase of the oxygen transport chain are cyanide poisoning, in which cellular cytochromes (key enzymes in the electron transport process) are inhibited, and septic shock. During sepsis there is failure of an often generous cardiac output to distribute appropriately and/or an inability of the tissues themselves to make use of O_2. As in failure of O_2 transport, lactic acidosis also occurs when there is failure of tissue uptake. However, the latter process is distinguished by *normal or high* values for mixed venous oxygen tension, saturation, and content. Thus, the indices which are so helpful in other forms of oxygenation failure, i.e., cardiac output, arterial O_2 tension, and mixed venous O_2 saturation ($S\bar{v}O_2$), may be quite misleading in the setting of impaired tissue O_2 uptake. Therapy directed at failure of the O_2 transport and uptake mechanisms is discussed in detail in other chapters. The present discussion focuses on the two problems that bear on the performance of the lung and thoracic pump: failure to oxygenate the arterial blood and ventilatory failure.

OXYGENATION FAILURE

Mechanisms of Arterial Hypoxemia

Six mechanisms cause arterial oxygen desaturation:

1. Inhalation of a hypoxic gas mixture or reduction of barometric pressure
2. Hypoventilation
3. Impaired alveolar diffusion of oxygen
4. Ventilation perfusion ($\dot{V}/\dot{Q}$) mismatching
5. Shunting of systemic venous blood to the systemic arterial circuit
6. Abnormally desaturated systemic venous blood

A *decrease in the partial pressure of inhaled oxygen* occurs at high altitude in response to reduced barometric pressure and in fires that consume O_2 in the burning process.

Hypoventilation causes the partial pressure of alveolar oxygen (P_AO_2) to fall when capillary flow carries O_2 away from the alveolus faster than it is replenished. Although PaO_2 may fall much faster than $PaCO_2$ rises during the initial phase of hypoventilation or apnea, the *steady state* concentration of P_AO_2 is predicted by the alveolar gas equation: $P_AO_2 = PIO_2 - PaCO_2/R$. In this equation, PIO_2 is the partial pressure of inspired oxygen at the tracheal level (corrected for humidification at body temperature), and R is the respiratory exchange ratio, i.e., the ratio of CO_2 production to oxygen consumption *at steady state*. Transiently, R can fall to very low values as oxygen is taken up faster than CO_2 is delivered to the alveolus. Such a mechanism explains post-hyperventilation hypoxemia and some forms of hypoxemia that accompany hemodialysis (see Ref. 5).

Impaired oxygen diffusion prevents complete equilibration of alveolar gas with pulmonary capillary blood. Although this mechanism has uncertain clinical importance, many of the factors which adversely influence diffusion are encountered clinically: increased distance between alveolus and erythrocyte, decreased O_2 gradient for diffusion, and shortened transit time of the red cell through the capillary.

Ventilation/perfusion ($\dot{V}/\dot{Q}$) mismatching is the most frequent contributor to clinically important O_2 desaturation. Lung units that are relatively poorly ventilated in relation to their perfusion cause desaturation; high $\dot{V}/\dot{Q}$ units contribute to physiologic deadspace, but not to hypoxemia. The relationship of O_2 content to PaO_2 is highly curvilinear. At normal barometric pressure little additional O_2 can be loaded onto blood with already saturated Hgb, no matter how high the O_2 tension in the overventilated alveolus may rise. Because aliquots of blood exiting from different lung units *mix gas contents (not partial pressures)*, overventilating some units in an attempt to compensate for others which are underventilated does not maintain PaO_2. Hence, when equal volumes of blood from well-ventilated and poorly ventilated units mix, the resultant blood will have an O_2 content halfway between them but a PaO_2 only slightly higher than that of the lower $\dot{V}/\dot{Q}$ unit.

Supplemental O_2 will impressively reverse hypoxemia when $\dot{V}/\dot{Q}$ mismatching, hypoventilation, or diffusion impairment is the cause. (The P_AO_2 of even poorly ventilated units climbs high enough to achieve full saturation.) After breathing 100% O_2 for a sufficient period of time, only perfused units which are *totally* unventilated (shunt units)

contribute to hypoxemia. However, when hypoxemia is caused by alveolar units with *very* low $\dot{V}/\dot{Q}$ ratios, relatively concentrated O_2 mixtures must be given before a substantial change in the PaO_2 is observed (Fig. 20.1).

Shunt refers to the bypass of venous blood from the right side to the left side of the circulation. Shunt can be intracardiac, as in cyanotic right-to-left congenital heart disease, or result from passage of blood through abnormal vascular channels within the lung, e.g., pulmonary arteriovenous communications. However, by far the most common cause of shunting is pulmonary disease that produces totally unventilated lung units that are unresponsive to oxygen therapy. After breathing 100% oxygen for 15 minutes, all alveoli are presumed to be filled with pure oxygen. Hence, the percentage of shunt can be calculated from the formula: $QS/QT = (CcO_2 - CaO_2)/(CcO_2 - C\bar{v}O_2) \times 100$. In this equation, C denotes content, and the lower case letters c, a, and $\bar{v}$ denote end-capillary, arterial, and mixed venous blood, respectively. In making such calculations, end-capillary and calculated alveolar oxygen tensions are assumed equivalent. For a patient breathing pure O_2, shunt fractions < 25% can be estimated rapidly by dividing the alveolar to arterial O_2 tension difference ($670 - PaO_2$) by 20, assuming that the $C\bar{v}O_2$ is normal.

At inspired oxygen fractions < 1.0, true shunt cannot be reliably estimated by an analysis of oxygen contents, but *"venous admixture"* or *"physiologic shunt"* can. Any degree of desaturation can be considered as if it all originated from true shunt units. To calculate venous admixture, CcO_2 in the shunt formula is estimated from the ideal P_AO_2 at that particular fraction of inspired oxygen (F_iO_2).

Many indices have been devised in an attempt to characterize oxygen exchange across the spectrum of F_iO_2 (see p. 49). Although none are completely successful, the PaO_2/P_AO_2 ratio and the alveolar to arterial oxygen tension difference (A-aDO_2) are perhaps the most widely utilized. Both of these, however, are affected by changes in $S\bar{v}O_2$, even when the lung tissue itself retains normal ability to transfer oxygen to the blood. Another imprecise but commonly used indicator of gas exchange is the P_AO_2/F_iO_2 ratio (the P/F ratio). In healthy adults this ratio normally exceeds 400, whatever the F_iO_2 may be. Even though measures such as the A-aDO_2 and the PaO_2/P_AO_2 ratio imprecisely quantify changes in oxygen exchange, their calculation is valuable in determining whether

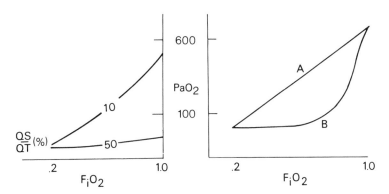

Figure 20.1 The effect of true shunt (QS/QT) and $\dot{V}/\dot{Q}$ mismatching on the relationship between PaO_2 and F_iO_2. Hypoxemia caused by true shunt (left panel) is refractory to supplemental oxygen once QS/QT exceeds 25%. A similar degree of hypoxemia responds to supplemental oxygen if caused by $\dot{V}/\dot{Q}$ mismatching (right panel). However, the F_iO_2 needed depends upon whether hypoxemia is caused by an extensive number of units with mildly abnormal $\dot{V}/\dot{Q}$ mismatch (A) or by a smaller number with very low $\dot{V}/\dot{Q}$ ratios (B).

or not lung pathology exists; hypoventilation and reduction in F_iO_2 do not cause abnormalities of these ratios.

The *admixture of abnormally desaturated venous blood* is an important mechanism acting to lower PaO_2 in patients with impaired pulmonary gas exchange and reduced cardiac output. $C\bar{v}O_2$, the product of Hgb concentration and $S\bar{v}O_2$, is influenced by cardiac output ($\dot{Q}$), arterial oxygen saturation (SaO_2), and $\dot{V}O_2$:

$$S\bar{v}O_2 \ \alpha \ SaO_2 \ - \ \dot{V}O_2/(Hgb \times \dot{Q}).$$

It is clear from this equation that $S\bar{v}O_2$ is directly influenced by any imbalance between $\dot{V}O_2$ and oxygen delivery. Thus, anemia uncompensated by an increase in cardiac output or a cardiac output too low for metabolic needs can both cause $S\bar{v}O_2$ and PaO_2 to fall. *Fluctuations in $S\bar{v}O_2$ exert a more profound influence on PaO_2 when the shunt is fixed, as in regional lung diseases* (atelectasis), than when the shunt varies with changing cardiac output, as in diffuse lung injury. Even when $S\bar{v}O_2$ is abnormally low, PaO_2 will remain unaffected if mixed venous blood gains access to well-oxygenated, well-ventilated alveoli.

Common Causes of Oxygenation Crises

The causes of oxygenation crises are conveniently categorized by their radiographic appearance. Lung collapse (atelectasis), diffuse parenchymal infiltration, volume overload, localized or unilateral infiltration, and a clear chest x-ray (CXR) are common patterns.

Atelectasis

There are several morphologic types and mechanisms of atelectasis. *Microatelectasis* naturally develops in a healthy lung when it is not periodically stretched beyond the normal tidal range. *Plate atelectasis* may be an exaggeration of this phenomenon due to regional hypodistention. *Lobar collapse* usually results from gas absorption in a plugged airway (e.g., by retained secretions, a misplaced endotracheal tube, or a central mass). External bronchial compression and regional hypoventilation are important in some patients.

Potential consequences of acute atelectasis are *worsened gas exchange*, *pneumonitis*, and *increased work of breathing*. PaO_2 drops precipitously to its nadir within hours of sudden bronchial occlusion, but then it improves steadily over hours to days as hypoxic vasoconstriction and mechanical factors increase pulmonary vascular resistance in the local area. Whether an individual patient manifests hypoxemia depends heavily on the vigor of the vasoconstrictive response, the abruptness of collapse, and the tissue volume involved. If small areas of atelectasis develop slowly, hypoxemia may never surface as a clinical problem.

Diffuse microatelectasis may be radiographically silent but detectable on physical examination by end-inspiratory rales which improve after several sustained deep breaths or coughs. Plate atelectasis yields similar physical findings plus tubular breath sounds and egophony over the involved area. Lobar atelectasis gives a dull percussion note and diminished breath sounds if the bronchus is occluded by secretions, but tubular breath sounds and egophony if the airway is patent. (The latter findings correlate well with the presence of air bronchograms on CXR.) Plate atelectasis most frequently develops at the lung base above a pleural effusion or above a raised, splinted, or poorly mobile hemidiaphragm. Lobar atelectasis most commonly occurs in patients with copious airway secretions and limited power to expel them. Acute upper lobe collapse is uncommon and tends to resolve quickly because of good gravitational drainage. Collapse of the left lower lobe is more frequent than collapse of the right lower lobe, perhaps because of its smaller caliber, retrocardiac position, and more sharply angulated bronchus. Lobar atelectasis may be complete or partial but in either case is radiographically recognized by opacified tissue, displaced fissures, compensatory hyperinflation, and obliterated air/soft tissue boundaries (see p. 99). Small amounts of pleural fluid are a natural concomitant of lobar collapse and do not necessarily signify an additional pathologic process.

Management of Atelectasis

Prophylaxis. Effective prevention of atelectasis in high-risk patients reverses shallow breathing and improves secretion clearance. Obesity, chronic bronchitis, neuromuscular weakness, pain, and advanced age are predisposing factors. High abdominal, thoracic, and lower abdominal incisions are associated with the highest incidence of postoperative atelectasis (in that order). Preoperatively, the airways should be maximally dilated and free of infection. Postoperatively, patients should be encouraged to breathe deeply, to sit upright, and to cough intermittently. Continuous positive airway pressure (CPAP) may be helpful, especially in intubated patients. Frequent turning and early mobilization are the most important prophylactic maneuvers. Respiratory therapy (RT) techniques such as airway suctioning, incentive spirometry, and chest physiotherapy are discussed in detail in *Respiratory Medicine for the House Officer* (Ref. 4).

Treatment. When possible, early *mobilization* is the best treatment. Periodic deep breathing effectively reverses plate and microatelectasis. *Sustained deep breaths* are particularly effective. Whether a higher lung volume is achieved by a positive airway pressure or by a negative pleural pressure is immaterial, assuming that similar distention occurs in both cases. Although rational, the place of positive end-expiratory pressure in treatment of established collapse has not been clar-

ified. *Relief of chest wall pain* helps to reduce splinting and enables more effective coughing. Intercostal nerve blocks with bupivacaine may be effective for 8–12 hours.

Dislodging secretions from the central airways is essential. This usually cannot be done effectively in the unintubated patient with blind tracheal suctioning alone. Vigorous RT initiated soon after the onset of lobar collapse can reverse most cases within 24–48 hours. As a general rule, *fiberoptic bronchoscopy* should be reserved for patients with symptomatic lobar collapse who lack central air bronchograms and who either cannot undergo RT or who fail to respond or tolerate 48 hours of vigorous RT. Even whole lung collapse deserves at least one RT treatment before bronchoscopy is performed. After re-expansion, a prophylactic RT program should be initiated to prevent recurrence. Adjunctive measures, e.g., bronchodilators, hydration, and frequent turning, should not be ignored.

Diffuse Pulmonary Infiltration

When fluid or cells cause alveolar flooding or collapse, severe refractory hypoxemia may result. Fluid confined to the interstitial spaces may cause hypoxemia as a result of peri-bronchial edema, $\dot{V}/\dot{Q}$ mismatching, and microatelectasis; however, interstitial fluid itself does not interfere with oxygen exchange.

Very few processes are confined exclusively to the air spaces or to the interstitium. Radiographic signs of alveolar filling include segmental distribution, coalescence, fluffy margins, air bronchograms, rosette patterns, and silhouetting of normal structures. If none of these are present, a diffuse infiltrate is likely to be largely interstitial, especially if it parallels the vascular distribution. Any diffuse interstitial process will appear more radiodense at the bases than at the apices, in part because there is more tissue to penetrate. Alveoli are also smaller at the bases, so the ratio of aerated volume to total tissue volume declines.

The major categories of disease that produce diffuse pulmonary infiltration and hypoxemia are *pneumonia, cardiogenic pulmonary edema, volume overload*, and the *adult respiratory distress syndrome (ARDS)*. From a radiographic viewpoint these processes may be difficult to distinguish; however, a few characteristic features are helpful.

Hydrostatic Edema

Perihilar infiltrates (sparing the costophrenic angles), a prominent vascular pattern, and a widened vascular pedicle suggest volume overload or very early cardiogenic edema. A gravitational distribution of edema is highly consistent with well-established left ventricular failure (or long-standing, severe volume overload), especially when accompanied by cardiomegaly and a widened vascular pedicle. Patchy peripheral infiltrates that lack a gravitational predilection and show reluctance to change with position are most suggestive of ARDS. Interestingly, septal (Kerley) lines and distinct peribronchial cuffing are very seldom seen in classical ARDS (see below). On the other hand, air bronchograms are common in permeability edema (ARDS) but are quite unusual with hydrostatic etiologies.

Variants of Hydrostatic Edema. Hydrostatic edema (HPE) may occur in multiple settings which have differing implications for prognosis and treatment. The most familiar form of HPE is that which accompanies left ventricular failure. In this setting, signs of systemic hypoperfusion and inadequate cardiac output often accompany oxygenation failure. However, HPE can develop even with a normally well compensated ventricle during transient heart dysfunction (ischemia, hypertensive crisis, arrhythmias). When the myocardium fails to fully relax during diastole ("diastolic dysfunction"), transient increases in the volume returning to the left heart or aberrancies of left heart function or rhythm may cause rapid, transient alveolar flooding—"flash pulmonary edema". In this setting, the radiographic appearance may be quite impressive but may resolve quickly.

Adult Respiratory Distress Syndrome (ARDS)

ARDS is an imprecise term, often applied to any acute diffuse parenchymal infiltration associated with severe hypoxemia and not attributable to HPE. However, the ARDS designation is most useful when restricted to acute noncardiogenic pulmonary edema with characteristic features:

1. delay between the precipitating event and the onset of dyspnea,
2. markedly diminished lung compliance,
3. reduced lung volume,
4. refractory hypoxemia, and
5. delayed resolution.

The precise pathogenesis of permeability edema remains unsettled but is almost certain to vary with the precipitating cause. The numerous synonyms for this syndrome previously in use ("shock lung", "post-pump lung", etc.) reflect the diversity of its causes. Despite a multitude of inciting events,

the pathophysiology is sufficiently similar to warrant a common treatment approach.

A prominent feature of all forms of ARDS is *injury to the alveolus-capillary membrane* from either the alveolar (e.g., smoke inhalation, aspiration of gastric acid or blood) or the capillary (e.g., sepsis, fat embolism) sides. Increased permeability allows seepage of protein-rich fluid into the interstitial and alveolar spaces. Surfactant production is inhibited, contributing to widespread atelectasis. Although wedge pressure is usually normal, increased pulmonary vascular resistance and pulmonary hypertension are almost invariable in the latter stages. Apart from the difference in hydrostatic pressure (measured by the wedge), permeability edema differs from HPE in that it *resolves more slowly, resists clearance by diuretic therapy,* and *produces proteinaceous edema fluid.* These distinctions are important, since similar patterns of diffuse pulmonary infiltration with a normal wedge pressure can be seen not only in ARDS but also in such problems as flash pulmonary edema and partially treated heart failure.

Rapidly Resolving Non-Cardiogenic Edema. A few disorders which fall loosely under the heading of "ARDS" are worth noting because of their fundamentally different pathophysiology and clinical course. In certain settings, transient disruption in the barrier function of the pulmonary capillary can occur without overt endothelial damage. For example, neurogenic and heroin-induced pulmonary edema are two problems in which a transiently elevated pulmonary *venous* pressure causes opening of epithelial tight junctions and leakage of proteinaceous fluid. However, resealing and resolution occur promptly without widespread endothelial damage. A similar process may be seen in settings such as severe metabolic acidosis and cardiopulmonary resuscitation. From the alveolar side, certain abrupt and unsustained inhalational injuries (e.g., limited chlorine gas or ammonia exposure) can produce a dramatic initial picture, only to clear rapidly over a brief period.

Hypoxemia with a Clear Chest X-ray

It is not uncommon for patients to present with life-threatening hypoxemia without major radiographic evidence of infiltration. In such cases, occult shunting and severe $\dot{V}/\dot{Q}$ mismatching are the most likely mechanisms (Table 20.1).

Intracardiac or intrapulmonary shunts, asthma and other forms of obstructive lung disease, low lung volume superimposed on a high closing ca-

Table 20.1
Causes of Hypoxemia with a "Clear" Chest X-ray

Intracardiac or pulmonary shunts	High "closing" volume / obesity
Microvascular shunts (cirrhosis)	Pneumothorax
Asthma/obstructive lung disease	Retained secretions
	Head injury
Pulmonary embolism	Low cardiac output / vasodilators

pacity (e.g., bronchitis in a supine obese patient), pulmonary embolism, and occult microvascular communications (such as occur in patients with cirrhosis) are likely explanations. Hypoxemia is amplified by profound desaturation of mixed venous blood, by reversal of hypoxic vasoconstriction with therapeutic vasodilators (e.g., nitroprusside), and by the severe $\dot{V}/\dot{Q}$ imbalance consequent to acute head injury. In our institution, acute oxygenation crises following head trauma has been termed "nonedematous respiratory distress syndrome" or "NERDS".

Unilateral Lung Disease

In the setting of severe hypoxemia, unilateral infiltration or marked asymmetry in radiographic density suggests a confined set of etiologic possibilities, most of which occur in highly characteristic clinical settings (Table 20.2). Marked asymmetry of radiographic involvement should prompt an especially careful search for a readily reversible cause for hypoxemia. Depending on the cause for unilaterality, precautions should also be taken against generalization of the process.

Table 20.2
Causes of Asymmetric Pulmonary Infiltration

Aspiration/foreign body	Pleural effusion
Contralateral pulmonary emboli	Trauma (contusion)
Ipsilateral pulmonary infarction	Re-expansion pulmonary edema
Mainstem bronchus intubation	Contralateral pneumothorax
Pulmonary hemorrhage	Lobar pneumonia
Drowned lung/massive atelectasis	Hydrostatic edema/ decubitus positioning

Techniques to Improve Tissue Oxygenation

Basic Therapeutic Principles

It is axiomatic that the underlying pathology must be reversed whenever possible. Although ate-

lectasis, fluid overload, and infection yield to specific measures, the treatment of diffuse lung injury is largely supportive. The primary therapeutic aims are to maintain oxygen delivery, to support the breathing workload, and to establish electrolyte balance while preventing further damage from oxygen toxicity, barotrauma, infection, and other iatrogenic complications. To these ends, the clinician should bear in mind a few fundamental principles.

1. *Apply minimal levels of potentially noxious therapies.* Positive airway pressure, oxygen, and vasoactive drugs are potentially injurious. Therefore, there should be frequent reassessment of the need for positive end-expiratory pressure (PEEP), the level of ventilator support, and F_iO_2. Toxic levels of F_iO_2 and PEEP may not always be necessary; an oxygen saturation of 85% may be acceptable if the patient has adequate oxygen-carrying capacity, has a strong heart, and shows no sign of critical oxygen privation (e.g., lactic acidosis). Similarly, allowing $PaCO_2$ to climb (buffering pH, if necessary, with $NaHCO_3$) may minimize the ventilatory requirement and reduce the risk of barotrauma. Mean intrathoracic pressure can be reduced by allowing the patient to provide as much ventilatory power as possible, compatible with comfort. (Dyspneic patients, however, must receive full support.)

2. *Prevent therapeutic disasters.* Patients must be kept under direct observation at all times. Paralyzed patients must be watched with special care, as ventilation is totally machine-dependent. Furthermore, the hands *must* be restrained in semi-conscious, agitated, confused or disoriented patients who receive mechanical ventilation; abrupt ventilator disconnections and extubations can produce lethal bradyarrhythmias, hypoxemia, asphyxia, or aspiration. In the setting of pulmonary edema, the interruption of PEEP for even brief periods (suctioning, tubing changes) may cause profound, slowly reversing desaturation as lung volume falls and the airways are rapidly flooded with edema fluid. Because air swallowing and ileus are common, the stomach should be decompressed in most recently intubated patients. The clinician must be ready to intervene immediately to decompress a tension pneumothorax. Prophylactic chest tubes may be indicated for patients who demonstrate tension cyst formation.

3. *Remember that oxygenation failure is often a multi-system disease.* Severe fluid restriction

may reduce lung water and improve oxygen exchange but compromise perfusion of gut and kidney. The routine use of corticosteroids is not justified; the systemic changes in metabolism and protein wastage far outweigh any potential therapeutic benefit, except perhaps in the setting of proven vasculitis, fat embolism, or allergic reactions. Appropriate levels of nutritional support and prophylaxis against gastrointestinal hemorrhage are important adjunctive measures.

Improving Tissue Oxygen Delivery

Oxygen delivery is the product of cardiac output and O_2 content of each milliliter of blood. Techniques for improving cardiac output are discussed in detail in Support of the Circulation, Chapter 3. The O_2-carrying capacity can be improved by increasing Hgb (Hgb) concentration and optimizing its dissociation characteristics. Both factors are important. For example, transfusion of stored blood can increase Hgb concentration, but low levels of 2,3-diphosphoglyceric acid (2,3 DPG) may impair its O_2 dissociation characteristics. Conversely, Hgb performance is improved by reversing alkalemia to facilitate O_2 offloading. As Hgb concentration rises, blood viscosity increases, retarding passage of erythrocytes through capillary networks. Thus, actual O_2 delivery can be impaired as hematocrit (Hct) rises over 50%. Although the optimal Hct in patients with an oxygenation crisis is unknown, it makes sense to restore Hct to $\simeq 3.^{-}$ -40%. More extensive supplementation increases transfusion related risks without proven benefit (see Chapter 13, Transfusion and Blood Component Therapy).

A very high percentage of the oxygen contained in blood is bound to Hgb; the proportion solubilized in plasma is very small ($\simeq 3\%$) at ambient pressure. In certain settings, however, dissolved oxygen can prove life-saving. For example, in severe anemia the Hgb-bound fraction is disproportionately small, so that total O_2-carrying capacity is significantly boosted when 100% O_2 is used. When Hgb is dysfunctional, as with carbon monoxide exposure, high partial pressures of O_2 (particularly those delivered under hyperbaric conditions) can deliver life-sustaining quantities of dissolved O_2.

In the setting of acute lung injury, attention focuses on maintaining an adequate oxygen delivery/consumption ratio while reversing underlying lung pathology. Although pulmonary edema and pneumonitis are treatable by specific measures, in the majority of cases the therapeutic approach centers on sustaining adequate O_2 delivery while allowing the lung tissue to spontaneously recover. Because extravascular water accumulates readily in the setting of permeability edema, fluids should be used judiciously to keep the wedge pressure as low as feasible, consistent with adequate oxygen delivery (see p. 23). Two basic tools are available to compensate for impaired oxygen exchange: supplemental O_2 and the use of positive pressure to recruit alveoli and redistribute lung liquid.

Oxygen Therapy

Increasing the F_iO_2 improves PaO_2 in all instances in which shunt is not responsible for desaturation. The goal is to increase the saturation of Hgb to at least 85–90% without risking O_2 toxicity. The incidence of O_2 toxicity is both concentration and time dependent. As a general rule, very high inspired fractions of oxygen can safely be used for brief periods as efforts are made to reverse the underlying process. However, sustained elevations in $F_iO_2 > 0.6$ result in inflammatory changes, alveolar infiltration, and eventual fibrosis in experimental models; therefore, every effort should be made to keep $F_iO_2 < 0.6$ during the support phase of acute lung injury.

PEEP, Positioning, and Other Techniques for Raising Lung Volume

PEEP and newer specialized techniques (e.g., inverse ratio ventilation) for increasing mean alveolar pressure are often successful in recruiting lung volume (see Chapter 8, Positive End-Expiratory Pressure). Virtually all patients benefit from low levels of PEEP (3–5 cmH₂O), helping to compensate for the loss of volume that accompanies the supine posture and translaryngeal intubation. There is no evidence, however, that PEEP helps in prophylaxis against the onset of ARDS. Although PEEP may be highly effective, its volume-recruiting effects can be negated by vigorous patient effort if expiratory muscle action forces the chest to a lung volume lower than the equilibrium position. When this happens, sedation or paralysis can prove very helpful. When infiltration is predominately unilateral, a common level of PEEP may prove ineffective or hazardous as compliant lung units are forced to overdistend. In this setting, the combination of selective intubation and independent lung ventilation allows individual tailoring of the pattern of lung inflation, F_iO_2, and PEEP, improves oxygenation, and reduces barotrauma.

The potential benefits of *position* changes are often overlooked. Patients should remain upright, if possible, and recumbent patients should be turned every few hours. (This is especially important in comatose or paralyzed patients.) Alternating lateral decubitus positions puts different regions of the lung on maximal stretch and improves secretion drainage. Intermittent shifts from the supine to the prone position may occasionally help dramatically in reversing hypoxemia in the setting of ARDS. When one lung is differentially affected, oxygenation may improve dramatically with the good lung in the dependent position. Care should be taken to ensure that secretions from the infiltrated lung are not aspirated into the airway of the dependent viable lung during this process.

Secretion Management and Bronchodilation

Although ARDS is often regarded strictly as a problem of parenchymal injury, airway edema, bronchospasm, and secretion retention often contribute to hypoxemia. (This is especially true in cases of ARDS caused or complicated by aspiration or bronchopneumonia). Retained secretions often pose an overlooked problem that increases endotracheal tube resistance and encourages bronchospasm and maldistribution of ventilation. In some patients with diffuse lung injury, profound bradycardia develops during ventilator disconnections, discouraging airway hygiene. Although hypoxemia occasionally contributes, this bradycardia is usually reflex in nature and responds to prophylactic (parenteral) atropine or re-application of positive airway pressure.

Reducing Oxygen Requirements

Reducing the tissue O_2 demand can be as effective as improving oxygen delivery. Fever, agitation, overfeeding, vigorous respiratory activity, shivering, sepsis, and a host of other commonly observed clinical conditions can markedly increase $\dot{V}O_2$. Aggressive steps should be taken to eliminate these stimuli. Fever reduction is an important therapeutic goal, but shivering must be prevented in the cooling process. Sedation and the use of antipyretics rather than cooling blankets make good therapeutic sense. (Although phenothiazines may prevent shivering, their use may inhibit the cutaneous vasodilation necessary for rapid heat loss.)

Paralysis is a valuable adjunct to reduce oxygen consumption and improves PaO_2 in patients who remain agitated or fight the ventilator despite more conservative measures. Although paralysis is helpful in the first hours of machine support, protracted paralysis must be avoided for several reasons. Paralysis places the entire responsibility for achieving adequate oxygenation and ventilation with the medical team. Furthermore, the patient is defenseless in the event of a ventilator disconnection. Paralysis also silences the coughing mechanism and creates a monotonous breathing pattern that encourages secretion retention in dependent regions.

VENTILATORY FAILURE

Definition

Ventilatory failure (VF) is the inability to sustain sufficient CO_2 elimination to maintain a stable pH without mechanical assistance, muscle fatigue, or intolerable dyspnea. Failure to maintain adequate alveolar ventilation is usually recognized by CO_2 retention and acidosis. Although a rise in $PaCO_2$ to a level > 50 mmHg has been suggested as a hallmark of VF, ventilatory failure can occur even when $PaCO_2$ falls to a value lower than its chronic level (which itself may exceed 50 mmHg). For example, a modest metabolic acidosis may exhaust the limited ventilatory reserve of a patient with quadriplegia or ARDS. In similar fashion, hypocapnic alkalosis may deteriorate to "normal" values for pH and $PaCO_2$ as ventilatory failure develops in a fatiguing asthmatic patient. Conversely, many patients maintain $PaCO_2 > 50$ mmHg on a chronic basis, without decompensation.

How is CO_2 Eliminated?

Pulmonary venous blood delivers CO_2 to the lungs, where it normally diffuses into the alveolar sacs. O_2 is replenished and CO_2 is eliminated by the pumping action of the chest muscles. If there is no blood flow to a particular air sac, work done to move fresh air in and out of that alveolus does not help with CO_2 elimination. Similarly, lung units that are meagerly perfused also contribute to the fraction of wasted ventilation—the *physiologic deadspace*. Normally, ventilatory drive adjusts the activity of the muscular pump to maintain pH within narrow limits. It is inadequacy of the ventilatory pump in relation to the level needed to prevent acute CO_2 retention that gives rise to clinical ventilatory failure.

To maintain effective ventilation, an appropriate signal must first be sent from the brain to the ventilatory muscles. The muscles must then contract forcefully and in a coordinated fashion to move the rib cage and generate the fluctuations of pleural pressure that drive airflow. Ventilatory work depends upon how difficult it is to move gas in and out of the chest and on how many liters of gas must be moved. Thus, there are three major mechanisms that can cause or contribute to VF: (1)

Respiratory drive can be insufficient; (2) the ventilatory workload can be too high, either because too many liters of gas must be moved or because it is too energy costly to move each liter of gas; (3) the ventilatory pump may be defective due to a structural problem in the chest wall, impaired muscle strength, or discoordination.

Determinants of Ventilatory Compensation

Ventilatory Drive

The sensitivity of the respiratory drive center to hypercapnia (and hypoxemia) is, in part, a congenital characteristic. The chemical drives to breathe tend to deteriorate with advancing age. However, many potentially reversible factors also affect ventilatory drive. In general, drive intensity varies with metabolic activity. Thus, for the same level of $PaCO_2$, minute ventilation ($\dot{V}_E$) will vary with $\dot{V}O_2$. Such conditions as hypothyroidism and malnutrition depress resting $\dot{V}O_2$ and the intensity of ventilatory drive. Other factors contributing to reduced drive include sedatives, depressed mental status, chronic loading of ventilation (e.g., with a prolonged asthma attack), sleep deprivation, and metabolic alkalosis.

Ventilatory Requirement

The $\dot{V}_E$ necessary to maintain a stable pH is influenced by the level of *CO$_2$ production*, by the *ventilatory deadspace*, and by the need to compensate for *metabolic acidosis*. (The factors contributing to each of these are discussed in detail in Ref. 4.) CO_2 retention may be an adaptive strategy to reduce the work of breathing and still accomplish effective alveolar ventilation. About the same quantity of CO_2 is eliminated when a patient with a $PaCO_2$ of 60 mmHg breathes 8 times a minute as when a patient with a $PaCO_2$ of 40 mmHg breathes 12 times a minute. Apart from $\dot{V}_E$ requirement, the work per liter of ventilation (the mean inspiratory pressure per breath) is the other major component that determines the total workload. Ventilatory work must be done primarily against frictional and elastic forces. Restrictive diseases of the lungs, pleural space, or chest wall increase the elastic component, whereas airflow obstruction increases the frictional component. In the acute setting, bronchospasm, mucosal edema, accumulated secretions, and bubbles from pulmonary edema froth are common causes of reversible obstruction. Restrictive disease is produced by any process that infiltrates the lung, causes loss of lung volume, e.g., atelectasis, or impedes the lung from expanding, e.g., pneumothorax, pleural effusion, and a stiff chest wall (obesity, abdominal operations, burn eschar, etc.).

Pump Function

For effective ventilation, pleural pressure must be developed by the respiratory muscles acting in a coordinated fashion on an intact rib cage. Diseases such as flail chest and kyphoscoliosis structurally impair the integrity of the chest wall and cause *inefficient coupling* between muscle contraction and pleural pressure generation. A similar problem can result when the inspiratory muscles of the diaphragm and rib cage do not act in concert, as during diaphragmatic paralysis, quadriplegia, or the acute phase of stroke. Discoordinated ventilatory patterns seen in many critically ill patients also contribute to the genesis and maintenance of ventilator dependence.

In many instances, neither the intensity of drive, the coordination of the respiratory muscles, the ventilatory requirement, or the structural integrity of the chest cage are defective, but the pump remains weak because of *reduced muscular power*. Total muscle bulk is a prime determinant of strength and endurance. Bulk relates not only to age, sex, and body size but also to nutritional status. Skeletal muscle loss from the respiratory system parallels that elsewhere in the body, so that malnutrition is a prime contributor to VF. Independently from muscle bulk, the performance of muscle fiber is determined by precontractile muscle *fiber length*, the *velocity of the shortening* process, and the *electrolytic environment*. Acid-base disturbances and deficiencies of phosphate, magnesium, potassium, chloride, calcium, and iron have been shown to impair fiber contractility. *Hyperinflation* seriously impairs the efficiency of the ventilatory pump in several ways. Not only are the inspiratory muscle fibers foreshortened so that they produce less force, but the elastic work that the muscles must do is also increased. Furthermore, the flattened diaphragm of hyperinflation produces a less effective vector of inspiratory force.

Endurance and Fatigue

As a general rule, patients can sustain for long periods a $\dot{V}_E$ of $\simeq$ 60% of their maximum level, or $\simeq$ 40% of the maximal inspiratory pressure that can be generated at functional residual capacity (see p. 59). The endurance of muscle fibers is determined by the balance of nutritional supply and demand. Therefore, muscles deprived of nutrients during hypotension or hypoxemia perform less efficiently. The primary physical signs of ventilatory fatigue are vigorous use of accessory ventilatory muscles, tachypnea, tachycardia, and paradoxical abdominal motion.

Management of Ventilatory Failure

VF is managed by defining its cause, correcting reversible factors, and providing mechanical support when necessary. If the cause of VF is not obvious, bedside measurements intended to define the mechanisms at work are especially important. Ventilatory workload is reflected in the $\dot{V}_E$ and in such indices of work of breathing as the mean and peak inspiratory pressures observed during passive machine inflation (see p. 52). In defining those factors which contribute to the ventilatory requirement, calculation of deadspace and measurements of core temperature may be very important. The impedance of chest inflation is best gauged by measures of chest mechanics (see p. 52). Neuromuscular function is evaluated by observing the ventilatory pattern, tidal volume, frequency, and maximal inspiratory pressure. The intensity of ventilatory drive is best assessed from an examination of the $PaCO_2$ in relation to the $\dot{V}_E$ requirement and signs of patient distress. (For example, if $PaCO_2$ is high and $\dot{V}_E$ is low, drive may be defective or mechanics may be impaired; evidence of patient agitation or distress argues for the latter.) The $P_{0.1}$ is just now emerging as a useful quantitative drive index, especially helpful when assessing the continuing need for machine support (see p. 58). Investigation of specific etiologies for VF is a topic too complex to be addressed in detail here. In general, this investigation should be guided by a systematic evaluation of ventilatory drive, $\dot{V}_E$, the work of breathing, and neuromuscular performance.

Correcting Reversible Factors

Therapy to reverse VF should be guided by knowledge of the underlying defect. For example, the $\dot{V}_E$ requirement may be diminished by reducing fever, agitation, and deadspace. Impedance can be optimized by relieving airway obstruction (bronchodilation, secretion clearance, placement of a larger endotracheal tube), by increasing parenchymal compliance (reduction of atelectasis, edema, and inflammation), and by improving chest wall

distensibility (drainage of air or fluid from the pleural space, relief of abdominal distention). Neuromuscular efficiency should be optimized by maintaining the patient as upright as possible, by relieving pain, and by correcting electrolyte disturbances, endocrine disorders, and nutritional deficiencies. Measures that improve cardiac output or arterial oxygenation will also improve neuromuscular performance. Treatable neuromuscular disorders (e.g., myasthenia) must be dealt with appropriately. Some problems of decreased ventilatory drive are self-limited, (e.g., sedative or opiate overdose); others improve with nutritional repletion or recovery of mental status. Few respond to such nonspecific ventilatory stimulants as progesterone. Unfortunately, many such problems are refractory to drug manipulation and must be treated by optimizing ventilatory mechanics with a goal of reducing the work of breathing sufficiently to achieve compensation.

Mechanical Support

Willingness to institute mechanical ventilation should be directly proportional to the risk of deterioration without support and inversely proportional to the anticipated difficulty of eventual weaning. The principles of intubation, mechanical ventilation with positive pressure, and weaning have been presented elsewhere (see Chapters 6–9). However, when trying to wean patients from mechanical ventilation, it should be emphasized that a relatively high $PaCO_2$ may be required to achieve compensation and that not every patient can be brought back to an arbitrary baseline $PaCO_2$ of 40 mmHg.

SUGGESTED READINGS

1. Bone RC (ed): Adult respiratory distress syndrome. *Clin Chest Med.* 1982.
2. Colice GL, Matthay MA, Bass E, et al: Neurogenic pulmonary edema. *Am Rev Respir Dis* 130:941–948, 1984.
3. Fallat RJ, Luce JM, (eds): Cardiopulmonary critical care management. *Clin Crit Care Med.* New York, Churchill Livingstone, 1988.
4. Marini JJ: *Respiratory Medicine for the House Officer,* ed 2. Baltimore, Williams & Wilkins, pp. 1–39, 1987.
5. Raimondi AC, Raimondi GA: Hypoxemia due to hyperventilation and reduced R value. *Chest* 81:391, 1982.
6. Rinaldo JE, Rogers RM: Adult respiratory distress syndrome. *N Engl J Med* 315(9):578–580, 1986.

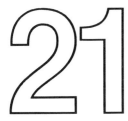

Life-threatening Infections

Three categories account for the majority of life-threatening infections seen in the intensive care unit (ICU): primary bacterial *infections that prompt admission* (meningitis, pneumonia, urinary tract infection, etc.); *nosocomial infections* such as catheter-related sepsis; and infections of the *immune-compromised host*. Because this broad, important topic cannot be addressed comprehensively in the space available, our discussion will center on principles fundamental to the management of the infected critically ill patient.

SEPSIS SYNDROME

Diagnosis

Tachypnea, *altered mental status*, and *hypotension* comprise the primary signs of the sepsis syndrome (SS). Although *fever* is almost universally present, it may be absent in patients with chronic renal failure or those receiving steroids or other anti-inflammatory drugs. The respiratory rate is a key vital sign, as tachypnea is one of the harbingers of SS. On the other hand, oliguria and metabolic acidosis develop later in response to critical perfusion deficits.

Disseminated coagulation, adult respiratory distress syndrome (ARDS), and purpura are also late hallmarks of the full blown syndrome. The differential diagnosis of SS includes hemorrhage, adrenal insufficiency, transfusion or drug reaction, and noninfectious causes of vascular instability.

In the early phase the laboratory is largely unhelpful; however, extreme leukocytosis or leukopenia supports the diagnosis. Rarely, overwhelming fungemia or bacteremia may be confirmed by Gram stain of the buffy coat of a centrifuged specimen of blood or tissue fluid.

Pathophysiology

Bacterial toxins, cell wall components (lipopolysaccharide), complement, monokines (e.g.,

interleukin 1 and tumor necrosis factor), and kinins all contribute to the pathophysiology of SS. Such products may be released into the bloodstream from localized sites of infection even when viable organisms do not circulate. Organisms are cultured from the blood in a *minority* of patients. Although gram-negative rods are the most common etiology, in recent years gram-positive cocci have been isolated with increasing frequency and may produce an identical clinical picture. The risk of SS is highest in patients with leukopenia, hematologic malignancies, cirrhosis, and a history of splenectomy.

Early cardiovascular manifestations include decreased systemic vascular resistance and increased cardiac output. However, if venous pooling and increased vascular permeability predominate, a low cardiac output may be seen. Therefore, in early SS the circulation may be hyper- or hypodynamic and the skin warm or cold. *Later*, systemic resistance rises and cardiac output falls in response to increased sympathetic tone. As vasomotor control deteriorates, maldistribution of blood flow produces perfusion defects that cause tissue hypoxia and anaerobic metabolism with lactate production.

Therapy

The speed with which appropriate treatment is begun is a crucial determinant of outcome. Delayed antibiotic therapy may inhibit bacterial growth too late to avert irreversible tissue damage. When the source of sepsis is unknown, protected interstitial foci in the abdomen or lung are likely. Translocation of organisms across the compromised gut wall frequently allows bacterial infection to become established in intra-abdominal lymph nodes, which then release mediators of sepsis. In cases in which the organism and site of origin cannot be identified, prognosis is poor. A similar phenomenon may account for the high incidence of positive lung cultures in patients who die with SS-

complicating ARDS. It is not surprising that the mortality of patients with hemodynamic alterations *and* bacteremia is 3–4 fold greater than those with isolated bacteremia.

Cardiorespiratory support and antibiotic therapy are the mainstays of treatment. The need for invasive monitoring, fluid replacement, and vasoactive drugs must be individualized. *Cultures of blood, sputum,* and *urine* should be obtained before initiating antibiotics. Unless the etiologic agent is known with certainty, *broad spectrum antibiotics*, including an extended spectrum penicillin or cephalosporin plus an aminoglycoside, are indicated until cultures return. Massive doses of *corticosteroids* have been advocated but there is little evidence to support their use. *Naloxone* may temporarily reverse hypotension but has not been shown to reduce mortality. *Non-steroidal anti-inflammatory agents* and *anti-endotoxin antibodies* hold promise.

URINARY TRACT INFECTIONS

Causes

Urinary tract infections (UTIs) are the most common ICU infections. Although usually inconsequential, the mortality rate for *bacteremic* UTI approaches 30%.

Risk factors include urinary catheters, female gender, and advanced age. *Colonization* of urinary catheters occurs at a rate of about 5% per day and most ICU-acquired UTIs occur in such patients. Teflon (rather than rubber) catheter construction reduces the infective risk. There is no evidence, however, that frequent catheter changes or application of antibiotic ointments decrease risk. Critical factors in preventing nosocomial UTI are *sterile insertion, early removal,* and *closed drainage.*

Diagnosis

The diagnosis of UTI is made when $> 10^5$ bacteria/ml are isolated from culture of freshly voided urine. The presence of > 1 organism per high-power field of unspun urine indicates a bacterial colony count $> 10^5$ organisms/ml. *Escherichia coli,* the most common isolate, occurs in $\simeq \frac{1}{3}$ of UTIs. Other enteric gram-negative rods, enterococci, and candida account for a large fraction of the remainder. Contrary to previous teaching, in many cases pure cultures of *Staphylococcus epidermidis* represent infection, not contamination. In the absence of frank pyuria, it is often difficult to differentiate *colonization* from *infection* in critically ill patients with indwelling catheters. Fluorescent antibody coating of bacteria may distinguish lower

from upper urinary tract infections, but it is not widely available.

Pyocystis, an infection of the bladder wall, may complicate oliguria or anuria, especially in patients requiring hemodialysis. In this setting, reduced urine flow allows bacteria to proliferate in the bladder. In oliguric patients with obscure fever, the bladder should be catheterized and the urine sediment examined. Murky, turbid urine establishes the diagnosis.

Treatment

When overtly symptomatic, the treatment of UTI includes the promotion of urinary flow and drainage, removal of catheters (when feasible), and antibiotic therapy. In seriously ill patients, an intravenous aminoglycoside plus an extended spectrum penicillin should be administered. Cephalothin or vancomycin may be substituted in penicillin-allergic patients. In stable patients, a simpler oral regimen may suffice (e.g., oral ampicillin, or trimethoprim-sulfa). Drainage bags provide important reservoirs for urinary pathogens. Therefore, manipulations of the closed drainage system should be undertaken only when necessary and conducted with appropriate sterile precautions.

PNEUMONIA

Pathogenesis

Organisms usually enter the lower respiratory tract in *aspirated* upper airway secretions. *Inhalation of an infective aerosol* and *hematogenous seeding* are other mechanisms. Unless the inoculum is massive, glottic closure, cough, and mucociliary clearance normally provide an effective *mechanical defense* (Table 21.1). Even when mechanical barriers fail, infection can be averted by effective *cellular and humoral immunity.* Unfortunately, both mechanical and immune defenses are commonly jeopardized in the critically ill. Con-

Table 21.1
Conditions Promoting Lung Inoculation

Aspiration
  Depressed consciousness
  Swallowing disorders
  Nasogastric and tracheal tubes
Hematogenous
  Bacteremia
Infected Aerosol
  Contaminated ventilator tubing and humidifiers

ditions allowing proliferation of pneumonia are listed in Table 21.2.

In the community, *Pneumococcus* and *Mycoplasma* are common pathogens in otherwise healthy adults. (The general problem of pneumonia is discussed in Ref. 7.) In the ICU, a different spectrum predominates. *Gram-negative rods* produce approximately 50% of all ICU pneumonias, with *Staphylococcus aureus* causing another 10–15% of infections. This difference in bacterial etiology is partially explained by the rapid rate at which the oropharynx of the critically ill patient is recolonized. (The environmental presence of multiply resistant bacteria also plays an important role.) Almost all patients are colonized with gram-negative bacteria by the third hospital day. All too often, a specific pathogen cannot be identified, despite good sampling methods and overt symptomatology compatible with acute pneumonia. *Mixed aerobic/anaerobic infection*, *Mycoplasma*, *Chlamydia*, *Legionella*, and *viral agents* are likely candidates to explain the process under these conditions. Fungal pneumonia (*Candida* or *Aspergillus*) is unusual in the immunocompetent patient, but when it occurs, is usually the result of hematogenous seeding. Furthermore, it is often difficult to distinguish bacterial colonization from true infection. The clinical picture is also clouded by the presence of non-infectious processes that mimic infectious pneumonitis (e.g., ARDS, pulmonary embolism, heart failure, chemical aspiration).

Diagnosis

The choice of initial therapy for a bacterial process is always accompanied by some uncertainty, even in the presence of a Gram stain "typical" of a specific organism. *Historical features* can help immensely in sorting through the diagnostic possibilities for community-acquired pneumonia. For example, the sudden onset of chills, pleurisy, rigors, and high temperature are characteristic features for pneumococcus in a young adult. On the other hand, these findings may be inconspicuous in an older person, in whom confusion or stupor often predominates. A history of seizures, drug abuse, alcoholism, or swallowing disorder focuses attention on the possibility of aspiration. Recent travel history, occupational exposure, and concurrent family illnesses can help to make the diagnosis of an unusual etiology (Table 21.3).

A pulse rate that fails to rise in proportion to fever (*pulse-temperature dissociation*) *suggests an intracellular infection*: Legionnaires' disease, *Mycoplasma*, Q fever, psittacosis, or tularemia. *Mycoplasma* often causes pharyngitis, myringitis, or conjunctivitis. Contrary to popular teaching, extrapulmonary symptoms (diarrhea, central nervous system disease) are no more common in Legionnaire's disease than in other bacterial pneumonias. Unlike community acquired pneumonia, nosocomial pneumonias offer few historical clues to diagnosis. Occasionally, however, a skin rash, gingival disease, or purulent sinus drainage help to narrow the possibilities.

Numerous classical *roentgenographic features* have been described, including lobar consolidation without air bronchograms (central obstruction), bulging fissures (*Klebsiella*), infiltrate with ipsilateral hilar adenopathy (histoplasmosis, tularemia, tuberculosis), widespread cavitation (*Staphylococcus*), and sequential progression to multi-lobar involvement (*Legionella*). These findings are not sufficiently consistent, however, to be of real value in confirming the diagnosis. For example, virtually any pneumonic infiltrate can imitate cavitation or pneumatocele formation in a patient with emphysema.

Laboratory studies are the cornerstone of the diagnostic workup. *Leukopenia*, an ominous prognostic sign, often results from overwhelming infections, particularly those due to *Staphylococcus*,

Table 21.2
Conditions Allowing Proliferation

Impaired Immunity	Mechanical Factors	Parenchymal Damage
Malnutrition	Secretion	Cytotoxic drugs
Steroids/	retention	Oxygen toxicity
cytotoxic	Atelectasis	ARDS
drugs	Smoking	Viral infections
Alcohol	Obstructive lung	
Diabetes	disease	
	Neuromuscular	
	weakness	

Table 21.3
Clues to Unusual Organisms

Diagnosis	History
Histoplasmosis	Excavation/bird exposure/ Ohio Valley
Coccidiomycosis	Travel to Southwest United States
Tularemia	Tick bite or exposure to skinned animals
Brucellosis	Slaughterhouse workers
Psittacosis	Exposure to pet birds
Q fever	Sheep contact

Pneumococcus, or gram-negative organisms. A *differential count* that is not significantly left shifted suggests the possibility of virus, *Mycoplasma*, or *Legionella*. When performed correctly, *stain and culture of pulmonary secretions* remain the most likely techniques to yield a diagnosis. Expectorated sputum is only appropriate for analysis and culture if there is a high ratio of inflammatory to epithelial cells. Apart from the Gram stain, agglutination tests (*Haemophilus influenzae*, *Pneumococcus*, *Klebsiella*) and direct immunofluorescent antibody staining (*Legionella*) are other useful methods for processing the expectorated sample that can yield an immediate, if only presumptive, diagnosis.

Inhalation of a hypotonic or hypertonic aerosol, particularly if given via an ultrasonic nebulizer, can stimulate a productive cough in patients otherwise unable or unwilling to expectorate. When adequate sputum cannot be obtained, nasotracheal or transtracheal catheterization can be helpful. Occasionally, more invasive methods are indicated, including bronchoscopy using the protected brush technique and/or lavage. In general, these procedures should be reserved for those who are seriously ill, immune compromised, or unresponsive to conventional therapy. *Transthoracic needle aspiration* often yields an adequate specimen but exposes the patient to attendant risks of pneumothorax and bleeding. Open lung biopsy is rarely necessary in patients with intact host defenses. *Cultures of the blood and pleural fluid* must be obtained and, when positive, are the most convincing evidence of the responsible organism. Unfortunately, such specimens are often negative, even in seriously ill patients.

Treatment

In the hospital, *nutritional*, *fluid*, *electrolyte*, and *oxygen* support of the patient with bacterial pneumonia are noncontroversial and universally applied. The initial choice of *antibiotic* must be guided not only by the nature of the suspected organism but also by the severity of illness. Thus, although treatment should be directed as specifically as possible in patients who are only moderately ill, the initial therapy of a compromised patient with serious illness should include ''broad spectrum'' coverage until culture results are available. There is no margin for error in critically ill patients with pneumonia. Therefore, regardless of the appearance of the Gram stain, empirical therapy in critically ill patients should include an extended spectrum penicillin plus an aminoglycoside. (Van-

comycin covers essentially all forms of gram-positive aerobic infection in penicillin-allergic patients.)

Erythromycin should be added if there is an ''atypical'' clinical or radiographic presentation or if fever persists despite usual therapy. In patients at risk of *H. influenza* or *Branhamella* infections (e.g., elderly, cirrhotics and patients with chronic obstructive pulmonary disease) initial therapy should include a third generation cephalosporin, providing effective treatment for strains which produce beta-lactamase. Patients likely to contract staphylococcal infection (e.g., recent influenza, neutropenia, or a suggestive sputum Gram stain) should receive an anti-staphylococcal penicillin or vancomycin. Recently, methicillin-resistant staphyloccci have surfaced as important pathogens in many institutions. In such hospitals, vancomycin represents first-line coverage.

Careful hand washing between patient contacts may also decrease the risk of nosocomial infection. Whenever suctioning intubated patients, gloves should be worn on *both hands* to prevent staff acquisition of herpetic infections.

INTRAVASCULAR CATHETER INFECTIONS

Risk Factors

Factors increasing the risk of intravascular catheter infection include: (1) placement under *emergency* conditions; (2) use of *plastic* rather than steel needles; (3) *catheterization of a central vein* (particularly the internal jugular); (4) *prolonged catheterization* at a single site; and (5) placement by surgical *cut-down*.

Most catheter infections can be prevented by using sterile technique when inserting, dressing, changing, and reconnecting catheters and by minimizing the frequency of catheter entry. *Antibiotic ointments* applied at the catheter entry site help to reduce local infections, but systemic antibiotics given prophylactically do not decrease the risk of bacteremia. Avoiding lower extremity catheterization and reducing motion at the skin-catheter interface also decrease the infection risk. Hypertonic fluids (peripheral total parenteral nutrition, TPN) or highly caustic drugs (e.g., amphotericin, diazepam, methicillin, erythromycin) may induce a chemical phlebitis, facilitating bacterial superinfection. Intravenous sites should be monitored daily and intravenous connecting tubing should be changed every 24–48 hours. Blood withdrawal increases the risk of infection, as does the filling of tubing systems in advance of their use. Even minute quantities of blood or fat provide nutrients adequate to support the growth of most bacteria; therefore, changing tubing after infusing blood or lipids reduces infection risk.

Continuous flush solutions and pressure monitoring devices attached to arterial catheters pose special hazards. Reducing the number of catheter entries for blood sampling will reduce infection risk. Glucose-containing fluids promote bacterial growth in the transducer dome, tubing, and flush solutions. It is especially important to avoid contamination during calibration.

Contamination of Swan Ganz catheters may be reduced by minimizing the number of cardiac output determinations and by using sterile precautions during preparation and introduction of the injectate. Because of the escalating risk of infection, arterial and Swan Ganz catheters should be removed within 3–5 days of their placement.

Diagnosis

Although redness, pain, and swelling around the insertion site strongly suggest infection, these signs are often *absent* in patients with catheter-related phlebitis. *Local* (soft-tissue) catheter infections may be confirmed by Gram staining and culturing the catheter and by "milking the wound" to provide material for Gram stain. Because intravascular infections usually produce continuous bacteremia, a positive blood culture withdrawn through a potentially contaminated intravenous line does not confirm catheter sepsis.

In patients with suspected "line" sepsis, the catheter, tubing, and fluids should be replaced with fresh components. Before catheter removal the skin should be cleansed with alcohol. The distal centimeter of the catheter tip should then be sent in a sterile container for culture and Gram stain. Semiquantitative culturing is performed by rolling the tip across a culture plate. If > 15 colonies of a single organism are isolated, *infection* is more likely than *colonization*. The catheter tip should *not* be placed into any solution for transport—doing so renders quantitative culturing impossible. Although probably acceptable for routine catheter changes, changing intravascular catheters over a guidewire is not rational in patients with sepsis or inflamed entry sites.

Common Organisms

Gram negative rods, *S. aureus*, *S. epidermidis*, and *Candida* account for the majority of catheter-related infections. Although uncommon, blood cultures growing *Enterobacter agglomerans*, *Pseudomonas cepacia*, and *Enterobacter cloacae* usually signify line sepsis. In patients with suspected line sepsis, an anti-staphylococcal penicillin and an aminoglycoside should be started after removal and culture of the catheter. Vancomycin may be substituted for penicillin in the allergic patient or if methicillin-resistant staphlococci are prevalent.

Persistent Bacteremia

In patients with persistent bacteremia, line sepsis must be distinguished from bacterial endocarditis. (The diagnosis of endocarditis usually obligates treatment with parenteral antibiotics for 4–6 weeks.) The following factors all favor a diagnosis of endocarditis: (1) a new or changing heart murmur; (2) valvular vegetations on echocardiogram; (3) physical stigmata of endocarditis; and (4) persistent bacteremia or fungemia following removal of the suspect intravenous catheter.

Persistent unexplained bacteremia, particularly when accompanied by pain, swelling, or redness of an intravenous site and a catheter-related organism, may signal *suppurative thrombophlebitis*. A low threshold for surgical exploration should be maintained because this often subtle and highly lethal disease will seldom be cured unless the suppurated vessel is excised, despite the use of appropriate antibiotics.

PSEUDOMEMBRANOUS COLITIS

Pathophysiology

Pseudomembranous colitis (PMC) is caused by a toxin produced by *Clostridium difficile*. This clostridial toxin directly attacks colonic cells, producing the areas of mucosal damage that form the characteristic "pseudomembrane". Although classically described following intravenous clindamycin therapy, *C. difficle* may overgrow the normal flora of patients receiving essentially any parenteral *or* oral antibiotic. Rarely, colonic overgrowth of other bacteria (e.g., staphylocci) in response to antibiotic therapy can give rise to a similar picture.

Signs And Symptoms

PMC typically presents with watery diarrhea on the fourth to ninth day of antibiotic therapy. Although usually guaiac positive, the stool is rarely bloody. However, bloody stools may result from one form of the disease localized to the hepatic flexure. Crampy periumbilical and hypogastric pain and low grade fever are common, whereas an "acute abdomen" is rare (see Chapter 34).

Diagnosis

No *routine* laboratory test is diagnostic, but leukocytosis occurs in ≃ 80% of cases. As with other forms of inflammatory colitis, red blood cells and leukocytes are usually detectable in the stool specimen. Diagnosis is confirmed by culturing *C. difficile* in profusion from the stool or by detecting bacterial toxin in a fecal specimen. The toxin assay is less sensitive but more specific than stool culture. (Some patients without PMC have small numbers of *C. difficile* cultured from stool.) Rigid sigmoidoscopy usually visualizes the colonic pseudomembranes, but in a small fraction of patients (about 10%) only the right colon is involved. In such cases, even *flexible* sigmoidoscopy may fail to disclose the mucosal lesions. Barium enema lacks sufficient resolution to be useful in diagnosis.

Treatment

The offending antibiotic should be discontinued and fluid and electrolyte support administered. Antidiarrheal agents should not be used because they may prolong colonic dwell time, thereby increasing the severity of the colitis. There is no evidence that using corticosteroids or that giving lactobacilli to change the fecal flora is beneficial. Because the toxin as well as the organism may be transmitted nosocomially, all patients with this disease should be placed on enteric precautions.

Given orally, vancomycin (0.5 to 2 gm/day) causes prompt cessation of diarrhea in 48–96 hours. Conversely, systemic vancomycin is ineffective. Treatment may fail due to *reinfection*, emergence of a *vancomycin-resistant* organism, or *bacterial tranformation* into a dormant spore phase. When therapy fails, relapses usually occur within 2 weeks of stopping treatment. In patients intolerant of vancomycin, oral metronidazole in doses of 1.2 to 1.5 gm/day for 7 to 14 days may be effective. (Recently, *intravenous* metronidazole has been reported effective.) Bacitracin has also been used in doses of 25,000 units orally, 4 times daily.

SINUSITIS

Although radiographic evidence of sinusitis can be demonstrated in most patients with nasogastric tubes, nasal packing, or nasotracheal tubes, sinusitis is commonly overlooked as a source for occult fever in the critically ill. Nosocomial sinusitis is usually *polymicrobial* with gram-negative rods and staphylococci predominating. Pseudomonas is not uncommon. Frequently, *cryptic fever* is the only clinical feature. *Headache and facial pain may be impossible to detect in comatose or intu-* bated patients. *Anterior nasal discharge is usually absent.* The paucity of overt clinical signs may allow purulent sinusitis to advance to a life-threatening infection of the central nervous system. Its remote position and contiguity to vital structures renders *sphenoid sinusitis* an unusually insidious process.

Because bedside sinus radiographs are usually of poor quality (particularly for visualizing the sphenoid sinus), *computed tomography of the head* with attention directed to the sinuses is the preferred method of diagnosis.

Most cases of sinusitis respond to tube removal, decongestants, and antibiotics. Empirical antibiotic selection should include an anti- staphylococcal penicillin and an aminoglycoside. More specific therapy is guided by Gram stain and culture of sinus cavity aspirates. In community-acquired sinusitis *H. influenzae* is a common etiologic organism that often requires therapy with a beta lactamase-resistant drug, such as a third generation cephalosporin. Surgical intervention may be necessary in patients with suppurative complications (e.g., retro-ortibal cellulitis, osteomyelitis, and brain abscess).

MENINGITIS

Bacterial meningitis should be suspected in patients with *mental status changes*, *fever*, and signs of *meningeal irritation*. When meningitis results from malignancy, tuberculosis, or fungal infection, the presentation is likely to be more subtle and may include focal neurological deficits.

Organisms

Etiology varies with site of acquisition (community versus hospital) and patient age. The *pneumococcus* is the most common organism in *community acquired*, *adult* meningitis. Sinusitis, otitis, pneumonia, or endocarditis frequently coexist. *Neisseria meningitidis* is the second most frequent cause of sporadic meningitis. Non-typeable strains of *H. influenzae* represent the third most likely organism. Although unusual in any setting, *Listeria* and enteric gram-negative rods are especially rare outside the hospital. In hospital-acquired meningitis, *S. aureus* or *epidermitis* and enteric gram-negative rods are the leading etiologies, particularly in the postoperative setting.

Diagnosis

Examination and culture of spinal fluid provide the only conclusive method of diagnosing meningitis. In the absence of papilledema or focal neurological deficits suggestive of a mass lesion, lumbar puncture may be safely performed without CT scan. Lumbar puncture (LP) may be technically impossible because of poor patient cooperation or lumbar disease. In such patients, cisternal puncture or LP under fluoroscopy may secure a specimen of spinal fluid. *Pleocytosis* with a granulocytic predominance is usually documented. The spinal fluid *glucose* level is usually < 50% of the peripheral blood glucose value and cerebrospinal fluid (CSF) *protein* concentration often exceeds 100 mg/dl. *Gram stain* of *spun* spinal fluid demonstrates the organism in 3 of 4 cases of bacterial meningitis. Culture establishes a definitive diagnosis. Although cultures of spinal fluid are positive in more than 90% of *untreated* cases of bacterial meningitis, the specimen may be rendered sterile by even a single oral dose of antibiotic. However, antibiotics rarely change the pattern of cells, CSF glucose, or protein measurements for 12–24 hours. If spinal fluid cultures are sterile, latex agglutination tests may reveal the etiology, especially when *pneumococcus* or *H. influenzae* are causative. However, because of wide cross-reactivity, agglutination tests are *least* helpful in establishing or ruling out *Neisseria* infections. Blood cultures, positive in ⅓ of patients with bacterial meningitis, should be obtained before instituting antibiotics. Once the diagnosis of bacterial meningitis has been established, the clinician should be careful to *exclude underlying pneumonia, abscess, or endocarditis* before deciding on the duration of treatment. Viral, neoplastic, fungal, and tuberculous organisms all cause meningitis but generally present less urgently than acute bacterial meningitis.

Treatment

Even if spinal fluid cannot be obtained, antibiotics *must* be administered within 1 hour of presentation. If lumbar puncture is contraindicated, empirical therapy should be initiated as efforts are undertaken to establish a delayed diagnosis by blood culture or latex agglutination testing.

Antibiotic therapy and its route of administration (intravenous, intrathecal) should be guided by Gram stain and culture of centrifuged spinal fluid. Although meningeal inflammation improves the penetration of most antibiotics into the CSF, certain drugs cross much more efficiently than others. For example, penicillin, chloramphenicol, and selected third generation cephalosporins cross the blood-brain barrier easily, whereas aminoglycosides and other cephalosporins may fail to achieve effective concentrations. Penicillin is the drug of choice for community-acquired meningitis when lancet-shaped gram-positive cocci are unequivocally present. Small gram-negative rods suggest *H. influenzae*, making a third generation cephalosporin (cefotaxime, ceftriaxone) the drug of choice. If Gram stain suggests an enteric (large) gram-negative rod or if there is evidence of a parameningeal focus (sinusitis, spinal osteomyelitis), an aminoglycoside should be added to a third generation cephalosporin. (Aminoglycosides are never sufficient therapy alone, and even when clearly indicated for gram-negative infections, consideration should be given to concurrent intrathecal administration.) In cases where spinal fluid cannot be obtained or is non-diagnostic, a third generation cephalosporin with or without ampicillin or penicillin is the safest alternative.

Complications of Meningitis

Four important complications of acute bacterial meningitis are (1) *cerebral edema*; (2) *inappropriate antidiuretic hormone (ADH) syndrome*; (3) *obstructive hydrocephalus*, and (4) *seizures*. Because 1 in 3 adults with meningitis experiences seizures, prophylactic anti-convulsant therapy is rational. Signs of increased intracranial pressure (e.g., lethargy, papilledema, 3d nerve palsy, hemiparesis) should prompt emergent evaluation for cerebral edema or hydrocephalus by CT scanning. Hyponatremia should raise concern for the syndrome of inappropriate antidiuretic hormone secretion (SIADH) syndrome.

Craniotomy patients are at particular risk of meningitis caused by staphlococci and gram-negative rods in the early postoperative period. Conversely, the pneumococcus is responsible for > 90% of *late* meningeal infections in patients with persistent post-traumatic CSF leakage. Septic *cerebral embolism* (e.g., from subacute bacterial endocarditis) or *parameningeal infection* (epidural abscess, brain abscess, sinusitis, and otitis media) are often confused with meningitis because they produce similar symptomatology and CSF pleocytosis. Paraspinal tenderness accompanied by radicular pain or weakness should be a clue to *epidural abscess*. *Staphlococcus aureus* is the causitive organism in more than ½ of such cases.

Brain abscess is most often a polymicrobial infection due to staphlococci, streptococci, and anaerobes. Abscess may develop by extension from the sinuses or ears, or by hematogenous seeding (infected dialysis shunts, heart valves) or long-standing purulent lung disease (abscess, bronchiectasis). Brain abscess is rarely confused with uncomplicated bacterial meningitis because it usually presents with a less toxic picture and focal neurological signs. Unless otherwise guided by results of culture, penicillin together with chloramphenicol or metronidazole should comprise the antibiotic treatment of brain abscess. In selected cases a third generation cephalosporin or antistaphylococcal agent may be indicated. Surgical intervention is generally reserved for lesions that compress vital structures, those unresponsive to medical management, and those for which malignancy is a strong alternative possibility.

GAS-PRODUCING SOFT TISSUE INFECTIONS

Gas-producing soft tissue infections usually develop in the setting of ischemia or gross contamination. Risk factors include diabetes, penetrating foot lesions, peripheral vascular disease, and open trauma. Gas-producing infections may be classical *gas gangrene* with myonecrosis, or a *mixed organism (synergistic) necrotizing fascitis*. Both may spread with alarming speed. A mixture of aerobic and anaerobic organisms (gram-positive cocci and gram-negative rods) cause most gas producing soft tissue infections. Classical clostridial gangrene is less common.

A combined medical/surgical treatment approach must be rapidly carried out. Cultures of blood should be obtained, in conjunction with biopsy or aspiration culture of the affected tissue. Although the choice of antibiotics should be guided by Gram stain and culture, empirical regimens usually include an anti-staphylococcal penicillin, *and* Penicillin G, with or without an aminoglycoside. Wide debridement or amputation is frequently required for control. If not up to date, tetanus immunization and toxoid should be administered.

INFECTION IN THE IMMUNE COMPROMISED HOST

Few problems present a greater diagnostic challenge than fever in the immune compromised host (CH). Because such patients often have impaired function of multiple organ systems or are under treatment with toxic agents, possible etiologies span a wide range of noninfectious and infectious agents. Multiple causes frequently coexist. Patients in this category have primary deficits of T-lymphocyte (cell-mediated), B-cell (antibody), or granulocyte (phagocytic) function. Knowledge of the type of deficit can narrow the differential diagnosis. For example, T-cell disorders predispose to viruses and fungi and B-cell disorders to bacterial pathogens.

Although loss of humoral immunity and T-cell function predispose to infection, profound neutropenia ($<$ 1000 granulocytes/mm^3) is the defect that represents the greatest risk to life. *Fever in such patients constitutes a true medical emergency.* In this setting, the speed with which appropriate therapy is begun determines outcome.

Unfortunately, establishing a specific diagnosis often proves difficult. Such patients frequently fail to produce suppuration or other localizing signs of inflammation. Regardless of the type of immune defect or site of inflammation, the etiologic organism is usually one that normally resides as a commensal in the host. Although any site may be the target of infection, a few problems are characteristic in the neutropenic patient. These include mucosal infections (e.g., gingivitis), "primary bacteremia", soft tissue phlegmons (e.g., perirectal abscess), and atypical pulmonary infiltration.

Infectious Pulmonary Infiltrates

The complex problem of pulmonary infections is addressed in detail in Ref. 7, Chapter 32. Only a few salient features can be covered here. In febrile neutropenic patients, infection must always be the leading diagnostic consideration. However, progression of the *primary neoplastic process*, *hemorrhage*, *edema*, *radiation*, and *drug reaction* are frequent causes of pulmonary infiltrates.

Although virtually any organism can cause pulmonary infiltration in the CH, the clinician can often integrate knowledge of the immune defect, epidemiology, and clinical and laboratory data to narrow the spectrum of likely possibilities and formulate a logical approach. As a first consideration, the underlying disease may give some clue to the nature of the pathogen.

For example, *acquired immune deficiency syndrome, (AIDS)*, a problem of helper T-lymphocytes, so predisposes to pneumocystis, mycobacteria, and cytomegalovirus (CMV) infections that a presumptive diagnosis is suggested by the radiographic and clinical pictures alone. Nonetheless, the spectrum of possibilities remains wide until confirmed by biopsy or fluid examination.

Epidemiological factors are also important to consider. The *duration of hospitalization* before the development of pneumonitis influences the microbiology. For example, *Pseudomonas*, *Candida*, and *Aspergillus* infections are most likely to develop after many days in the hospital, whereas the likelihood of routine (community prevalent) pathogens wanes rapidly after the first few days of confinement. *Renal transplant* recipients are unusually prone to CMV, Herpes simplex, *Crypto-coccus*, *Aspergillus*, and *Pneumocystis carinii* infections during the period of maximal T-cell suppression, 1–6 months after operation. *Neutro-penic* patients are highly susceptible to gram-negative bacteria and fungal infections (*Aspergillus*, zygomycetes). (*Aspergillus* becomes a common infecting organism if neutropenia is sustained longer than 3 weeks).

Concurrent infection with two or more organisms occurs commonly in patients with AIDS and in those undergoing renal or marrow transplantation. CMV, *Cryptococcus*, and *Nocardia* are frequently recovered in conjunction with other pathogens. (CMV and *Pneumocystis* are commonly associated.) Superinfections also occur frequently in immune-suppressed patients, particularly during sustained neutropenia, and prolonged high-dose immunosuppressive therapy.

Certain clinical findings are especially noteworthy. *Legionella*, *Strongyloides*, and *Cryptosporidium* may cause diarrhea and pulmonary infiltration. Concurrent infiltration of lungs and skin may result from *Pseudomonas*, *Aspergillus*, *Candida*, and varicella-zoster. Hepatic and pulmonary disease tend to coexist during infections with CMV, *Nocardia*, mycobacteria, and necrotizing bacteria (Pseudomonas, Staphylococcus).

Workup and Therapeutic Approach to Pulmonary Infiltrates

Unfortunately, these problems often defy easy diagnosis, and a tissue biopsy is frequently needed. The pace of the disease may be very rapid, so that the objective is to cover broadly while attempting to establish a specific etiologic diagnosis expediently and safely.

Two important questions must be answered to deal effectively with a life-threatening pulmonary process in a CH. First, given that the process appears to be infectious and that the course cannot be easily determined, *does a precise diagnosis need to be established?* (Is empirical therapy sufficient?) Second, if a precise diagnosis is required, *what is the most efficacious technique in a fragile, critically ill patient?* These questions are not straightforward and remain the subject of intense controversy. In general, the approach should vary with the severity of illness, the pace of advancement, coagulation and ventilation status, the strength of ancillary information, and the experience of available personnel with specific invasive procedures. If a diffuse pattern on chest x-ray cannot be confidently distinguished from pulmonary edema,

a brief trial of diuresis may be prudent before proceeding to invasive diagnostic measures. Unless contraindicated, *"diuresis before biopsy"* is a good rule of thumb. Sputum examination, when possible, is an obvious first step. Transtracheal aspiration and transthoracic needle biopsy are dangerous, low-yield procedures in this setting and should be withheld.

Ancillary Data

Both the characteristics of the chest x-ray at any single point in time and its rate of progression can provide helpful diagnostic clues. Localized infiltrates, either consolidated or nodular, are most consistent with bacterial or fungal infection, hemorrhage, or thromboembolic disease. Bilateral "interstitial" infiltrates, on the other hand, suggest volume-overload, *Pneumocystis*, mycobacteria, or virus. Serious lung infections may develop without causing pulmonary infiltrates, particularly in neutropenic patients. A fulminant evolution suggests a bacterial process or a non-infectious etiology (fluid overload, embolism, adult respiratory distress syndrome, ARDS). Conversely, a process requiring 1–2 weeks for full expression calls to mind mycobacterial, parasitic, or systemic fungal diseases. The severity of hypoxemia is another key observation. Life-threatening depressions of blood oxygen tension are typical for bacterial, viral, and *Pneumocystis* infections but are less common with indolent fungal and mycobacterial processes.

Examination of body fluids from extrapulmonary sources can suggest a presumptive diagnosis for the chest infiltrate. Spinal fluid may demonstrate *Cryptococcus* but does not prove that the roentgenographic infiltrates are related. Nonetheless, in the appropriate setting, pleural and joint fluids should be tapped, examined, and cultured and a stool specimen sent for parasite detection. Whereas blood cultures are unquestionably important, serologic testing rarely provides definitive information in an appropriate time frame.

Pulmonary Secretions and Tissue

Sputum is less frequently produced by the CH than by immune competent patients, especially when neutropenia is present. Nonetheless, when sputum can be obtained, its careful examination may reveal the responsible pathogen. Apart from the routine Gram stain, a direct fluorescent antibody test for *Legionella*, a phase contrast or cytological preparation for *blastomycosis*, an acid-fast stain for *mycobacteria* and *Nocardia*, and a silver stain for *Pneumocystis* and fungal elements are highly worthwhile. Concentrated specimens may reveal *Strongyloides*. Patients with AIDS harbor such a profusion of *Pneumocystis* organisms that expectorated specimens often reveal them. Unfortunately, cultures of many pathogens require days to weeks for growth.

The Need for Biopsy

If a specific diagnosis is not in hand after review of clinical data and laboratory results, the next step should be guided by the strength of clinical suspicion and the urgency of making the correct diagnosis. In most instances, bronchoscopy should be the first invasive procedure. Although coagulopathy and the need for mechanical ventilation are moderate contraindications to forceps biopsy, lavage and gentle brushings can be safely obtained when care is taken to administer platelets and/or missing clotting factors beforehand. Bronchoscopic yield varies greatly with the disease process and with the method of conducting this procedure. For example, when all specimen-gathering techniques (biopsy, brushings, and lavage) are used, a specific diagnosis can be established about 50% of the time. In special instances, such as AIDS, the yield is considerably higher.

The decision to undertake an *open lung biospy* is often delayed because of the perceived morbidity and expense. In fact, open biopsy conducted *early* in the course of the illness is well tolerated, safe, and often helpful. Open biopsy is a procedure that can be completed within 20–40 minutes. It is the most reliable means of securing tissue for histologic diagnosis while establishing effective hemostasis in patients at high risk for bleeding. Its expense should be considered alongside the high cost of empirical multi-antibiotic therapy. The empirical antibiotics commonly used—trimethoprim/ sulfa (TMP-SMX), aminoglycosides, amphotericin—are not without associated toxicity for kidneys and bone marrow. Whatever the value of open lung biopsy may be when undertaken early in the course of disease, it is clearly less valuable after broad spectrum antibiotics have been given for a prolonged period. In such instances, it is unusual for open biopsy to add sufficient new information to warrant its attendant drawbacks. Failure to define a specific etiology does not mandate withdrawal of empirical antibiotics.

Antibiotic management can be streamlined when a specific diagnosis has been made. However, the clinician must remain alert to *superinfection*. Furthermore, if a patient fails to improve with specific therapy directed against a known pathogen, a *second organism* is commonly present. For example, AIDS patients with confirmed *Pneumocystis* pneumonia who fail to respond to TMP/SMX often have coexistent CMV infection. When no specific diagnosis has been made and the clinician is forced to choose a regimen, it should be remembered that *Legionella* and *Pneumocystis* are among the most lethal and common pathogens. In addition to a third generation cephalosporin and an aminoglycoside, erythromycin and TMP-SMX are usually chosen. In centers where fungi present a major problem, amphotericin is often begun very early in the course. The recent introduction of ultra-broad spectrum antibiotics (such as imipenem) may help to greatly simplify initial coverage.

Non-pulmonary Sites of Infection

Neutropenia most frequently is an iatrogenic complication of antineoplastic chemotherapy. These same drugs profoundly impair host ability to maintain the integrity of tissues having rapid cellular turnover (e.g., bowel wall and the mucosa of gingiva and rectum). Therefore, it is not surprising that *diffuse necrotizing colitis*, *anorectal cellulitis*, and *typhlitis* (a severe bacterial infection of the cecum mimicking appendicitis) are frequent sources of infection. Violation of the normally intact integument by intravenous catheters, surgical incisions, or decubitus ulcers also opens a portal for bacterial entry. Therefore, in febrile neutropenic patients physical examination should routinely include catheter entry sites and the gingival and perirectal regions. Lack of tenderness with gentle palpation of the anal verge usually suffices to exclude this as a site of infection. All too often no site is found for bacteremia or the sepsis syndrome.

General Principles

Survival of neutropenic patients is dependent upon *early empirical therapy with more than one antibiotic effective against the infecting organism*. The most common organisms include: gram-negative rods (particularly *Pseudomonas*), *Staphylococci*, and fungi (e.g., *Aspergillus* and *Candida*). Patients with impaired cell-mediated immunity are more likely to be infected with *Pneumocystis* or *Candida*. When a site of infection is clearly definable, antibiotics should be chosen against the likely organisms. However, neutropenic patients frequently lack localizing signs of inflammation and no likely source is found in most cases (even with careful examination). In such cases, cultures of blood, urine, sputum, and skin lesions should be obtained. Even though pyuria may be absent, microscopic examination of the urine may reveal large numbers of organisms. Broad spectrum antibiotics including an *extended spectrum penicillin* (e.g., ticarcillin) or *third generation cephalosporin* plus an *aminoglycoside* should be initiated. The empirical use of vancomycin is unwarranted unless there is a penicillin allergy or reason to suspect a methicillin-resistant staphylococcal infection. In many centers amphotericin is begun if the patient remains febrile for more than 72 hours following institution of broad spectrum antibiotics.

POST-SPLENECTOMY INFECTIONS

Serious infections following splenectomy are usually due to *encapsulated bacteria* (e.g., pneumococcus, *Salmonella*, *Haemophilus*). The spleen provides a critical period of bacterial control until adequate circulating antibodies are elaborated. Loss of this phagocytic function allows unchecked bacterial proliferation. Similarly, loss of hepatic phagocytic function in patients with cirrhosis makes them subject to overwhelming infection. *Salmonella* and *Vibrio* species are two unusual pathogens seen in such patients. Therefore, in patients without a spleen, the *prevention* of infections and the early institution of antibiotics are essential.

SUGGESTED READINGS

1. Brewer NS, MacCarty CS, Wellman WE: Brain abscess: a review of recent experience. *Ann Intern Med* 82:571–576, 1975.
2. Caplan ES, Hoyt NJ: Nosocomial sinusitis. *JAMA* 247:639–641, 1982.
3. Garibaldi RA, Burke JP, Dickman ML, et al: Factors predisposing to bacteriuria during indwelling urethral catheterization. *N Engl J Med* 291:215–219, 1974.
4. Graybill JR, Marshall LW, Charache P, et al: Nosocomial pneumonia. *Am Rev Respir Dis* 108:1130–1140, 1973.
5. Maki DG, Weise CE, Sarafin HW: A semiquantitative culture method for identifying intravenous-catheter-related infection. *N Engl J Med* 296:1304–1309, 1977.
6. Maki DG: Nosocomial bacteremia. *Am J Med* 70:719–732, 1981.
7. Marini JJ: *Respiratory Medicine for the House Officer.* Baltimore, Williams & Wilkins, 1987.
8. Nishijima H, Weil MH, Shubin H, et al.: Hemodynamic and metabolic studies on shock associated with gram-negative bacteremia. *Medicine* 52:287–294, 1973.
9. Rosenow EC, Wilson WR, Cockerill FR: Pulmonary disease in the immunocompromised host. (Parts 1 and 2) *Mayo Clin Proc* 60:473–487, 610–631, 1985.
10. Stone HH, Martin JD: Synergistic necrotizing cellulitis. *Ann Surg* 175:702–711, 1972.

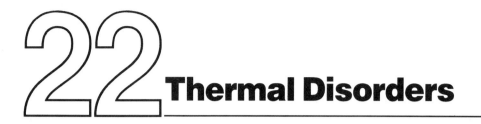

Thermal Disorders

TEMPERATURE MEASUREMENT

Types of Measuring Devices

The *technique* used to measure temperature is critical in detecting fever or hypothermia. Mercury thermometers are usually unable to detect temperatures < 94°F or > 105°F and fail to record values below the initial "shaken" level. Mercury thermometers respond rather slowly to temperature changes, making use of an electronic device or thermocouple (e.g., on a pulmonary artery catheter) preferable when recording temperature extremes and rapid fluctuations. Plastic strip thermometers have limited accuracy and recording range.

Sites of Measurement

Recorded *oral* temperatures are reduced below true core values when respiratory rates exceed 18 breaths/minute. *Rectal* temperatures avoid artifacts arising from varying respiratory rates, poor thermometer-patient contact, and aberrations of regional temperature caused by smoking or oral consumption of hot or cold liquids. Although usually accurate, rectal temperatures may spuriously indicate hypothermia in patients with colonic impaction or intense mucosal vasoconstriction.

Axillary temperatures often underestimate core temperature due to poor thermometer-skin contact and wide differences between skin and core temperature. *Esophageal* temperature measurement is an effective "non-invasive" way to measure core temperature, but it requires specialized equipment. Similarly, although *tympanic membrane* probes directly record temperature of blood perfusing the hypothalamic regulation center, technical sophistication limits their clinical application to the operative setting.

The temperature of *pulmonary artery blood* may be continuously monitored using the thermistor-tipped pulmonary artery catheter. *Freshly voided urine* also provides a source for on-line measurement of central temperature by specialized collection systems.

HYPOTHERMIA

Definition and Problems in Detection

Patients with *uremia, hypothyroidism, malnutrition,* and *congestive heart failure* often have mildly reduced (1–3°F) basal temperatures. In these patients "normal" or slightly increased temperature may represent fever. *Clinical hypothermia* (HT), a core temperature below 35°C (95°F), frequently escapes detection because symptoms are non-specific and because most thermometers fail to record in the appropriate range.

Etiology

Most HT occurs in an urban setting and is multifactorial in origin. (Environmental exposure subsequent to intoxication or a primary neurological event is a common sequence.) HT may be caused by medications that (1) alter the perception of cold; (2) increase heat loss through vasodilation; or (3) inhibit heat generation. (Phenothiazines and barbiturates are frequent offenders.) Common contributing metabolic conditions include *adrenal insufficiency, hypoglycemia,* and *myxedema.* Hypothyroidism decreases heat production, blunts the shivering response, and impairs temperature perception. Consequently, myxedema is an etiologic factor in up to 10% of cases of hypothermia. *Hypopituitarism, diabetic ketoacidosis, malnutrition,* and mass lesions of the *central nervous system* may also induce hypothermia. An intact skin covering and the ability to vasoconstrict are essential to the regulation of core temperature. Hence, *burns* and *spinal cord injuries* both impair the ability to conserve heat. For similar reasons, HT is commonly observed during and immediately after general anesthesia.

Clinical Manifestations

Vasoconstriction to conserve heat and shivering to generate heat are important initial compensatory mechanisms to prevent HT. Unfortunately, both responses may be blunted by a variety of underlying diseases or drugs and are blunted by profound HT. HT depresses metabolism, affecting essentially all organ systems. The key physiologic events occurring during HT are illustrated in Figure 22.1.

Cardiovascular

Hypothermia decreases cardiac conduction and slows repolarization prolonging all measured electrocardiograph (ECG) intervals eventually causing atrioventricular (AV) nodal blockade. Characteristic deformations of the J-point (Osbourn waves) may be seen on the ECG, but are neither sensitive nor specific indicators of core temperature. Myocardial irritability is increased at temperatures < 86°F. Conversely, asystole may supervene at temperatures < 60°F. Disproportionate reductions of cardiac output and blood pressure often result in metabolic acidosis.

Neurological

Cerebral oxygen consumption is roughly halved for each 10°C (18°F) decline in temperature, mak-

ing the central nervous system (CNS) more tolerant of reduced perfusion during HT. Initial CNS responses to HT include decreased respiratory drive, lethargy, and fatigue. Coma usually develops when core temperatures fall below 80° F. Concurrent with the loss of consciousness, deep tendon reflexes disappear and the pupils become fixed. Asymmetric cranial nerve dysfunction rarely results from HT, unless an independent CNS event (trauma or stroke) has occurred. Complete neurological recovery is possible following an hour or more of asystolic cardiac resuscitation of patients with HT.

Renal

Early in HT, tubular dysfunction produces a "cold diuresis" of large volumes of dilute urine (often with an osmolarity < 60 mOsm/liter.) Late in the course of HT, volume contraction and arterial vasoconstriction profoundly decrease renal blood flow. At temperatures < 81°F, most patients become anuric.

Respiratory

Hypercarbic respiratory drive generally decreases parallel to reductions in temperature and metabolic rate. Hence, a suppressed hypercarbic drive often allows respiratory acidosis to develop, even though hypoxic drive is preserved. Altered consciousness and an increased volume of respiratory secretions warrant a low threshold for intubation to protect the airway. Furthermore, special caution must be exercised when interpreting arterial blood gas values in this setting. It is important always to record patient temperature on the requisition and to inquire from the laboratory whether the reported values are temperature corrected.

Correction of Arterial Blood Gas Values

When analyzed under standard conditions, the uncorrected *pH is falsely depressed* by ≈ 0.01 units per 1°F fall in core temperature, whereas *arterial carbon dioxide tension (PaCO$_2$) and arterial oxygen tension (PaO$_2$) are falsely elevated* by 2–4% per 1°F. Artifactual increases in gas tensions occur because higher partial pressures are required to keep CO_2 and O_2 in solution as cold blood is warmed to 37°C during analysis. Furthermore, oxygen binds less avidly to warmed hemoglobin, releasing more into solution. If unaccounted for, these artifacts may prompt poor clinical decisions: (1) the use of sodium bicarbonate to treat an artifactual acidosis; (2) overventi-

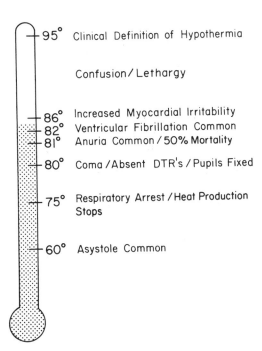

95°   Clinical Definition of Hypothermia

Confusion / Lethargy

86°   Increased Myocardial Irritability
82°   Ventricular Fibrillation Common
81°   Anuria Common / 50% Mortality
80°   Coma / Absent DTR's / Pupils Fixed

75°   Respiratory Arrest / Heat Production Stops

60°   Asystole Common

Figure 22.1 Benchmarks in hypothermia.

lation in response to artifactual hypercarbia; (3) withholding supplemental oxygen because reported PaO$_2$ values appear adequate.

Hematologic

Hypothermia-induced diuresis decreases plasma volume, causing *hemoconcentration* and *increased serum viscosity*. The resulting sluggish blood predisposes to deep venous thrombosis. The oxyhemoglobin dissociation curve shifts to the left in hypothermia, further decreasing tissue oxygen delivery. Total leukocyte counts are usually normal or slightly increased, but isolated granulocytopenia may be seen. Thrombocytopenia, a common finding, is believed to result from platelet sequestration.

Other Complications

Counter-regulatory hormones, including cortisol and growth hormone, are increased in HT, frequently causing *hyperglycemia*. Skeletal and cardiac muscle enzymes may increase in response to membrane dysfunction or *rhabdomyolysis*. *Pancreatitis*, *ileus*, and *deep venous thrombosis* are common. Although deep venous thrombosis often complicates HT, subcutaneous heparin is poorly absorbed and full anticoagulation is risky. Coexisting or precipitating *infections* (particularly pneumonia and meningitis) complicate as many as 40% of HT cases. Cold-induced stiffness of the abdominal wall or neck often confounds clinical interpretation by simulating acute abdomen or meningitis.

Treatment

General Principles

Many HT deaths are iatrogenic. Overly aggressive treatment (excessive catecholamines, prophylactic pacemakers) must be avoided; *rewarming*, *close observation*, and *gentle patient handling* are key factors in successful therapy.

Fluids should be replaced as necessary to maintain blood pressure and vital organ perfusion. *Central venous catheters* are preferred for fluid and drug administration because peripheral intravenous lines are difficult to place (due to vasoconstriction) and allow only sluggish infusion. Delivery of vasoactive drugs to the central circulation may be significantly delayed if peripherally administered. Central venous catheters *must not* be advanced into the right atrium or ventricle where they may stimulate life-threatening arrhythmias.

Serum *amylase* determinations should be routine to detect pancreatitis - a common complication of HT. A gently inserted *nasogastric tube* is useful in management, not only to counter gut hypomotility but also to enable gastric lavage for rewarming. Because many medications undergo prolongation of action in HT, all drugs must be given cautiously, particularly those that are hepatically degraded.

Finally, it should be emphasized that prolonged resuscitative efforts (hours) can prove successful in hypothermia. Therefore, patients with HT must be rewarmed to temperatures exceeding 85°F before death is declared.

Rewarming

The aggressiveness with which HT is reversed depends not only on the depth of temperature depression, but also on the physiologic manifestations. Caution must be exercised in reversing well-tolerated HT. *Passive external rewarming* with ordinary blankets is usually adequate if the temperature is > 91°F. *Active external rewarming* may shunt blood away from deep vital tissues to the body surface, producing visceral hypoperfusion and hypotension. Active external rewarming has been associated with higher mortality than passive external or *active internal rewarming* and is therefore not recommended.

Internal rewarming may be performed by several methods. *Cardiopulmonary bypass* and *mediastinal lavage* are the most rapid methods but for logistical and safety reasons are not the techniques of choice. *Peritoneal lavage* with warmed fluid is an attractive option because it may raise core temperature as quickly as 4°C per hour and can be instituted rapidly. *Warmed, fully humidified oxygen* (via an endotracheal tube at temperatures up to 46°C) delivers heat more slowly, raising core temperature ≃ 1°C per hour. *Warm gastric lavage* may be an adjunctive technique but is not particularly effective alone and increases the risk of aspiration in the non-intubated patient. Although insufficient by itself, infusion of *warmed intravenous fluids* may augment other rewarming methods.

Unstable Cardiac Patients

The primary therapeutic goal in patients with life-threatening arrhythmias should be *rewarming the core* quickly to temperatures > 85°F, a threshold below which defibrillation and antiarrhythmic therapy are often ineffective. *Bretylium* has been reported more helpful than lidocaine or procainamide for suppressing ventricular arrhythmias in HT, but no controlled trials have been performed.

Digitalis preparations should be *avoided*. *Pacemakers* increase myocardial irritability and the risk of *ventricular fibrillation*. Therefore, they should not be used in the absence of a clear indication.

Diagnosis of Death

Prolonged resuscitative efforts (hours) can prove successful in hypothermia. Therefore, patients with HT must be rewarmed to temperatures exceeding 85°F before death is declared.

HYPERTHERMIA

Causes of Temperature Elevation

In the intensive care unit (ICU) sudden temperature elevations usually signal infection, making it prudent to perform a directed physical examination and, if indicated, *obtain appropriate cultures* and *institute empirical antibiotics*. Although infection is the most common explanation, several life threatening non-infectious causes of fever are frequently overlooked.

Non-infectious Causes of Fever

Heat stroke	Malignancy
Neuroleptic malignant syndrome	Stroke or CNS hemorrhage
Malignant hyperthermia	Alcohol withdrawal
Drug or transfusion reaction	Crystalline arthritis (gout and pseudogout)
Autonomic insufficiency	Vasculitis
	Alpha-agonists

Syndromes of Extreme Hyperthermia

Even brief episodes of extreme hyperthermia (core temperature > 105°F) may permanently injure the central nervous system and must be reduced to safer levels as quickly as possible. Apart from thyroid storm (see p. 221), three non-infectious conditions producing high fever include: (1) heat stroke (HS); (2) neuroleptic malignant syndrome (NMS); and (3) malignant hyperthermia (MH). All are associated with dramatic elevations in core temperature and demand immediate recognition and therapy. Clinical features, etiology, and treatment of these diseases are contrasted in Table 22.1.

Heat Stroke

Causes and Mechanisms

Heat stroke (HS) is a potentially lethal disorder that should be suspected in all patients exposed to high ambient temperatures who develop altered mental status. HS is a triad of: 1) *fever* > 105° F,

2) *hot dry skin*, and 3) *CNS dysfunction*. Other organ systems (renal, hematologic) are frequently affected, but their involvement is not necessary for diagnosis.

Evaporation of moisture from the skin surface is the primary mechanism of heat dissipation. High humidity and poor air circulation impair the efficiency of this process. Classical (non-exertional) HS occurs most commonly among the elderly because of an *impaired ability to dissipate heat* due to: *decreased sweat production, decreased skin blood flow, impaired hypothalamic regulation*, and the use of *drugs impairing heat loss*. Impaired heat loss may also be seen with extensive burns or skin diseases (e.g., scleroderma) and with the use of occlusive dressings or ointments that cover large surface areas. Low cardiac output, dehydration, and use of beta blockers, diuretics, or peripheral vasoconstrictors reduce cutaneous perfusion and may contribute to HS by this mechanism. CNS tumors, stroke, and certain drugs (e.g., cocaine, lysergic acid diethylamide (LSD), amphetamines) may disrupt hypothalamic heat regulation. Other drugs may produce HS through increased heat production (e.g., cocaine, tricyclics, lithium, or alcohol withdrawal), by impairing heat loss (e.g., anticholinergics, phenothiazines, diuretics, and tricyclics), or by a combination of these two mechanisms.

Laboratory studies are commonly abnormal in HS. Arterial blood gases must be corrected for temperature (see p. 197). The most common acid-base pattern is respiratory alkalosis, but metabolic acidosis is commonly superimposed. Outcome correlates poorly with the degree of acidosis. Rhabdomyolysis is often responsible for the hypocalcemia, hypokalemia, and elevations in creatinine phosphokinase (CPK) and serum glutamic oxaloacetic transaminase (SGOT) that commonly attend HS. Abnormal coagulation studies are seen in about 10% of patients and hyponatremia occurs in about half of all cases.

Complications and Prognosis

Renal damage from HS is the result of dehydration, hyperuricemia, and rhabdomyolysis. Renal failure is much more common in *exertional* HS than classical HS, a difference based on the higher incidence of volume depletion and rhabdomyolysis. HS may also result in "high output" heart failure. Prolonged fever, exceedingly high temperature, and elevated serum lactate values portend CNS damage and death.

Table 22.1

Clinical Features, Etiology, and Treatment of Heat Stroke, Neuroleptic Malignant Syndrome, and Malignant Hyperthermia.

Feature	Malignant Hyperthermia	Neuroleptic Malignant Syndrome	Classical Heat Stroke
Usual age (yr)	< 30	< 30	> 60
Common precipitants	Succinylcholine, halogenated anesthetics	Neuroleptics (e.g., anti-psychotics)	Diuretics, tricyclics, anticholinergics
Mechanism	Increased heat production ? Impaired muscle reuptake of Ca^{2+}	Increased heat production ? Central dopamine receptor blockade	Impaired heat loss
Therapy	Remove offending agent, dantrolene	Dantrolene, bromocryptine	External cooling

?, questionable mechanism.

Treatment

With the exception of therapy to rapidly lower temperature, the treatment of HS is supportive. Core temperature should be lowered to $< 103°F$ as quickly as possible. The most effective method of cooling is through the use of convection and evaporation, *not conduction*. Spraying unclothed HS victims with tepid water and using a fan to encourage evaporation cools most patients to less than $103°F$ within 60 minutes. Ice packing or ice water immersion produces heat loss rapidly by conduction but has major limitations, apart from the difficulty of implementation. Immersion causes intense peripheral vasoconstriction, encouraging maintenance of the core temperature. Furthermore, rebound elevations of temperature may be more common after ending treatment.

Fluid deficits in HS average $\simeq 1.5$ liters, but the extent of dehydration is highly variable. Alpha-agonists and atropine in support of the circulation should be avoided whenever possible because drug-induced peripheral vasoconstriction further impairs heat loss.

Malignant Hyperthermia

Causes

Malignant hyperthermia (MH) is a rare but dramatic disorder caused by *excessive heat generation*, probably a result of altered calcium kinetics. MH is most commonly a disease of young people in which the temperature may rise as fast as $2°C$ $(3.6°F)$/min within minutes of drug exposure. Predisposition to MH is an autosomal dominant trait usually expressed following exposure to anesthetic drugs. Halothane and succinylcholine precipitate more than 80% of all cases of MH, although other halogenated anesthetics, neuromuscular blockers, ketamine, and phencyclidine (PCP) can be responsible.

Diagnosis

The diagnosis must be a clinical one recognized by the occurrence of: (1) *muscular rigidity*; (2) *high and rapidly developing fever*; and (3) *tachycardia*. Extreme muscle activity causes increased oxygen consumption and CO_2 production. MH produces hypoxia, hypercarbia, and metabolic acidosis that may cause arrhythmias and skin mottling. The differential diagnosis of MH includes thyroid storm and pheochromocytoma. Neither lumbar puncture nor electroencephalogram (EEG) is helpful in explaining the altered mental status. Phosphate, uric acid, and muscle enzymes (CPK, lactic dehydrogenase, LDH, aldolase) are routinely elevated as a result of rhabdomyolysis.

Complications

Massive increases in metabolic rate cause hypercapnia, hypoxemia, and hypoglycemia in a large percentage of cases. When not promptly treated, MH can produce severe muscle damage with necrosis and soft tissue calcification. Circulating myoglobin may produce renal failure. In such cases renal damage may be averted by alkalinizing the urine and by maintaining blood pressure and tubular flow.

High cardiac output with low systemic vascular resistance may result in hypotension, but dopamine or alpha agonists should be used cautiously because vasoconstriction may retard heat loss. Tissue hypoxia is more intense in MH than in HS or NMS, accounting for a higher incidence of cardiac arrhythmias and muscular damage.

Direct thermal toxicity may cause neuronal death. The hippocampus and the Purkinje cell layer of the cerebellum are particularly vulnerable, accounting for a high incidence of movement disorders after recovery. Prophylactic anticonvulsants may prevent the seizures that occur almost universally in MH.

Prophylactic use of histamine blockers or antacids is indicated to counteract the tendency for GI hemorrhage. Hepatic necrosis and cholestasis are infrequently seen.

Late hematologic effects include increased leukocyte and platelet counts, coagulopathy resulting from impaired liver function, and direct thermal activation of platelets and clotting factors.

Treatment

The mortality of MH relates directly to the magnitude and duration of peak temperature. Even brief delays in therapy may prove fatal. Anesthesia must be immediately terminated and breathing circuit elements changed out. Direct external cooling and specific treatment with *dantrolene* (2–10 mg/kg) should be initiated as soon as possible. Dantrolene may uncouple excitation-contraction mechanisms to stop heat generation but response to dantrolene is not diagnostic (HS and NMS may also respond).

Corticosteroids do not improve outcome and should not be used. Drugs believed safe in MH include nitrous oxide, barbiturates, diazepam, pancuronium, and opiates. Patients with MH usually have normal circulating volume, unlike patients with exertional heat stroke who are frequently dehydrated.

Neuroleptic Malignant Syndrome

Definition

As with MH, NMS is a drug-induced hyperthermic syndrome characterized by *fever*, *muscle rigidity*, *altered mentation*, and frequently by *pulmonary dysfunction*, and *autonomic instability*. It differs, however, regarding precipitating factors, underlying mechanism, time course, prognosis, and patient substrate. Laboratory abnormalities all are non-specific and include elevated CPK, leukocytosis, and elevated liver function tests. Lumbar puncture and head computed tomography (CT) are not helpful. Other diseases in the differential diagnosis of NMS include heat stroke, pheochromocytoma, anticholinergic toxicity, and monoamine oxidase (MAO) inhibitor crisis.

Causes

NMS occurs in < 1% of all patients receiving neuroleptic drugs (e.g., haloperidol). The vast majority of patients develop symptoms within 2 weeks of initiating therapy or increasing drug dosage. However, the syndrome may occur after a single dose of neuroleptic drug or at any time during therapy. NMS has also been reported when antiparkinsonian (dopaminergic) drugs are abruptly discontinued. Regardless of etiology, symptoms develop over 24–72 hours and usually last about 12 days. (A longer duration may accompany longer acting neuroleptics.) The cause of NMS is unknown, but its predominance in patients receiving drugs with the most potent anti-dopaminergic properties and anticholinergic effects (haloperidol, fluphenazine, and chlorpromazine) implies *dopamine and acetylcholine receptor blockade* as potential mechanisms. Dehydration and muscular exhaustion predispose to NMS.

Laboratory

Laboratory abnormalities all are nonspecific and include elevated CPK, leukocytosis, and elevated liver function tests. Lumbar puncture and head computed tomography (CT) are not helpful.

Complications

NMS is fatal in 20–30% of cases and is frequently complicated by rhabdomyolysis, acute myocardial infarction, and persistent movement disorders. Not all patients with NMS relapse when rechallenged with similar neuroleptic drugs. Although the degree of crossover between MH and NMS is unknown, some patients who have had *malignant hyperthermia* undergo uneventful therapy with neuroleptic drugs, suggesting that MH and NMS have different etiologies, despite a similar clinical appearance.

Treatment

As with MH, the treatment of NMS requires *stopping the offending drug* and administering *dantrolene* in intravenous doses up to 10 mg/kg. *Bromocriptine*, *amantadine*, and *neuromuscular paralysis* with pancuronium may also be useful in controlling the muscular rigidity.

SUGGESTED READINGS

1. Gallant EM, Ahern CP: Malignant hyperthermia: responses of skeletal muscles to general anesthetics. *Mayo Clin Proc* 58:758–763, 1983.
2. Guzé BH, Baxter LR: Neuroleptic malignant syndrome. *N Engl J Med* 313:163–166, 1985.
3. Hudson LD, Conn RD: Accidental hypothermia. *JAMA* 227:37–40, 1974.
4. Kelman GR: Nomograms for correction of blood PO_2, PCO_2, pH and base excess for time and temperature. *J Appl Physiol* 21:1484–1487, 1966.

5. Kurlan R, Hamill R, Shoulson I: Neuroleptic malignant syndrome. *Clin Neuropharmacol* 7:109–120, 1984.
6. Nelson TE, Flewellen EH: The malignant hyperthermia syndrome. *N Engl J Med* 309:416–418, 1983.
7. Reuler JB: Hypothermia: pathophysiology, clinical settings, and management. *Ann Intern Med* 89:519–527, 1978.
8. Welton DE, Mattox KL, Miller RR, et al: Treatment of profound hypothermia. *JAMA* 240:2291–2292, 1978.
9. Weyman AE, Greenbaum DM, Grace WJ: Accidental hypothermia in an alcoholic population. *Am J Med* 56:13–20, 1974.
10. Wong KC: Physiology and pharmacology of hypothermia. *West J Med* 138:227–232, 1983.

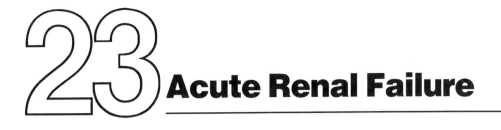

Acute Renal Failure

INDICES OF RENAL FUNCTION

Because the kidney is the primary excretor of nitrogenous waste, blood concentrations of urea nitrogen (BUN) and creatinine (Cr) track renal function. The extreme variation of urea load and the ability of the tubule to absorb filtered urea renders BUN less reliable than Cr for this purpose. As general guidelines, the BUN increases 10–15 mg/dl/day and creatinine by 1–2.5 mg/dl/day after abrupt renal shutdown. The serum potassium usually rises less than 0.5 mEq/l/day and HCO_3^- falls by $\simeq$ 1 mEq/l/day. Under the catabolic stress of burns, trauma, steroids, sepsis, or starvation, the rates of change of these parameters may be doubled.

In contrast to BUN, daily Cr production is relatively constant. A rising Cr indicates that the rate of production exceeds clearance by glomerular filtration. Therefore, a *stable* elevation of Cr implies a new steady state has been achieved at a decreased rate of glomerular filtration (GFR). Until Cr stabilizes the severity of acute renal dysfunction and Cr clearance cannot be reliably assessed. If shutdown continues, Cr usually levels out at $\simeq$ 12–15 mg/dl, depending on catabolic state. (Rhabdomyolysis can cause Cr to transiently exceed this value.) Ketones and cefoxitin are the only common causes of an artifactually elevated Cr.

Urine volume usually reflects *kidney perfusion* while *urine specific gravity* parallels concentrating ability (*tubular function*). Therefore, renal blood flow is probably adequate in non-oliguric patients. Furthermore, patients producing concentrated urine are unlikely to have significant tubular damage. Certain calculated indices may be helpful in separating problems of perfusion from those of tubular dysfunction (Table 23.1).

ETIOLOGY OF ACUTE RENAL FAILURE

Approximately 20% of critically ill patients develop acute renal failure (ARF). ARF may be clas-

sified as *oliguric* ($<$ 15 ml/hr) or *non-oliguric*. The mortality of oliguric failure is at least twofold greater. ARF may result from a variety of causes that produce (1) hypoperfusion (*pre-renal*); (2) outlet obstruction (*post-renal*); or (3) parenchymal disease (*intra-renal*) (Fig. 23.1).

Pre-renal Failure

Because hypoperfusion is the most common cause of ARF, the initial step in management is to ensure that renal blood flow is adequate. Renal hypoperfusion results from circulatory failure, hypotension, vascular obstruction (e.g., vasculitis, cholesterol embolization), hypovolemia, or maldistribution of cardiac output (as in sepsis). Certain forms of renal insufficiency (e.g., the hepatorenal syndrome and the renal response to positive endexpiratory pressure, PEEP) mimic pre-renal physiology by redistributing blood flow away from the filtering glomerulus. Prolonged *renal ischemia* may lead to ARF. In general, mean arterial pressures below 60–70 mmHg for longer than 30 minutes risk renal injury.

Indicators of Intravascular Volume Status

Orthostatic blood pressure is a helpful clinical measure of intravascular volume status in healthy persons. However, few critically ill patients can be tested in this fashion and autonomic insufficiency may render such changes less reliable in patients who are diabetic, elderly, or bedridden. Dry mucous membranes, skin laxity, and absence of axillary moisture may also be clues to hypovolemia. Unfortunately, these signs, too, prove unreliable in patients with hyperpnea or advanced age.

Because non-invasive laboratory methods to assess fluid status (chest x-ray and echocardiogram) are not sensitive tests of intravascular volume, invasive monitoring is often required (see Chapter 20).

203

Table 23.1
Laboratory Indices in ARF

	Prerenal	Renal
BUN/Cr	> 10:1	≈ 10:1
Urinary Na$^+$ concentration	< 20 mEq/1	> 40 mEq/1
Urine osmolality	> 500 mOsm/1	< 300–400 mOsm/1
Urine [Cr] /plasma [Cr]	> 40	< 20
Urine Na/Cr clearance	< 1	> 2
Na clearance/Cr clearance	< 1	> 1
Sediment	Normal	Active

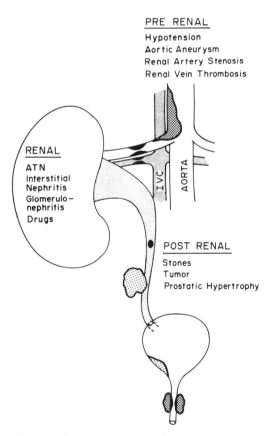

PRE RENAL

Hypotension
Aortic Aneurysm
Renal Artery Stenosis
Renal Vein Thrombosis

RENAL

ATN
Interstitial
Nephritis
Glomerulo–
nephritis
Drugs

IVC

AORTA

POST RENAL

Stones
Tumor
Prostatic Hypertrophy

Figure 23.1 Common causes of acute renal failure in the intensive care unit.

In pre-renal failure the *urinalysis is normal* or minimally abnormal with non-specific sediment. A pre-renal state prompts the tubule to reabsorb sodium [Na$^+$] and water, yielding a *concentrated urine with low [Na$^+$]* and an *elevated ratio of urine to plasma Cr*. Diuretics render urine [Na$^+$] determinations useless for 24 hours following administration. Osmotic agents (glucose and mannitol) may also confuse interpretation of urine chemistry

by producing dilute urine. In pre-renal states the *BUN/Cr ratio is usually elevated (> 10:1)*. Although the BUN may be disproportionately high because of increased urea production resulting from tetracycline, steroids, or gastrointestinal (GI) bleeding, an elevated BUN/Cr ratio more commonly results from reduced tubular urine flow and increased tubular reabsorption of urea nitrogen. The renal tubules cannot absorb Cr; therefore, reduced tubular flow rates have no effect on the [Cr] when GFR is preserved. Comparing urea clearance to creatinine clearance will determine whether increased urea production or decreased excretion is the cause of an elevated BUN; if the urea/creatinine clearance ratio is > 1, increased production is the likely etiology.

Post-renal Failure

Once pre-renal causes have been excluded, obstructive (post-renal) causes (e.g., urinary calculi, tumor, prostatic hypertrophy, blood clot, retroperitoneal hemorrhage) should be considered. While post-renal disease accounts for only 1–10% of cases of ARF, this reversible problem should not be overlooked. (Obstruction is the most common cause of total *anuria*.) Upper tract obstruction produces anuria only if bilateral or if it occurs in a patient with a single kidney or drainage pathway.

Urethral obstruction may be immediately excluded or confirmed by the attempt to place a *Foley catheter* into the bladder. Because of the high incidence of urinary collecting system abnormalities, Foley catheterization alone never excludes the possibility of more proximal obstructive uropathy. *Renal ultrasonography* can detect hydronephrosis and urinary obstruction within or proximal to the bladder.

In obstructive uropathy the *urinalysis is usually normal* and *urine chemistries* are seldom helpful. *Computed tomography (CT) scan* may demonstrate lesions obstructing the ureters or bladder, and *nuclear renal scans* assess flow or tubular function.

The intravenous pyelogram (IVP) is not likely to be useful in obstructive uropathy unless stones or trauma are suspected. Furthermore, IVP contrast is potentially nephrotoxic.

Intra-renal Failure

Urinalysis and urinary chemistry provide vital clues to distinguish prerenal from intrarenal causes for ARF (Table 23.1). There are three intra-renal categories of acute renal failure (1) *tubular disorders*; (2) *interstitial nephritis*; and (3) *glomerulonephritis* and *small vessel vasculitis*.

Tubular Disorders

After pre-renal azotemia, nephrotoxic drugs are the most common cause of ARF. Elderly, dehydrated, and diabetic patients, and those with myeloma are at particular risk of drug-induced renal insufficiency. Aminoglycosides, contrast agents, and non-steroidal anti-inflammatory drugs are the most common agents causing ARF.

Aminoglycosides (AGs) cause renal insufficiency in 10–20% of all individuals who receive them. AGs bind to cellular proteins in the proximal tubule, resulting in acute tubular necrosis when toxic trough levels of drug are sustained. The incidence of ARF differs only modestly among the most commonly used AGs. Volume depletion and concomitant use of other nephrotoxins (e.g., cephalosporins) accentuate the injury. *Prolonged usage* and *pre-existant renal disease* predispose to toxicity. Most patients with AG-induced renal failure recover sufficient renal function to obviate long term dialysis. A frequent mistake is to administer AGs empirically to high risk patients and to continue them without a clear therapeutic endpoint. Although loading doses need no modification, maintenance doses of AGs should be reduced in proportion to GFR. (For example, a patient with 50% of predicted GFR should receive approximately 50% of the standard *maintenance* dose). Serum peak and trough levels should be determined after steady-state concentrations are achieved (after approximately five half-lives).

Radiographic contrast agents rarely cause renal insufficiency in patients with normal baseline renal function but frequently produce ARF in patients with underlying renal disease, diabetes mellitus, or paraproteinemia. The toxicity of radiographic contrast may be reduced by prophylactic fluid loading, loop diuretics, and mannitol.

Non-steroidal anti-inflammatory agents (NSAIAs) impair renal function in patients with pre-renal azotemia, shock, heart failure, cirrhosis, and nephrotic syndrome. Prostaglandin E2 (PGE_2), an endogenous vasodilator, is pivotal in maintaining renal blood flow in high renin/angiotensin states. NSAIAs block PGE_2 formation, decreasing renal blood flow. If a NSAIA must be used, *aspirin* should be the first choice. *Sulindac* appears to be the next best option. NSAIAs encourage sodium and fluid retention and inhibit diuretic action. The combination of angiotensin converting enzyme (ACE) inhibitors and NSAIAs is unusually detrimental to renal function. Even when used alone ACE inhibitors may precipitously lower the GFR, especially in patients with bilateral renal artery stenosis.

Myoglobin and hemoglobin may cause ARF when released into serum during hemolysis or rhabdomyolysis. These compounds precipitate in the renal tubules, obstructing them. Rhabdomyolysis does not always result from trauma and may be relatively asymptomatic. (Half of all patients have no complaints of muscle pain, tenderness, or weakness). Clues to rhabdomyolysis include *rapidly increasing creatinine* with *disproportionate rises in potassium, phosphate*, and *uric acid*. Volume loading, osmotic diuretics, and alkalinizing agents may help to keep these compounds in solution, thus encouraging their elimination and preventing renal failure.

Interstitial Nephritis

Acute interstitial nephritis (AIN) is a common but frequently unrecognized allergic reaction in the renal interstitium, usually in response to a specific drug. Penicillin, rifampin, furosemide, and cimetidine are reported causes. AIN presents with *fever, eosinophilia, rash*, and *ARF*. Laboratory clues to diagnosis include *eosinophilia* and *eosinophiluria*. Hansel's stain documents urinary eosinophilia. (Wright's stain is pH dependent and often fails to demonstrate eosinophils in the urine.) Removal of the offending drug and high dose corticosteroids are accepted treatments.

Glomerulonephritis and Vasculitis

Although glomerulonephritis (GN) and vasculitis often produce subacute and chronic renal disease, they are an uncommon cause of abrupt renal failure in the intensive care unit. The diverse spectrum of these disorders includes post-streptococcal GN, rickettsial infection, subacute bacterial endocarditis, systemic lupus erythematous (SLE), malignant hypertension, and drug-related vasculitis.

Urinalysis reveals an active sediment containing

leukocytes, protein, and the hallmark of GN-red blood cell (RBC) casts. Diagnosis may be aided by analysis of serum complement, antinuclear antibody (ANA), rheumatoid factor latex agglutination, hepatitis B surface antigen and blood culture. Therapy is directed at the underlying condition (e.g., antibiotics for endocarditis, steroids for SLE, and cytotoxic therapy for polyarteritis).

COMPLICATIONS AND TREATMENT OF ARF

With the widespread use of dialysis, morbidity and mortality in ARF usually result from non-uremic causes (Table 23.2). Avoiding circulatory crises and recognizing urinary obstruction can prevent the majority of cases of ARF. Careful use of nephrotoxic drugs in appropriate doses is the next most important preventative measure. Volume expansion is effective prophylaxis against ARF induced by contrast agents, rhabdomyolysis, cis-platinin, methotrexate, or cyclophosphamide.

The initial approach to ongoing ARF should be to exclude obstructive uropathy, eliminate pre-renal factors, and, whenever possible, reverse oliguria. After pre-renal and post-renal causes have been excluded, careful review of the history, physical examination, and laboratory and medication records may give clues to the cause.

Unfortunately, ARF often occurs in the setting of multi-organ failure. Combined renal and respiratory insufficiency is particularly ominous, with mortality exceeding 90% in several published series. Supportive care must be meticulous to ensure survival. It is most important to avoid such iatrogenic complications as infection related to monitoring devices, fluid and electrolyte imbalances, drug toxicity, and inappropriate nutritional support.

Fluid Management

Non-oliguric ARF is associated with lower mortality than oliguric ARF. Therefore, it is possible that restoring urine flow reduces mortality. Attempts to convert oliguric to non-oliguric ARF are most successful when undertaken shortly after the onset of oliguria. When 8 or more hours have elapsed, efforts to restore urine flow by volume loading routinely fail. In attempting to reverse oliguria, a fluid challenge should first be performed (unless there are obvious signs of intravascular congestion). Volume loading should then be followed by a large dose of loop diuretic (e.g., furosemide, 1 mg/kg). Although osmotic agents (mannitol, 25–50 gm) may also be effective, these risk volume overload. Invasive monitoring should be considered in patients with tenuous cardiovascular or pulmonary status.

Dopamine may be a useful adjunct in the treatment of ARF due to hypoperfusion, or maldistribution of renal blood flow. At low doses < 5 mcg/kg/min dopamine has renal vasodilating and natriuretic effects that complement the action of loop diuretics and may help reverse oliguria.

Electrolyte Disorders

Hyperkalemia, hyponatremia, hypermagnesemia, and hyperphosphatemia are the major electrolyte disturbances of ARF. The primary approach to each disorder is to modify input and/or enhance removal of solute or fluid, as detailed in Fluids and Electrolytes, Chapter 12. It should be emphasized here, however, that oral phosphate binders (aluminum-containing antacids) usually suppress

Table 23.2
Complications of Acute Renal Failure

Metabolic	Cardiovascular	Neurological
Hyponatremia	Fluid overload	Neuropathy
Hyperkalemia	Hypertension	Dementia
Hypocalcemia	Arrhythmias	Seizures
Hyperphosphatemia	Pericarditis	
Hyperuricemia		
Hematologic	**Gastrointestinal**	**Infectious**
Anemia	Nausea and vomiting	Urinary tract
Coagulopathy	GI bleeding*	Sepsis
		IV catheter*
		Pneumonia

*GI, gastrointestinal; IV, intravenous.

serum phosphate sufficiently to prevent hypocalcemia. Because magnesium excretion is impaired in patients with ARF, products containing magnesium (particularly cathartics) should be avoided.

Water, sodium, and potassium intake should be adjusted to match measured urinary output and normalize serum values. In the resolution of acute tubular necrosis, patients frequently undergo a polyuric phase 3–4 weeks after onset. Fluid losses may be life-threatening unless appropriately replaced to maintain circulating volume. The cause of the polyuric phase is not known with certainty, but probably results from tubular dysfunction in the face of recovering GFR and excess total body water.

Bleeding Disorders

Bleeding is common in ARF due to the inhibitory actions of uremic toxins on platelets and factor VIII. Replacement of factor VIII with cryoprecipitate or fresh frozen plasma (FFP) may help to correct bleeding defects (see Transfusion and Blood Component Therapy, Chapter 13). Arginine vasopressin (DDAVP) increases serum levels of factor VIII complex, improving bleeding time in uremic patients. Platelet transfusions may also be helpful to improve hemostasis before invasive procedures.

Nutrition

The production of uremic toxins is limited by minimizing catabolism and providing sufficient calories to prevent protein wasting. Except in AIN and some forms of renal vasculitis, corticosteroids should be avoided because of their catabolic effect and impact on immune function. Sufficient carbohydrate ($>$ 100 gm/day) or fat calories should be provided to prevent the catabolism of protein for energy production. In patients who do not require dialysis (i.e., Cr $<$ 8–10 mg/dl) protein intake should be limited to 40–50 gm/day, the majority of which is of high biological value. In dialyzed patients, protein intake may be liberalized, (80–100 gm/day). However, it should be recognized that higher protein intake may necessitate more frequent dialysis. Folate and pyridoxine must be supplemented because they are lost through hemodialysis.

Total parenteral nutrition (TPN) using hypertonic glucose, and l-amino acids can reduce the mortality of ARF and hasten recovery of renal function. If TPN is used, a formulation low in Na, Mg, PO_4, and K is mandatory.

Drug Therapy

The need for *all* drugs should be questioned in ARF. Any drug that may impair renal function should be discontinued or the dosage modified. Renally metabolized or excreted drugs usually require reductions in dosage.

As a general guideline, the dosage needs revision in proportion to its percentage of elimination by the kidney and the degree of renal impairment. Dosing of each drug susceptible to renal excretion should be guided by published nomograms (Ref. 1). Even when dosage is precisely calculated, serum levels of drugs with a low therapeutic index must be followed.

Dialysis

In the setting of ARF the indications for dialysis or hemofiltration are:

1. *fluid overload,*
2. *refractory hyperkalemia,*
3. *life-threatening acidosis,*
4. *symptomatic uremia.*

Characteristics of blood purification methods are provided in Table 23.3. Although *hemofiltration* can remove excess volume, *hemodialysis* and *peritoneal dialysis* are the only practical methods of removing uremic toxins. Dialysis is almost always instituted when the serum Cr exceeds 8 mg/dl or the BUN approaches 100 mg/dl. In catabolic patients, early dialysis (to maintain Cr $<$ 4 mg/dl and BUN $<$ 50 mg/dl) improves outcome. Access to the circulation for hemodialysis or hemofiltration may be achieved by a multi-lumen central venous catheter or by establishing an arteriovenous communication. Peritoneal dialysis can be undertaken in most patients with a freely communicating and uninflamed peritoneal cavity, but it is considerably less efficient than hemodialysis in removing toxins or correcting electrolyte imbalance.

Complications of Dialysis

Certain complications of dialysis are important to emphasize in the critical care setting. Although more efficient than the peritoneal approach, hemodialysis requires *cardiovascular stability*—rapid shifts of fluid between intracellular and extracellular compartments are not well tolerated by hemodynamically unstable patients. Furthermore, intra-neuronal tonicity may not track the abrupt shifts in fluid/solute composition that occur in the extracellular compartment, producing the ''*dialysis disequilibrium*'' syndrome. Depending on choice of dialyzing membrane and dialysate, *hy-*

Table 23.3
Charactertistics of Blood Purification Methods

	Efficiency of Solute Removal		Incidence of Disequilibrium Syndrome	Cardiovascular Instability	Hypoxemia	Protein Losses
	Small	Large				
Intermittent peritoneal dialysis	Low	Medium	Rare	Rare	High volume	Present
Hemodialysis	Very high	Low	Frequent	Frequent	Acetate/ cellophane	Absent
Intermittent hemofiltration	High	High	Frequent	Rare	None	Absent
Continuous hemofiltration	Low	Very high	None	None	None	Absent

poxemia during hemodialysis may result from leukostasis within the pulmonary capillaries (cuprophane membrane) or from hypoventilation (acetate buffer). Hypoventilation occurs as CO_2 diffuses into the dialysate, reducing the stimulation of ventilatory chemoreceptors.

Although hemodynamically well-tolerated, peritoneal dialysis is not risk-free. Abdominal distention during high volume peritoneal dialysis may drive the diaphragm cephalad, causing atelectasis, hypoxemia, and increased work of breathing. Electrolyte imbalance, hyperglycemia and peritonitis are commonly encountered.

Continuous Hemofiltration

Recently, continuous ultrafiltration (CUF; Amicon filtration) has been used to *remove excess circulating volume* from critically ill patients. CUF establishes an arteriovenous anastomosis through a cartridge of highly permeable hollow fibers to produce an ultrafiltrate of plasma.

Because filtration is driven by the gradient of arterial to venous pressure CUF is generally ineffective when mean arterial pressure falls below 60 mmHg. The rate of filtration may be increased by restricting venous outflow (raising venous pressure), by increasing the arterial pressure, or by increasing the transmembrane filtration pressure. Filtration pressure can be augmented by applying suction to the shell surrounding the permeable fibers or by lowering the collection bag if suction is not applied. Filtration rate may be decreased by restricting the arterial inflow (by clamping the arterial line). Local anticoagulation is useful in pre-

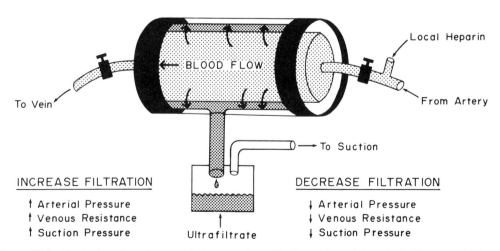

Figure 23.2 Mechanism of continuous arteriovenous hemofiltration and regulation of ultrafiltrate production.

venting clotting of the cartridge and does not usually impair systemic hemostasis. (Avoiding systemic anticoagulation is another advantage in the fluid-overloaded patient with central nervous system disease, coagulopathy, or recent hemorrhage.)

Ultrafiltration is appropriate when removal of intravascular volume (salt and water) is a primary objective. For example, CUF has been used successfully to treat metabolic acidosis, replacing filtered fluid with $NaHCO_3$. Unfortunately, uremic toxins are inefficiently removed. Hence, CUF is sometimes used in conjunction with intermittent dialysis.

SUGGESTED READINGS

1. Bryan CS, Stone WJ: Antimicrobial dosage in renal failure: a unifying nomogram (updated version). *Clin Neph* 7:81, 1977.
2. Cameron JS: Acute renal failure—the continuing challenge. *Q J Med* 228:337–343, 1986.
3. Dixon BS, Anderson RJ: Nonoliguric acute renal failure. *Am J Kidney Dis* 6(2):71–80, 1985.
4. Kaplan AA, Longnecker RE, Folkert VW: Continuous arteriovenous hemofiltration. *Ann Intern Med* 100:358–367, 1984.
5. Miller TR, Anderson RJ, Linas SL, et al.: Urinary diagnostic indices in acute renal failure. *Ann Intern Med* 89:47–50, 1978.
6. Misson RT, Cutler RE: Radiocontrast-induced renal failure. *West J Med* 142:657–664, 1985.

24 Coagulation Disorders

Vascular endothelium, clotting proteins, and platelets comprise the key components of the hemostatic mechanism. Only when 2 or more of these hemostatic components are defective is spontaneous or uncontrollable hemorrhage likely; impairment of any single factor seldom provokes clinical bleeding.

APPROACH TO THE BLEEDING PATIENT

History

The history provides important clues to the etiology of bleeding. With few exceptions, *hereditary* disorders produce deficiency or dysfunction of a single clotting factor, whereas the much more common *acquired* disorders usually cause multiple factor abnormalities. All congenital bleeding disorders are *autosomal*, except for the sex-linked recessive hemophilias. The hemophilias are the most common congenital bleeding disorders. Deficiencies of factors VIII and IX account for 85% and 12% of congenital bleeding diatheses, respectively. Von Willebrand's disease, the next most common category, is an autosomal dominant disorder producing platelet and/or vessel wall dysfunction. All other inherited factor deficiencies are very rare; therefore, a negative *family history* virtually excludes a diagnosis of hereditary coagulopathy.

A coagulation history must include more than just a report of "easy bleeding" or "bruising". Specific answers to the following questions should be sought. (1) Has there been prior *life threatening hemorrhage*? (2) Has bleeding required *transfusion or re-operation*? (3) If *oral surgery* has been performed, was there excessive bleeding? (4) What *drugs* are currently taken? Particular attention should be paid to those affecting platelet function (aspirin, alcohol, and non-steroidal anti-inflammatory agents)

or synthesis of vitamin K-dependent clotting proteins (warfarin and antibiotics).

Physical Examination

The examiner should search for evidence of petechiae (especially in dependent, high-venous-pressure areas), purpura, and persistent oozing from skin punctures or mucosal sites. Such findings are most characteristic of *platelet disorders*. *Palpable purpura* is a sign of small artery occlusion usually associated with vasculitis due to collagen-vascular disease (polyarteritis, systemic lupus erythematosus, SLE), endocarditis, or sepsis (especially with gram-negative rods and the meningococcus). Larger vessel occlusions from disseminated intravascular coagulation (DIC) may cause the extensive echynoses of *purpura fulminans*. In contrast, factor deficiencies most often cause deep muscle and joint bleeding that results in echymoses, hematomas, and hemarthroses.

Laboratory Tests

Clotting tests are indicated for patients undergoing *surgery* or *invasive procedures* and for those with a *history that suggests a bleeding disorder*. Clotting tests are also useful in patients undergoing *massive transfusion*, *anticoagulation*, or *thrombolytic therapy*.

Platelet count, prothrombin time (PT), and partial thromboplastin time (PTT) usually suffice to exclude clinically important bleeding disorders, but a bleeding time (BT) should be added when platelet dysfunction is suspected.

INTERPRETATION OF ABNORMAL CLOTTING TESTS

Prothrombin Time

The PT is a test of the *extrinsic* clotting pathway in which factors II, V, VII, and X are activated by adding thromboplastin and calcium to the blood sample. Because the endpoint of the prothrombin test is clot formation, deficiencies of factor VII (or any factor below factor X in the clotting cascade) can prolong the PT (Fig. 24.1). A normal PT requires each factor in the sequence to have ≥ 30% of normal activity. Common causes of a prolonged PT are listed in Table 24.1.

The combination of a normal PTT with a prolonged PT can be explained by selective deficiency of factor VII. This rarely occurs as a chronic condition, but because factor VII has the shortest half-life of all vitamin K-dependent clotting proteins, isolated prolongation of PT can occur in *early* vitamin K deficiency, hepatic failure, or warfarin (Coumadin) therapy.

Activated Partial Thromboplastin Time

The PTT tests the *intrinsic* pathway by adding kaolin and phospholipid to activate coagulation. It tests all clotting proteins *except* factor VII (Fig. 24.1). Although the PTT is the *most sensitive* test of clotting factor abnormalities, it is *less specific* than the PT for the same reason. The combination of a normal PT and a prolonged PTT indicates deficiency or dysfunction of factors VIII, IX, XI, or XII. When both PT and PTT are abnormal, an acquired bleeding disorder is almost always responsible. Common causes of an activated PTT are listed in Table 24.2.

Thrombin Time

The thrombin time (TT) is performed by adding thrombin to an anticoagulated sample, thereby converting fibrinogen to fibrin. The TT measures *only* this final step in coagulation (See Fig. 24.1) and therefore can detect only a small number of clotting abnormalities. *Fibrinogen levels < 100 mg/dl* (DIC, thrombolytic therapy) or *dysfunctional fibrinogen* may prolong the TT. *Heparin, fibrin degradation products*, and abnormal *immunoglobins* also prolong the TT by interfering with thrombin-induced fibrinogen conversion.

Bleeding Time

The *bleeding time* (BT) is primarily a test of *platelet function* but can also be influenced by platelet number and tissue turgor. The BT will always be prolonged if platelets number fewer than 50,000/mm³. Together, platelet count and BT effectively screen for platelet problems by testing platelet number, adhesion, and aggregation. The BT is often abnormal in patients with *uremia* and

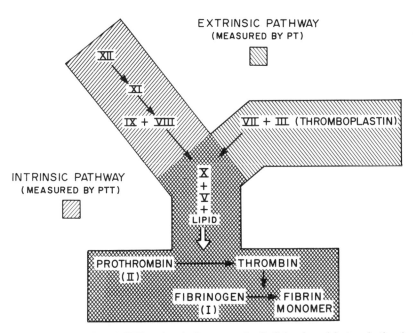

Figure 24.1 Relationship of PT and PTT to the clotting cascade. Deficiencies of factors in the doubly cross-hatched region (the intersection of intrinsic and extrinsic pathways) produce abnormalities of both tests. The thrombin time tests only the final conversion of fibrinogen to fibrin monomer. Factor XIII (not shown) stabilizes the linkup of fibrin monomers into organized clot.

Table 24.1
Common Causes of a Prolonged PT

Liver disease	Aspirin
Vitamin K deficiency	Circulating anticoagulants
Warfarin	Dilutional coagulapathy
Excessive heparin	DIC

Table 24.2
Common Causes of a Prolonged PTT

Spurious results (underfilled tube)	Heparin
	Hemophilia
A delay in performing the test	Von Willebrand's disease
Circulating anticoagulants	

in those receiving *drugs* that impair platelet function (aspirin, nonsteroidal anti-inflammatory agents). Although abnormal platelet function will be detected by a BT, prolongation correlates only very roughly with the tendency to bleed.

Inhibitor Testing

Only ≃ 30% activity of each factor is needed for normal clotting assays. Hence, combining equal portions of normal plasma and plasma from a patient with a clotting factor deficiency will yield normal PT and PTT results, unless a factor *inhibitor* (e.g., lupus anticoagulant, heparin) is present.

Fibrinogen and Fibrin Degradation Products

Fibrinogen levels may be reduced as a result of impaired production or increased consumption. Since fibrinogen is an acute phase reactant released from the liver, it may be elevated in hepatitis or other infections. Therefore, even if consumption is increased, fibrogen levels may remain in the normal range.

Fibrin degradation products (FDPs), fibrin monomers, D-dimers, and fibrinopeptide A are all products resulting from the lysis of fibrinogen. Although the fibrin monomer and D-dimer tests are the most sensitive and specific, FDP measurements are the most widely available.

PLATELET DISORDERS

Causes of Platelet-related Bleeding

Bleeding occurs when *platelet number* or *function* is inadequate. If platelet counts are normal but the BT is prolonged, the next step is to determine whether the problem is the platelet itself or caused by the circulating plasma. *Platelet defects*

are assayed by aggregation studies. *Plasma* of such patients should be evaluated for factor VIII activity. (Humoral factors impairing platelet function usually result from Von Willebrand's disease.)

Problems of Platelet Function

Drug effects, uremia, DIC, leukemia, Von Willebrand's disease, or paraproteinemias can explain a prolonged BT with normal platelet count. The most common drugs to impair platelet function are listed below (Table 24.3).

Significant drug-induced abnormalities of platelet aggregation may not be reflected by the BT. Platelet function may be impaired by drug combinations even when any single one acting alone would be well tolerated. (The most common combination leading to platelet dysfunction is aspirin and alcohol.) Platelet function requires at least 24 hours to recover after discontinuing the responsible medication. Some drugs (like aspirin) injure platelet function irreversibly, so that hemostasis is restored only by tranfusion or formation of new platelets over a period of days. *Aspirin* should be avoided in patients with bleeding disorders. It is important to ask specifically about salicylate containing over-the-counter medicines. *Alcohol* inhibits platelet production and action in several ways. Heavy alcohol usage predisposes to trauma, encourages nutritional deficiency, and directly injures the marrow. Given in high doses, most *penicillins* bind to the platelet surface, preventing interaction with Von Willebrand's factor. (This does not occur with methacillin or cephalosporins.) *Uremic toxins* diminish factor VIII/VWF activity and, like *paraproteinemias*, interfere with interaction between the platelet and the vessel wall.

Therapy of Platelet Dysfunction

Bleeding rarely occurs in patients with *isolated* platelet dysfunction. Unless sequestered or destroyed, transfused platelets quickly restore coagulation competency. Platelet transfusions effectively correct dysfunction induced by aspirin or the cardiac bypass pump. Platelet transfusion is also *transiently* useful when the platelet environment is abnormal (uremia, paraproteinemia, high-dose penicillin, dextran). However, it is better to

Table 24.3
Drugs Inhibiting Platelet Function

Aspirin	High-dose penicillin or ticarcillin
NSAIAs*	Moxalactam
Alcohol	Heparin

*NSAIAs, nonsteroidal anti-inflammatory agents

correct the underlying defect, for example by dialysis, plasmapheresis, or discontinuing the offending drug. Defects caused by uremia and Von Willebrand's disease may be corrected with fresh frozen plasma, DDAVP, or cryoprecipitate. Corticosteroids often decrease the BT when antiplatelet antibodies produce thrombocytopenia.

Problems of Platelet Number— Thrombocytopenia

The BT is seldom prolonged until the count of normal platelets falls below $80,000/mm^3$ (≤ 8 platelets per high power field on peripheral blood smear). Although counts $> 50,000/mm^3$ are acceptable for most types of operation, levels $> 100,000/mm^3$ are preferred for cardiac procedures or neurosurgery. Spontaneous bleeding is rare with a count of $> 20,000/mm^3$ normally functioning platelets, but at this level bleeding may occur even with minor trauma. When counts fall below $20,000/mm^3$, spontaneous bleeding is possible. Normally, $\approx 10\%$ of platelets appear large on the peripheral smear, reflecting recent production. Young platelets produced by an active marrow are more hemostatically effective. Therefore, at any given count, bleeding is more likely to occur if thrombocytopenia results from impaired platelet production (rather than increased destruction).

Mechanistically, thrombocytopenias are usually classified as disorders of *production and destruction. Idiopathic thrombocytopenia (ITP), acute leukemia*, and *aplastic crisis* are the most likely causes of severe thrombocytopenia ($< 10,000/mm^3$).

Impaired Production

Isolated production defects are rare; when inadequate production accounts for thrombocytopenia, anemia and leukopenia usually coexist. In such cases, *platelets are small* and bone marrow examination shows a *decreased number of megakaryocytes*. Marrow failure may result from alcohol or radiation, a deficiency of Vitamin B_{12} or folate, high dose chemotherapy, or marrow infiltration with tumor, fibrosis, or granuloma. Selective failure of platelet production may occur with the use of gold, sulfa, and thiazides.

Increased Consumption

Excessive platelet consumption may be due to immunologic or non-immunologic mechanisms. Non-immunologic platelet consumption occurs in DIC, sepsis, microangiopathic hemolysis, thrombotic thrombocytopenic purpura (TTP), hemolytic

uremic syndrome, and splenic sequestration. Anemia, leukopenia and a normal or hyperplastic marrow usually accompany thrombocytopenia due to hypersplenism. *Laboratory* clues to platelet *consumption* include disproportionate numbers of large (young) platelets on peripheral smear and an increased number of marrow megakaryocytes. Antiplatelet antibodies stimulated by drugs (e.g., quinidine, sulfa, digoxin, methyldopa, heparin, and morphine) may all lead to complement mediated platelet destruction. Removal of the offending drug elevates platelet counts substantially within 5 days, but full recovery may take 3–4 weeks. Platelet transfusions and steroids may help restore platelet counts rapidly once the offending drug is removed.

In *acute* ITP, immunologic platelet destruction usually follows a *childhood* viral illness. Steroids are frequently helpful if thrombocytopenia persists more than several weeks. In *adults* ITP usually presents as a *chronic disease*, with counts ranging from 20 to 80 thousand. The spleen is the major site of platelet destruction. Splenectomy is indicated in the 10–20% of patients who fail to respond to steroids. Vincristine may be useful in patients who fail steroids and splenectomy. Anemia in ITP is secondary to blood loss, not immune hemolysis.

Heparin also commonly causes the formation of antibodies that may cross-react with platelets causing thrombocytopenia. This syndrome has been associated with both hemorrhage and large vessel thrombosis. Withdrawal of heparin is the treatment of choice.

SPECIFIC CLOTTING DISORDERS

Hemophilias

The hemophilias are sex-linked recessive diseases producing clinical bleeding in affected males. Spontaneous hemorrage in hemophilia A (factor VIII deficiency) or hemophilia B (factor IX deficiency) usually occurs only when factor levels dip below 5% of normal (most commonly $< 1\%$). Therefore, female carriers possessing 50% of normal factor VIII or IX levels are spared bleeding complications. Despite these guidelines, a less than ideal correlation exists between factor levels and bleeding tendency.

Laboratory examination most commonly reveals a prolonged PTT, with normal PT, platelet count, BT, and thrombin time. Specific levels of factors VIII and IX are required to distinguish hemophilia A from B.

The urgency of therapy must be guided by the amount and location of bleeding; massive hemorrhage or bleeding into the brain or upper airway are most urgent. Surgery and invasive procedures in hemophiliacs require maintenance of factor levels > 50% for 14 days following the procedure. In critical operative sites (e.g., brain, spinal cord), activities approaching 100% are desirable. Topical aminocaproic acid (Amicar) may be effective at controlling localized mucosal or venipuncture bleeding.

Although factor VIII is present in fresh frozen plasma (FFP) and cryoprecipitate, specific factor VIII concentrate is usually the most practical replacement vehicle because of cost and fluid volume considerations. However, cryoprecipitate is safer than specific factor concentrate because it carries a lower risk of hepatitis and acquired immune deficiency syndrome (AIDS). In factor IX deficiency (hemophilia B), replacement of the deficient factor can be accomplished with FFP or factor IX complex (Konyne). (For recommendations on the replacement of factors VIII and IX see Chapter 13, Transfusion and Blood Component Therapy.)

Liver Disease

Apart from its role in clearing FDPs the liver produces albumin and all clotting factors except factor VIII/VWF. Therefore, a low serum albumin concentration supports hepatic insufficiency as the etiology of the coagulation disorder. Laboratory examination reveals *decreased fibrinogen, increased circulating levels of FDPs, prolonged PT and PTT*, and *an increased thrombin time (due to FDPs)*. Such a laboratory pattern is identical to that seen with DIC; however, detecting D-dimers and fibrin monomers favors a diagnosis of DIC.

Liver disease and vitamin K deficiency decrease levels of factor VII (the vitamin K dependent factor with the shortest half life). This reduction leads to early increases in PT. Because multiple factors (II, VII, IX, and X) are deficient in liver disease, FFP is the replacement product of choice if immediate correction is necessary. In less urgent situations, vitamin K will usually suffice. Vitamin K should also be given empirically to virtually all patients with liver-related coagulopathy because it is difficult to distinguish liver disease from pure vitamin K deficiency. Parenteral vitamin K should usually be injected subcutaneously. Intravenous administration carries the risk of anaphylaxis, and intramuscular injections can cause hematoma formation. Platelet counts are usually normal in liver disease, unless there is co-existing hypersplenism or DIC. When platelet counts are significantly decreased

($< 50,000/mm^3$), platelet concentrates may be administered. Unfortunately, these are often ineffective.

Vitamin K Deficiency

Vitamin K deficiency may develop in any patient deprived of a balanced diet for 7–14 days. Because broad spectrum antibiotic therapy may eliminate the enteric bacteria required for the production of vitamin K when intake is insufficient, malnourished patients and those receiving *broad spectrum antibiotic therapy* are at particular risk. Fat soluble vitamin K is incompatible with many total parenteral nutrition (TPN) preparations and, if omitted, must be given separately. Warfarin compounds can produce vitamin K deficiency by preventing carboxylation to the active form. Malabsorption (from pancreatic insufficiency) and bile salt deficiency (from ductal obstruction) may also prevent vitamin K absorption.

Vitamin K is required for the formation of factors II, VII, IX, and X. Although depletion of vitamin K usually extends both the PT and PTT, prolongation of the PT is more marked and occurs earlier because factor VII (extrinsic pathway) has the shortest half-life of all clotting proteins. (Vitamin K deficiency may also stop production of the *anti-clotting proteins*, proteins C, S, and antithrombin III, a problem which may cause seemingly paradoxical *thrombosis*.) FFP corrects the clotting disorder of vitamin K deficiency very rapidly (2–3 bags usually suffice). Parenteral vitamin K usually corrects the deficiency within 24–48 hours if liver function is normal.

Disseminated Intravascular Coagulation

Disseminated intravascular coagulation (DIC) should be strongly considered in any patient with the combination of *diffuse bleeding or clotting, elevations in PT and PTT*, and *a decreased platelet count*. DIC is not self-perpetuating but requires continuous activation of the clotting mechanism. Such stimulation most frequently results from vascular damage or sepsis. In DIC, thrombin activation stimulates plasmin-mediated thrombolysis. Fibrin split products are formed in this process. With concurrent clotting and fibrinolysis, factors V, VII, fibrinogen, and platelets are rapidly consumed. Bleeding occurs if consumption outstrips production. The causes of DIC are numerous but usually relate to tissue *inflammation* from infection, tumors, or release of the products of conception into the circulation. Cytotoxic drugs, heat stroke, and shock, as well as vascular disruption (aortic aneurysm) may also cause DIC.

Diagnosis of DIC is usually straightforward. *Early in the course the PTT may be shortened* as thromboplastin is released into the circulation. *Later the PT and PTT are prolonged due to depletion of fibrinogen, factors V and VII*, and the anticoagulant action of *FDPs*. The platelet count is usually < 150,000/mm^3 and fibrinogen usually < 150 mg%. (Fibrinogen concentration may be in the normal range if levels were initially elevated, as in hepatitis.) The hallmark of DIC is an increase in the titers of fibrin degradation products (FDPs) or fibrin monomers to > 1:40. Large platelets are usually seen on peripheral smear along with fragmented red blood cells (RBCs) suggestive of microangiopathic hemolysis. A laboratory picture similar to DIC may be seen in dilutional coagulopathy or in hepatic failure if complicated by thrombocytopenia from splenic sequestration or platelet destruction.

The *treatment* of DIC is to *reverse the underlying cause* and to *supplement consumed clotting factors*. FFP may be used to replace factors V and VII. Platelets should be administered for severe thrombocytopenia. Cryoprecipitate may be used to replace fibrinogen if levels are markedly depressed. There is no clear evidence that heparin is beneficial, except in acute promyelocytic leukemia.

Dilutional Coagulopathy

Dilutional coagulopathy occurs during massive hemorrhage, when replacement of a substantial fraction of the circulating volume leads to washout of platelets and clotting factors. After 10 units of packed red blood cells are given, it is generally recommended to give 2 units of FFP and 6 units of platelets for every 4–6 units of packed RBCs. The major diagnostic dilemma is to separate dilutional coagulopathy, (increased PT and PTT, decreased platelet count) from DIC, a distinction that is reliably made by FDP or fibrin monomer assay. While awaiting laboratory confirmation, the best strategy is to administer 2 units of fresh frozen plasma; if the clotting disorder is dilutional, FFP will correct the defect.

Circulating Anticoagulants

Circulating anticoagulants are immunoglobins that inhibit the action of clotting proteins. Sources include *hemophilia, AIDS, advanced age*, and *drugs* (e.g., penicillin and chlorpromazine). The most notable circulating anticoagulant occurs in *systemic lupus*, in which the action of factors II, V, IX, and X are impaired. Although termed the "lupus anticoagulant", such antibodies are much more commonly associated with thrombosis than hemorrhage. Screening for a circulating anticoagulant is done by performing a PT and PTT on a mixture of equal parts of normal and patient plasma. If a simple factor *deficiency* is the cause of abnormal clotting, the addition of normal plasma will provide 50% activity and will normalize clotting tests. However, if an inhibitor is present, clotting tests tend to remain abnormal. Circulating anticoagulants often increase only the PTT mimicking the laboratory findings of hemophilia. In urgent circumstances, therapy may include massive replacement of the affected factors or the use of activated factor X.

Von Willebrand's Disease

Von Willebrand's disease (VWD), an autosomal dominant trait, decreases the activity of factor VIII/VWF, thereby reducing the adherence of platelets to sites of vascular injury. VWD usually presents with hemorrhage after trauma, mucosal bleeding, or menorrhagia. Laboratory findings include an *increased bleeding time with a normal platelet count and a prolonged PTT*. Cryoprecipitate is superior to factor VIII concentrate for treatment because it contains all forms of the factor (including more factor VIII/VWF polymers and fibrinogen) and carries a lower risk of hepatitis. The vasopressin analog DDAVP may be used to transiently increase the endogenous *release* of factor VIII, thereby avoiding transfusion in patients requiring only temporary normalization of hemostasis (e.g., patients undergoing brief invasive procedures).

Paraproteinemias

When present in large amounts, serum proteins of the IgG, IgM, and IgA classes may impair clotting. Such problems usually occur in patients with *myeloma* or *Waldenström's macroglobulinemia*. Plasmapheresis reduces the serum protein level and reverses the coagulopathy.

Bleeding During Thrombolytic Therapy

Almost any clotting test will confirm the presence of a "lytic state" during the administration of thrombolytic agents (streptokinase, urokinase, or tissue plasminogen activator). The *thrombin time* directly monitors the effect of thrombolytic drugs by examining the final step in the clotting cascade (the conversion of fibrinogen to fibrin). The TT should be maintained 2–5 times the baseline value when assessed 4 hours after the initiation of thrombolytic therapy. When bleeding occurs, cryoprecipitate and FFP can rapidly correct the clotting abnormalities (see p. 128). Because hemorrhage during thrombolytic therapy is usually a consequence of poor patient selection (e.g., elderly, traumatized) or the result of invasive procedures during the lytic period, most bleeding episodes can be avoided.

Anticoagulant-Induced Bleeding

Bleeding during anticoagulation usually indicates a coexisting disturbance of vascular integrity or platelet function. Gastrointestinal or genito-urinary tract hemorrhage that occurs at therapeutic levels of anticoagulation usually indicates an underlying *structural lesion*. Risk factors for anticoagulant-induced bleeding include *advanced age*, *alcohol and aspirin use*, and *female gender*.

Warfarin (Coumadin) inhibits production of vitamin K dependent proteins prolonging the PT to a greater degree than the PTT. The goal of warfarin therapy is to maintain PT 1.5–2.5 times baseline. However, recent evidence suggests that PT values 1.25–1.5 times control are adequate for most conditions. Changes in previously stable levels of anticoagulation are often due to fluctuations in warfarin metabolism or protein binding induced by the addition or discontinuation of other drugs (e.g., erythromycin, phenobarbital, or phenytoin). The intensity of anticoagulation is also increased by drugs that compete with warfarin for albumin binding (sulfas, sulfonureas, indomethacin, and phenylbutazone).

In patients with warfarin-induced bleeding and firm indications for chronic anticoagulation (prosthetic heart valves, recurrent embolism), interruption of warfarin for 2–4 days is usually uneventful. If more precise control of anticoagulation is needed, heparin may be temporarily substituted. Vitamin K is usually sufficient to reverse the anticoagulant effect of warfarin in patients with an excessively prolonged PT *without bleeding*. However, vitamin K does not provide ideal reversal because its effect may be delayed 6–24 hours and re-anticoagulation may be difficult if greater than 1 mg of vitamin K is given. In more urgent cases, FFP will promptly (but temporarily) reverse anticoagulation.

Heparin is a poorly understood, complex drug with a half life of about 90 minutes. Used subcutaneously in prophylactic doses (5000 units every 8–12 hr), the PTT usually remains unaffected and bleeding is very rare. The goal of full dose anticoagulation with heparin is to prolong the PTT to 1.5–2 times control. There is little evidence to suggest anything more than a weak correlation between therapeutic PTT elevations and bleeding tendency during heparin therapy. However, if the PT or PTT are "infinitely" prolonged, the tendency for unprovoked bleeding may be increased. The therapy of heparin overdose includes discontinuation of the drug and the administration of protamine (1 mg/unit of circulating heparin). Interruption of a continuous infusion of heparin for more than 3 hours almost always results in a subtherapeutic PTT, except in the setting of massive overdosage.

SUGGESTED READINGS

1. Bachmann F: Diagnostic approaches to mild bleeding disorders. *Semin Hematol* 1980;17(4):292–305.
2. Bowie ESW, Owen CA, Jr: Hemostatic failure in clinical medicine. *Semin Hematol* 1977;14(3):341–364.
3. Counts RB, Haisch C, Simon TL, et al: Hemostasis in massively transfused trauma patients. *Ann Surg* 1979;190(1):91–99.
4. Deykin D: The clinical challenge of disseminated intravascular coagulation. *N Engl J Med* 1970;283:636–644.
5. Feinstein DI: Diagnosis and management of disseminated intravascular coagulation: the role of heparin therapy. *Blood* 1982;60:284–287.
6. King DJ, Kelton JG: Heparin-associated thrombocytopenia. *Ann Intern Med* 1984;100:535–540.
7. Malpass TW, Harker LA: Acquired disorders of platelet function. *Semin Hematol* 1980;17:242–258.

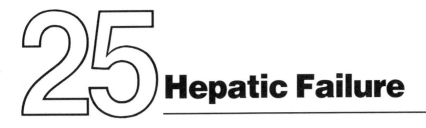

Hepatic Failure

CLASSIFICATION OF ACUTE HEPATIC FAILURE

Acute hepatic failure (AHF) can arise as a primary process in a previously healthy person, as an exacerbation of a chronic liver disease (cirrhosis, chronic active hepatitis), or as part of the "multiorgan failure syndrome" of critical illness. Whatever the cause, certain key manifestations of AHF are shared. All forms of AHF disrupt one or more of the 5 major functions of the liver: (1) Maintenance of *acid-base balance* through the metabolism of lactate; (2) *Drug metabolism* and detoxification; (3) *glucose and lipid metabolism*; (4) *synthesis of proteins* (including immunoglobins, clotting factors, and albumin), and (5) *phagocytic clearance* of organisms and injurious debris.

Fulminant Hepatic Dysfunction as a Primary Process

When fulminant hepatic failure develops as a primary process, the manifestations evolve over a period of < 4 weeks in a previously healthy person. The most advanced form of this syndrome, massive hepatic necrosis, is produced by a wide variety of noxious insults and proves fatal in 75–90% of cases. Etiologies of massive hepatic necrosis are listed in Table 25.1

AHF as a Secondary Process

Although fulminant liver failure occurs only rarely as a primary process, life-threatening hepatic dysfunction often develops in patients with limited reserves, in whom relatively minor insults can tip the balance. Severe liver injury also occurs when nutritional flow is compromised (congestive heart failure, shock) or when hepatocytes are damaged by circulating mediators of inflammation (sepsis syndrome).

Table 25.1
Etiologies of Massive Hepatic Necrosis

Viral	Drug Ingestion
Hepatitis A	Halogenated anesthetics
Hepatitis B	Acetaminophen
(+/- Δ agent)	Tetracycline
Non-A, non-B	Isoniazid
Cytomegalovirus	Rifampin
Chemical Hepatotoxins	**Miscellaneous**
Carbon tetrachloride	Reye's syndrome
Benzene	Toxemia of pregnancy
Ethylene glycol	Toxic mushrooms
Ethanol	

DIAGNOSIS OF AHF

The clinical diagnosis of AHF is seldom made until biochemical signs of liver *and* central nervous system (CNS) dysfunction are present. Irritability, confusion, and vomiting are all *early* signs of CNS involvement. Fever is common early in the course, whereas hypothermia is more frequent later. Ascites and peripheral edema reflect portal hypertension and hypoalbuminemia but are not necessary for diagnosis. Hypoxemia is present in most patients, and the adult respiratory distress syndrome (ARDS) complicates about ⅓ of all cases.

Laboratory Features

Leukocytosis with neutrophilia and hepatic transaminase elevations are usually present. Marked hyperbilirubinemia commonly precedes a fall in serum albumin and prolongation of the prothrombin time, both late signs of hepatic failure. Extensive hepatic destruction may impair gluconeogenesis, giving rise to hypoglycemia. Low-grade disseminated intravascular coagulation (DIC) commonly results from decreased synthesis of clotting factors, together with failure of the liver to clear fibrin degradation products (see p. 214). Deficient production of anti-thrombins may predispose to thrombosis. In AHF with encephalopathy arterial ammonia concentrations are usually elevated; a normal ammonia level in a patient with altered mental status may help to exclude the diagnosis of hepatic encephalopathy. (Ammonia levels may be spuriously elevated by venous rather than arterial sampling, or improper specimen handling. Conversely, ammonia levels may be artifactually low in patients with severe protein malnutrition.)

THERAPY AND COMPLICATIONS

There is no specific therapy for AHF. Supportive care includes maintenance of adequate nutrition and hemodynamic support as well as monitoring for the most frequent complications: (1) hepatic encephalopathy; (2) cerebral edema; (3) bacterial infection; (4) gastrointestinal bleeding; (5) coagulopathy; and (6) renal failure.

Hepatic Encephalopathy

Etiology

Hepatic encephalopathy or porto-systemic encephalopathy (PSE) is the most frequent fatal complication of AHF. However, it is important to exclude other reversible causes of altered mental status: (1) hypoglycemia; (2) infection; (3) electrolyte imbalance; (4) drug overdosage (particularly sedatives); (5) hypoxemia; and (6) vitamin deficiency.

PSE develops in patients whose severe liver disease causes shunting of portal blood around the liver directly to the systemic circulation. PSE results from toxins produced by gut bacteria uncleared by the damaged liver. Ammonia, fatty acids, mercaptans, and other false neurotransmitters have been implicated as causative, but there is no concensus. PSE may produce fixed neurological deficits as well as alter consciousness, intellectual performance, and personality. In salvagable cases, mental status changes usually respond to appropriate therapy within several days.

Regardless of the specific biochemical cause, a number of precipitating factors are known to worsen PSE. *Gastrointestinal hemorrhage* increases the gut protein load and ammonia production. *Intravascular volume depletion* (from bleeding or diuretics), *alkalosis*, and *hypokalemia* are also common precipitating factors. *Hypokalemia* and *alkalosis* both predispose to the formation of ammonia and worsen mental status. Excessive withdrawal of ascitic fluid may cause translocation of fluid from the vascular space to the peritoneal cav-

ity, thereby decreasing hepatic perfusion. Weight lost through the use of diuretics or fluid restriction must not exceed 1 to 2 pounds per day. All *drugs* (but particularly sedatives and narcotics) must be used with extreme caution in the setting of impaired hepatic metabolism. Histamine blockers should also be used cautiously because of the likelihood of impaired mentation in patients with liver disease. *Failing renal function* accentuates the accumulation of ammonia and other toxins. Almost any *systemic infection* may alter mental status, but the most common infection precipitating PSE is spontaneous bacterial peritonitis.

Diagnosis of PSE

The diagnosis of PSE is made on clinical grounds and supported by specific electroencephalogram (EEG) findings, elevated blood ammonia levels, or increases in spinal fluid glutamine. Hyperpnea and hyperventilation are common. While computed tomographic (CT) scanning of the brain can only reveal non-specific cerebral edema in PSE, an EEG occasionally demonstrates characteristic abnormalities (high amplitude delta and triphasic waves). Unfortunately, the EEG usually demonstrates only non-specific, diffuse slowing. Evoked potential testing has been advocated as a specific and sensitive marker of PSE, but whether it offers an advantage over the EEG is not yet clear. In patients with subtle PSE or in cases in which the diagnosis is in doubt, a therapeutic trial should be undertaken. (Other causes of reversible encephalopathy must first be excluded.) Response to therapy usually occurs within 3–4 days if the diagnosis is correct.

Treatment of PSE

Correction of precipitating causes (bleeding, drugs, infection, alkalosis, hypovolemia) are key to improvement. However, once PSE is established, restricting protein intake and preventing gastrointestinal (GI) bleeding reduce the substrate available for the production of cerebral toxins. Aromatic amino acids (phenylalanine, tyrosine) have been implicated in PSE. Ideally, protein supplements should be rich in branched chain amino acids (valine, leucine, and isoleucine), and contain normal amounts of aromatic amino acids.

Laxatives or enemas decrease fecal generation of nitrogenous toxins, but severe or protracted diarrhea sufficient to cause fluid depletion and electrolyte abnormalities must be avoided. *Neomycin*, given in 2–4 gm oral doses or administered as an enema once or twice daily, reduces the number of intestinal bacteria forming these toxic compounds. Because as much as 5% of the drug may be absorbed systemically, renal insufficiency may occur when large doses are given to patients with impaired renal function. Rarely, neomycin causes reversible diarrhea, nephrotoxicity, and ototoxicity.

Lactulose, a synthetic non-absorbable and poorly digestible disaccharide, is broken down by colonic bacteria to lactic and acetic acids. These compounds induce an acidic diarrhea that renders nitrogenous toxins less absorbable. Initially, lactulose is administered hourly until a laxative effect is produced. It is then continued in doses sufficient to produce 1–2 soft stools per day. Excessive lactulose-induced diarrhea may deplete intravascular volume, worsening hepatic encephalopathy and precipitating the hepatorenal syndrome. Occasionally patients respond to neomycin but not to lactulose, or vice versa. Experimental therapy of PSE with *L-dopa or bromocryptine* is of unknown effectiveness.

Spontaneous Bacterial Peritonitis

Spontaneous bacterial peritonitis (SBP) is a common complication of AHF in which bacteria seed the peritoneal cavity. In most cases, bacteria cross directly into the ascitic fluid through the bowel wall. Hypoperfusion often precipitates SBP, presumably by impairing bowel wall integrity. In patients with ascites, sudden deterioration of renal function or mental status, rapid weight gain, or ascites that becomes resistant to diuretic therapy should all prompt consideration of SBP. Untreated SBP is fatal in 60–90% of cases and even with early antibiotic treatment the fatality rate remains ≃ 40%. High mortality despite treatment may be due to delayed diagnosis and institution of therapy or may reflect the high incidence of debilitation and multiple organ disease. Classically, SBP may be recognized by the triad of *fever, abdominal pain*, and *PSE*. However, SBP differs from peritonitis of other causes in that fever, abdominal pain, and tenderness are often minimal. About 25% of all patients with SBP have *no abdominal* symptoms, and 5% of patients are *entirely asymptomatic*.

Nothing short of obtaining peritoneal fluid can exclude the diagnosis of SBP. A peritoneal fluid pH < 7.31, a gradient in pH between the serum and acidic fluid of > 0.1 unit, or a lactic acid level > 32 mg/dl are suggestive. Diagnosis is confirmed when bacteria are seen on Gram stain or grow in culture. An absolute leukocyte count in the ascitic

fluid that is > 500/mm³ should prompt immediate therapy (particularly if polymorphonuclear leukocytes predominate).

Enteric gram-negative rods are the most common organisms, but 15% of patients with SBP have polymicrobial infections and 5% grow anerobes. The single most likely organism is *E. coli*, but pneumococcal infections are also prevalent. Because bacteremia occurs in ≃ 50% of cases, blood cultures should be obtained. An aminoglycoside together with an extended spectrum penicillin or cephalosporin is appropriate initial coverage.

Cerebral Edema

Cerebral edema, another cause of altered mental status in AHF, generally fails to respond to usual forms of treatment. Surgical decompression and dexamethasone appear to be of little or no benefit. Mannitol may reduce edema, but there is no evidence that survival is increased. The physical examination is rarely helpful in detecting cerebral edema. Furthermore, there is no evidence that mortality is improved through direct monitoring of CSF pressure. Death due to cerebral herniation may be sudden and unexpected.

Infection

Ten to 20% of patients with AHF die of bacterial infection. Prophylactic antibiotics offer no benefit. SBP, aspiration pneumonia and catheter-related sepsis are especially common infections, largely preventable with proper supportive care.

GI Bleeding

Because GI bleeding frequently produces shock, PSE, or hypoperfusion that initiates acute renal failure. It often the proximate cause of death in these patients. Coagulopathy frequently accentuates the tendency for GI blood loss. Although antacids and histamine (H_2) blockers are both effective in preventing stress ulceration, H_2 blockers are difficult to use safely in AHF because of impaired drug metabolism and CNS side effects.

Coagulation Disorders

All clotting factors are produced by the liver, with the exception of factor VIII-VWF (see p. 214). Thrombocytopenia is common, usually related to DIC. Vitamin K safely augments production of certain clotting factors (II, VII, IX, X). Because renal as well as liver function is often impaired, volume overload is a common complication when fresh frozen plasma is used to reverse clotting factor deficiencies.

Renal Failure

Two types of renal failure may accompany AHF: acute tubular necrosis (ATN) and the hepatorenal syndrome, (HRS). The diagnosis and therapy of ATN is outlined elsewhere (see p. 205). HRS is a unique form of oliguric renal failure seen in patients with liver failure. It is characterized by increasing serum creatinine, oliguria, and failure to respond to fluids or diuretics. Urinary sodium values are typically very low (< 10 mEq/l). Because of its high fatality rate and failure to respond to treatment, HRS must be prevented. It is especially important to avoid nephrotoxic drugs and the intravascular volume depletion that results from untreated GI hemorrhage, overzealous paracentesis, or excessive diuretic usage. The role of low-dose dopamine in the treatment of HRS is not yet defined.

Nutrition

Adequate nutrition is important to the survival of patients with AHF. Although adequate calories and protein of high biologic value must be provided, high protein loads should be avoided. Vitamin K, thiamine, and folate are required by most patients. Sufficient glucose should be given to provide protein sparing effects (see p. 136). It may be advantageous to use branched chain (rather than aromatic) amino acids in total parenteral nutrition (TPN) preparations to minimize PSE. Restoring a positive nitrogen balance is a major goal of nutritional repletion and may be assessed by standard tests of urine urea nitrogen. Lipid infusions are of limited usefulness because the failing liver cannot process fats readily.

Miscellaneous Complications

Many hepatically metabolized *drugs* are potentially lethal in AHF. Because narcotics, sedatives, and anesthetics severely depress mental status and glottic reflexes in these sensitive patients, indiscriminant use may have a fatal outcome; careful dosing and patient monitoring are mandatory. Long-acting sedatives given frequently or in large doses should be avoided because of cumulative drug effects. If sedation is necessary, small doses of short acting drugs without active metabolites (e.g., oxazepam) should be used.

Ascites is frequently present in AHF and on occasion, a pleuro-peritoneal communication may allow ascitic fluid to enter the chest, producing a symptomatic *pleural effusion*. The development of ascites with or without pleural fluid may impair ventilation and increase the work of breathing.

Experimental Treatment

All published studies using corticosteroids in AHF demonstrate increased protein catabolism, and a higher incidence of infection without hepatic improvement. There is no evidence that plasmapheresis, exchange transfusion, hyperimmune globulin, or cross-species circulation improves survival. In survivors of fulminant AHF, combined therapy with insulin and glucagon may cause the remaining liver to regenerate at a faster rate.

SUGGESTED READINGS

1. Conn HO, Fessel JM: Spontaneous bacterial peritonitis in cirrhosis: variations on a theme. *Medicine* 50:161–197, 1971.
2. Dunn GD, Hayes P, Breen KJ, et al: The liver in congestive heart failure: a review. *Am J Med Sci* 265:174–189, 1973.
3. Hoyumpa AM, Desmond PV, Arant GR, et al: Hepatic encephalopathy. *Gastroenterology* 76:189–195, 1979.
4. MacDougall BRD, Williams R: H$_2$-receptor antagonists and antacids in the prevention of acute gastrointestinal hemorrhage in fulminant hepatic failure. Two controlled trials. *Lancet* 1:617, 1977.
5. Rizzetto M, Verme G: Delta hepatitis—present status. *J Hepatol* 1:187–193, 1985.
6. Williams R: Fulminant hepatic failure. *Postgrad Med J* (59 Suppl) 4:33–41, 1983.
7. Williams R, Gimson A: Management of acute liver failure. *Clin Gastroenterol* 14:93–104, 1985.

26 Endocrine Emergencies

THYROID DISEASE

Severe Hyperthyroidism and Thyroid Storm

Definitions

It is often difficult to distinguish thyroid storm (TS) from severe hyperthyroidism. Apart from accentuated signs and symptoms of hyperthyroidism, TS is typified by *fever* exceeding 100°F and *tachycardia* (pulse greater than 100/min). Ancillary features include congestive heart failure, arrhythmias, tremor, diaphoresis, diarrhea, elevated liver function tests, and psychosis.

Etiology

Historically, *surgery* performed on large goiters with poor preoperative preparation was the most common cause of TS, but currently, TS usually results from an acute *infection, withdrawal of antithyroid drugs,* or *non-thyroid surgery.* Recognizable Graves disease is present in most patients with severe hyperthyroidism. *Iodine ingestion* initially increases thyroxine (T4) production but suppresses T4 release. After 10–14 days, serum levels of iodine decline, allowing discharge of large amounts of T4 into the circulation. Therefore, radioactive iodine, cardiac catheterization dye, intravenous pyelogram (IVP) contrast, and oral iodinated contrast may precipitate delayed TS in predisposed individuals. *Exogenous T4* rarely leads to TS except in massive ingestions.

Laboratory Tests

In the critically ill patient with TS, the diagnosis *must* be a clinical one because the results of thyroid function tests are often delayed. Thyroid function tests are not predictably different in patients with clinically mild and severe hyperthyroidism, except that *free T4* levels trend higher in patients with TS. Elevated hepatic transaminases often indicate life-threatening disease. Rarely, hypercalcemia may be present. In TS, the leukocyte count is usually normal or slightly elevated, but *relative lymphocytosis* is common, a feature that may help to differentiate thyroid disease from infectious causes of fever.

Treatment

The treatment of TS is four-fold: (1) *block T4 formation*; (2) *prevent T4 release*; (3) *prevent peripheral conversion* of T4 to T3; and (4) *inhibit the tissue effects* of T4 (Fig. 26.1). Propylthiouracil (PTU) and methimazole both block T4 synthesis, an effect which develops its full clinical impact over days. Of the two choices, PTU is preferred because of its additional ability to block the conversion of T4 to its biological active form (T3) in peripheral tissues. (Inhibition of T4 to T3 conversion may also be accomplished by dexamethasone and to a minor degree by propranolol.) Release of preformed T4 into the circulation is rapidly blocked by a supersaturated oral solution of iodine but circulating T4 has a long half-life. Because PTU and iodine only are available as oral preparations, administration may prove difficult in the critically ill. PTU and methimazole must be administered at least 2 hours before iodine therapy because iodine inhibits thyroid uptake of these drugs. Beta blockers blunt the tissue actions of thyroid hormone, but the need for such therapy is questionable. In extreme cases plasmaphoresis or peritoneal dialysis may be used to remove thyroid hormone from the circulation.

Complications

Hypertension may respond to beta blockade. Clinical heart failure occurs in half of patients with TS. Although classically described as a "high output" state, many patients have *normal cardiac outputs* and *elevated wedge pressures* and may be

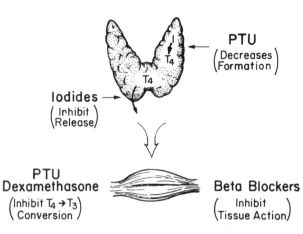

Figure 26.1   Sites of action of anti-thyroid medications.

harmed by the use of beta blockers. Fever from increased metabolic rate may be controlled by direct external cooling but salicylates should be avoided because of their tendency to displace T4 from serum proteins, worsening TS. Therapy of TS must include nutritional support because of increased caloric requirements. Folate and B vitamins are also rapidly consumed and should be supplemented. TS increases the metabolism of many drugs including some of those useful in its treatment (beta blockers and dexamethasone), making larger doses of these drugs necessary on a more frequent schedule.

Severe Hypothyroidism (Myxedema Coma)

Definition

Hypothermia, central nervous system (CNS) dysfunction, and *hypotension* differentiate myxedema coma from simple hypothyroidism. Myxedema is a rare but reversible cause of several common syndromes precipitating intensive care unit (ICU) admission: (1) *ileus* suggestive of bowel obstruction; (2) *respiratory failure*; (3) *heart failure*; and (4) *coma*.

Etiology

Hypothyroidism usually results from primary failure of the thyroid gland, not from pituitary insufficiency. Severe myxedema usually does not become manifest until some intercurrent illness complicates preexisting hypothyroidism (e.g., infection, surgery, hypothermia, trauma, and drugs, particularly opiates).

Diagnosis

The physical signs of hypothyroidism include: (1) *dry puffy skin*; (2) *characteristic facies*; (3) *bradycardia*; (4) decreased relaxation phase of *deep tendon reflexes*; and (5) *non-pitting edema*.

Laboratory Tests

Hyponatremia, hypoglycemia, and hypercapnia are common in hypothyroidism but are not diagnostic. The laboratory hallmark of hypothyroidism is an *elevated serum concentration of thyroid-stimulating hormone (TSH)* accompanied by *low total and free T4 levels* (Table 26.1). Many nonthyroidal illnesses decrease the total T4 without impairing thyroid function, the so-called "*sic-euthyroid*" state. In this syndrome decreased T4 binding protein and altered T4 metabolism lead to a decreased total T4 with normal or slightly depressed free T4 and normal TSH. Rarely, dopamine infusions may inhibit pituitary release of TSH, inducing a *false* sic-euthyroid state in the truly hypothyroid patient.

Treatment

Because orally administered drugs are poorly absorbed in myxedema, *T4 should be administered intravenously*. No controlled studies have been

Table 26.1
Laboratory Analysis of Hypothyroidism

	Total T4	Free T4	TSH
Sic euthyroid	↓	→ or ↓	Normal
Hypothyroidism	↓	↓ ↓	↑

↓, decreased; ↑, increased.

conducted to guide dosing, but initial daily doses of thyroxine in myxedema range from 0.2 to 0.5 mg intravenously. Commonly, 0.5 mg of T4 is given intravenously in the first 24 hours, followed by 0.1 mg each day thereafter. Clinical response is usually seen within 6–12 hours. T4 doses should be *reduced* in patients with known ischemic heart disease or angina because abrupt elevation of thyroxine may precipitate cardiac ischemia. In normotensive, euthermic patients the initial dose may be as low as 0.1 mg.

If hypothyroidism is suspected, adrenal function must also be tested because an adrenal crisis may be precipitated if T4 is administered to patients with adrenal insufficiency. Hypoglycemia occurs frequently enough to warrant urgent evaluation in acutely ill patients with altered mental status and suspected hypothyroidism. Arterial blood gases should be analyzed because suppressed ventilatory drive leading to hypercapnic respiratory failure is common. Hyponatremia may be effectively treated by water restriction. Hypotension and hypoperfusion should be treated with thyroxine and corticosteroids as well as the fluids and vasopressors as dictated by usual hemodynamic parameters. Many patients will have concomitant hypothermia requiring treatment (see p. 196).

ADRENAL DISEASES

Adrenal Insufficiency

Etiology

The physiologic effects of adrenal insufficiency (AI) result from deficiencies of cortisol and/or aldosterone. *Primary* adrenal insufficiency may result from adrenal destruction by tuberculosis, fungal disease, surgery, infarction, metastatic malignancy, or hemorrhage. Yet, in most cases the etiology remains obscure.

In *secondary* AI pituitary secretion of adrenocorticotrophic hormone (ACTH) is insufficient to maintain normal levels of cortisol, but aldosterone secretion remains normal because it is not regulated by ACTH. Secondary AI may result from direct trauma, tumor growth, or pituitary infarction. Abrupt withdrawal of exogenous steroids mimics secondary AI. Because aldosterone levels remain normal, secondary AI seldom results in dehydration or hyperkalemia. Conversely, primary AI frequently demonstrates these features. In most patients adrenal crisis is precipitated by a intercurrent illness that causes volume depletion (vomiting/diarrhea). Surgery increases the risk of adrenal

crisis by increasing cortisol clearance and by predisposing to volume depletion.

Signs and Symptoms

Weakness, *fatigue*, *anorexia*, *fever*, and *nausea* are the most common presenting signs of AI, regardless of etiology. *Shock* may be the initial presentation in adrenal failure complicated by infection or dehydration. In anticoagulated patients, flank pain may be a presenting sign of adrenal hemorrhage. Cutaneous hyperpigmentation is seen only in primary AI. (A functioning pituitary gland is necessary to produce the ACTH-like melanocyte stimulating hormone, responsible for hyperpigmentation).

Laboratory Examination

Urinary *sodium wasting* and *hyperkalemia* are seen predominately in primary AI as a result of *aldosterone deficiency*. Conversely the isolated *cortisol deficiency* of secondary AI impairs free water excretion but rarely causes hyperkalemia. Hypercalcemia may be seen in either form of AI because cortisol is required to regulate gastrointestinal absorption and renal excretion of calcium. Although the total leukocyte count is usually normal, the percentage of eosinophils and lymphocytes is often increased. Hypoglycemia may be the presenting manifestation of either primary or secondary AI.

Tests of Adrenal Function

Because AI is life threatening, it is important to institute cortisol replacement *before* laboratory confirmation of the diagnosis. The following protocol may be used to both diagnose and treat adrenal failure simultaneously. (1) Draw baseline blood cortisol and ACTH levels. (2) Administer an ACTH analog (intravenous Cortrosyn, 250 mcg). (3) Obtain cortisol levels 30 and 60 minutes after ACTH injection. 4) Begin empirical glucocorticoid therapy. A baseline cortisol level exceeding 25 mcg/dl or a brisk ($\simeq$ 2-fold) rise after stimulation in an acutely ill patient makes a diagnosis of AI unlikely. The usual response to ACTH stimulation is illustrated in Table 26.2.

Treatment

Glucocorticoids and *salt-containing fluid* are the essence of therapy. If adequate amounts of salt-containing crystalloid are infused, *mineralocorticoid* hormones are not immediately necessary in either form of AI. Cortisol levels may rise 10 fold above baseline levels under periods of maximal

Table 26.2
Usual Response to ACTH Stimulation

	ACTH Level	Cortisol Level	
		Baseline	Post-ACTH Stimulation
Normal	Normal	Normal	Increased
Primary adrenal failure	Marked increase	Low	Low
Secondary adrenal failure	Low or normal	Low	Increased
Post-steroid withdrawal	Low	Low or normal	Mild increase*

*Requires 24-hour ACTH infusion for confirmation.

stress to a daily equivalent of 300–400 mg of hydrocortisone; therefore, patients with acute AI require large doses of corticosteroids. Although hydrocortisone (100 mg every 6–8 hr) is often given intravenously because of its mineralocorticoid effects, dexamethasone (2–5 mg every 8 hr) is a useful alternative because it does not interfere with serum cortisol assays. Intravenous steroid administration avoids potential problems of delayed or incomplete absorption.

Although mild hyperkalemia is commonly seen, potassium concentrations seldom rise to dangerous levels in AI. Hyperkalemia is usually rapidly corrected with volume expansion and glucocorticoids alone. Because AI impairs gluconeogenesis, intravenous fluids should include adequate glucose supplementation.

Withdrawal of Exogenous Steroids

Partial or complete adrenal suppression from exogenous corticosteroids may occur with as little as 5 days of low-dose prednisone (20–30 mg). Prolonged steroid use may impair adrenal responsiveness for as long as 1 year after withdrawal of exogenous steroids (Fig. 26.2). The ACTH response returns first, (usually within 90 days); however, several months often pass before normal cortisol response to ACTH is restored. Patients who demonstrate a normal cortisol response to ACTH stimulation are unlikely to have subnormal adrenal response to stress. If the adrenal responsiveness of a critically ill patient is questionable, adrenal function should be tested and cortisol given.

Excessive Corticosteroid Administration

Excessive corticosteroids predispose to infection and produce protein wasting, poor wound healing, and glucose intolerance. Long-term exogenous steroids may also cause intracranial hypertension, bone loss, aseptic necrosis, glaucoma, pancreatitis, and cataract formation. Adverse steroid effects are

minimized by: (1) using the *lowest effective dose*; (2) using a *short-acting* steroid preparation such as hydrocortisone; (3) administering the full daily requirement in a *single morning dose*; and (4) using *alternate day therapy*.

DISORDERS OF GLUCOSE METABOLISM

General Care of the Critically Ill Diabetic Patient

Several important principles apply to treatment of glucose abnormalities in the intensive care unit. (1) Critical illness induces a state of relative insulin resistance due to release of stress hormones (glucagon, epinephrine, cortisol). (2) Starvation, sepsis, and drug therapy complicate diabetes management by unpredictably altering the effectiveness of insulin.

The following suggestions comprise a rational approach to managing the critically ill, nonketotic diabetic patient:

1. *Withhold oral hypoglycemic agents.*
2. *Avoid interruption of feedings.*
3. Eliminate or significantly *reduce* the proportion of *long-acting insulin*. (Instead, monitor blood glucose values frequently and treat with small doses of regular insulin.)
4. Do not substitute *urine* tests for serum tests of glucose. (At best urine tests are time-delayed measures of serum levels and are less precise.)

Hypoglycemia

Blood glucose should be rapidly determined in patients with altered mental status to rule out hypoglycemia, even if focal neurological deficits are present. The symptoms of hypoglycemia depend not only upon the absolute level of serum glucose but also upon the *rate of its decline*.

Insulin Reactions

Insulin reactions are common in the ICU largely because renal insufficiency impairs insulin clear-

ACTH AND CORTISOL FOLLOWING STEROID WITHDRAWAL

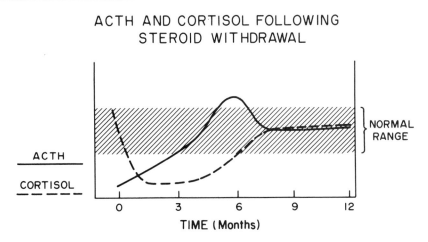

Figure 26.2   ACTH and cortisol levels following abrupt termination of prolonged glucocorticoid therapy at time 0.

ance and because hospitalized diabetics frequently do not receive regular feedings. (Long acting insulins amplify this risk.) Insulin-induced hypoglycemia may also occur when insulin injected into underperfused tissues is later absorbed following reestablished perfusion. High insulin levels and low C-peptide levels in the hypoglycemic patient suggest intentional or inadvertant insulin overdosage.

Oral Hypoglycemic Agents

Oral hypoglycemic agents are a poor choice for glucose control in the hospitalized diabetic because of their long half-life and frequent interactions with other drugs. Patients with hypoglycemia due to these agents should be observed closely because of the potential for prolonged or recurrent symptoms. Hypoglycemia due to oral agents is often refractory to glucose alone and may require combined therapy with *hydrocortisone*, *diazoxide*, and *glucagon*. Renal failure prolongs the half-life of these drugs and their attendant toxicity. Hypoglycemic action of these agents is also potentiated by butazolidin, sulfonamides, probenecid, and salicylates. Furthermore, oral hypoglycemics interact with such commonly used medications as phenytoin, phenothiazines, rifampin, and thiazides.

Other Causes of Hypoglycemia

Overwhelming infection may produce hypoglycemia by multiple mechanisms including hepatic hypoperfusion or failure, renal insufficiency, depletion of muscle glycogen, and starvation.
Alcohol suppresses gluconeogenesis, restricts

nutrient intake, and induces a low insulin state that favors free fatty acid release and ketone production. Consequently alcoholics may present with hypoglycemia, a mixed ketosis, and lactic acidosis. By the time such patients seek medical attention, alcohol has usually been completely metabolized. Glucose, thiamine, and fluids comprise the key elements in the treatment of alcoholic acidosis with hypoglycemia. Although ketoacids are present, insulin *does not* speed resolution of the acidosis and may exacerbate hypoglycemia. Sodium bicarbonate is necessary only to maintain the pH above 7.15.

Other causes of hypoglycemia include *hepatic failure* (due to cirrhosis, tumor infiltration, or massive hepatic necrosis), *renal failure*, *salicylate poisoning*, and *insulin secreting tumors*.

Surgery and other states of major stress blunt the effect of insulin while stimulating the release of counter-regulatory hormones. Imbalance of these effects may cause circulating glucose to *rise or decline* unpredictably to dangerous levels. To prevent hypoglycemia in the surgical patient it is prudent to monitor glucose closely and to decrease (but not discontinue) preoperative insulin. A useful strategy is to administer one-half of the regular insulin dosage before surgery despite the fasting state. The key to preventing hypoglycemia is frequent *intraoperative* and *postoperative glucose testing*.

Treatment of Hypoglycemia

Unless otherwise contraindicated, intravenous glucose should be empirically administered to all patients with abruptly altered and undiagnosed disorders of mental status or neurological function (even focal). Two ampules of D50W (100 gm glucose) are sufficient to acutely raise the serum glucose levels above 100 mg/dl. Larger doses simply increase serum osmolarity. When hypoglycemic patients of unknown or questionable nutritional status are treated with glucose, 100 mg of thiamine should be given concurrently to prevent Wernicke's encephalopathy. In all cases of hypoglycemia it is prudent to closely monitor the patient and recheck the serum glucose frequently during the acute period.

Diabetic Ketoacidosis

Precipitating Factors

Diabetic ketoacidosis (DKA) is a common, serious condition, the mortality of which remains at 5–15%, despite aggressive therapy. DKA is most commonly precipitated by *infection* or *non-compliance* with diet or medications. However, *stroke*, *myocardial infarction*, *trauma*, *pregnancy*, *pancreatitis*, and *hyperthyroidism* are also frequent precipitants.

Physical Features

The most prominent physical features of DKA (hypotension, hypoperfusion and tachypnea) are the result of the two major metabolic derangements—volume depletion and metabolic acidosis. Deep and rapid "Kussmaul" respirations are an attempt to compensate for metabolic acidosis. Recognition of DKA is not difficult, but some "classic" features are seldom seen. For example, whereas obtundation is frequent, frank coma is rare. Fever is not a part of DKA in the absence of infection. Common but unexplained features of DKA include pleurisy and abdominal pain. Therefore, patients with undiagnosed acute abdominal pain should have glucose and ketone determinations before undergoing other diagnostic procedures.

Laboratory Features

Metabolic acidosis, resulting from accumulated ketones and lactic acid is the hallmark of DKA. *Ketone* measurements should be made in all patients with hyperglycemia. Three ketones are present in chemical equilibrium: acetoacetate (ACAC); acetone; and beta-hydroxybutyrate (BHB). Only ACAC is measured by the nitroprusside reaction commonly used to detect ketones. Normally, BHB exceeds ACAC by a 3:1 ratio, but in severe acidosis BHB may be present in concentrations 12-fold greater than ACAC. *As the acidosis improves*,

the dynamic equilibrium shifts in favor of ACAC, and *ketone concentrations may appear to worsen*.

Glucose levels typically range between 400 and 800 mg/dl, but they may be lower in young, well-hydrated patients whose preserved glomerular filtration facilitates glucose clearance. Leukocytosis ($> 20,000/mm^3$) with a predominance of granulocytes may occur even in the absence of infection. Loss of free water due to osmotic diuresis may lead to *hyperosmolarity* and *hemoconcentration*; therefore, even mild reductions of packed cell volume in patients with DKA suggest severe underlying anemia or active bleeding.

The osmotic effects of glucose translocate water from the intracellular to the extracellular space, producing *hyponatremia*. Sodium concentration declines approximately 1.6 mEq/l for each increase of 100 mg/dl of glucose. Because serum glucose seldom exceeds 1000 mg/dl, it is unlikely for the serum sodium to fall below 120 mEq/l on an osmotic basis alone. Artifactual depressions of sodium concentration may be seen in DKA when triglycerides contribute substantially to plasma volume.

Because acidosis shifts *potassium* from the intracellular to the extracellular compartment, most patients with DKA have normal or elevated potassium values despite sizeable total body deficits ($\simeq$ 200–700 mEq). Disturbances of other vital electrolytes (Mg^{2+}, PO_4^{3-}) occur with sufficient frequency to warrant analysis.

Serum creatinine is commonly elevated by dehydration induced decreases in glomerular filtration rate (GFR). (With colorimetric assays, ketones may cause artifactual elevations in creatinine.) For obscure reasons the serum amylase (particularly the salivary isoenzyme) may be elevated.

Treatment

The most important components in DKA therapy are adequate *fluid replacement* and *careful record keeping*. Total body deficits of fluid range between 5 and 10 liters. Adequate circulating volume should be replenished rapidly with normal saline in patients with evidence of hypoperfusion. After immediate stabilization, the aim should be to restore 50–75% of the deficit within 24 hours. Physical examination, urine output, and frequent electrolyte measurements should guide subsequent fluid and electrolyte administration.

In patients with DKA and hypotension refractory to repletion of volume and pH correction, one should consider: (1) bleeding (particularly gastrointestinal or retroperitoneal); (2) adrenal insufficiency; (3) hemorrhagic pancreatitis; (4) myocardial infarction; and (5) septic shock (particularly as a result of urinary tract infection (UTI) or pneumonia).

Low-dose regular *insulin* should be titrated by pump infusion to allow accurate delivery. Glucose measurements at 1–2 hour intervals should guide the rate of insulin and fluid administration. An initial bolus of 0.1–0.5 units/kg followed by an infusion of 0.1 units/kg/hr should suffice for most patients. Insulin infusions should be *continued until serum ketones are cleared* and the *anion gap is normalized*, even if supplemental glucose must be used to prevent hypoglycemia. Insulin infusions may be discontinued when the serum glucose reaches approximately 200 mg/dl *if ketonemia has resolved*. Premature termination of insulin infusions is the most common cause of ''relapsing DKA''. Failure of glucose to decline significantly within 2–3 hours indicates insulin resistance and should prompt increased insulin dosage and consideration of the use of recombinant human insulin.

Bicarbonate is usually needed in DKA only if the pH is below 7.1 or the patient demonstrates *refractory* hypotension or respiratory failure. (pH correction helps reduce ventilatory requirement and improve diaphragmatic function.) When insulin is provided to the patient with adequate hepatic perfusion, the liver regenerates bicarbonate from ketones and lactate. Therefore, patients receiving a bicarbonate load frequently develop ''rebound'' alkalosis. The osmolality of a 50-ml ampule of $NaHCO_3$ is nearly 5–fold greater than normal saline; therefore, aggressive bicarbonate therapy may exacerbate hyperosmolarity. In addition, rapid reversal of acidemia shifts the oxyhemoglobin curve leftward, exacerbates hypokalemia, and may cause paradoxical CNS acidosis.

Arrhythmias induced by acid-base and electrolyte disturbances (primary or iatrogenic) are a major preventable cause of morbidity in DKA. For example, insulin and bicarbonate can drive potassium across the cell membrane, dramatically decreasing the serum K^+. Therefore after adequate urine flow is re-established, *potassium* should be administered to almost all patients. Other critical electrolytes (Mg^{2+}, PO_4^{3-}) should be monitored. *Hypophosphatemia* may decrease 2,3-diphosphoglyceric acid (2, 3-DPG) levels and muscle strength, but phosphate administration has yet to be shown to improve outcome. Risks of phosphate therapy include acute hypocalcemia and precipitation of calcium-phosphate complexes, inducing acute renal failure.

Hypoglycemia (a common complication of DKA therapy) may be prevented through vigilant monitoring.

Hyperglycemic Hyperosmolar Coma

Insulin levels in hyperosmolar non-ketotic coma (HHNC) are sufficient to prevent ketone formation but insufficient to prevent hyperglycemia. Such patients generate fewer ketones than patients in DKA because they tend to have lower levels of lipolytic hormones (i.e., growth hormone and cortisol). Glycosuria, (a method of limiting increases in serum glucose) is tightly linked to GFR, therefore, HHNC is particularly common in the elderly and in those underlying renal dysfunction. Patients with impaired perception of thirst (e.g., the elderly) and/or deprived of access to free water are also predisposed.

Laboratory features of HHNC are similar to those of DKA except *ketoacidosis is absent or minimal*, whereas *glucose values are often extremely elevated* (> 1000 mg/dl). Marked hyperglycemia produces the hyperosmolarity that characterizes this disorder (See Chapter 12, Fluids and Electrolytes).

Although *intravascular volume* is usually better preserved than in DKA, it is at the expense of the intracellular compartment. This effect is responsible for the primary clinical expression of HHNC—life-threatening depression of neurological function. *Marked depletion of total body water* is present in HHNC, due largely to osmotic diuresis. Nonetheless, the osmotic effects of high glucose levels help maintain intravascular volume. Insulin administration before expansion of circulating volume with isotonic saline may produce rapid shifts of glucose and water into cells causing *sudden and profound hypotension*. As with DKA, potassium and phosphorus abnormalities are common. Correction of HHNC must be cautious, as abrupt reversal of serum hyperosmolarity may produce intracellular water intoxication manifested by dysphoria and seizures.

Despite differences in pathophysiology the treatment of HHNC is similar to that of DKA: initial restoration of circulating volume with normal saline. (In such patients normal saline represents a relatively *hypotonic* fluid.) Low-dose insulin therapy and repletion of free water should be guided by serial electrolyte and glucose determinations.

SUGGESTED READINGS

1. Fischer KF, Lees JA, Newman JH: Hypoglycemia in hospitalized patients: Causes and outcomes. *N Engl J Med* 315(20):1245–1250, 1986.

2. Gordon EE, Kabadi UM: The hyperglycemic hyperosmolar syndrome. *Am J Med Sci* 271:252–268, 1976.
3. Levy GS: The heart and hyperthyroidism: use of beta-adrenergic blocking drugs. *Med Clin N Am* 59:1193–1201, 1975.
4. Refetoff S: Thyroid hormone therapy. *Med Clin N Am* 59:1147–1162, 1975.
5. Sullivan JN: Saturday Conference: steroid withdrawal syndromes. *South Med J* 75:726–733, 1982.
6. Nicoloff JT: Thyroid storm and myxedema coma. *Med Clin N Am* 69:1005–1017, 1985.
7. Baruh S, Sherman L, Markowitz S: Diabetic ketoacidosis and coma. *Med Clin N Am* 65:117–132, 1981.

27 Drug Overdose and Poisoning

Overdose (OD) and poisoning account for $\simeq$ 15% of all intensive care unit (ICU) admissions. Despite a myriad of potential toxins, only 20 drugs account for more than 90% of all OD cases. In *adults, OD is usually a deliberate ingestion of multiple drugs.* In *children, poisoning is usually an accidental ingestion of a single agent.* Most poisonings occur in patients under age 35, which is fortunate because few have chronic underlying diseases. The in-hospital mortality of drug OD is < 1%. (Most fatalities occur from hypoventilation-induced anoxic brain damage before patients reach the hospital.)

DIAGNOSIS OF DRUG OVERDOSE

Clinical History

Although often erroneous, detailed historical information is important to secure. Many patients overestimate the dose ingested; others have taken a drug they do not report. Suicidal patients may attempt to conceal the nature of the ingested poisons, and patients ingesting illicit drugs often lack accurate knowledge of these substances or fail to provide information, fearing prosecution. In the drug history it is important to seek the following information: (1) type of drug or toxin; (2) quantity consumed; (3) time since ingestion; (4) initial symptoms, including a history of vomiting or diarrhea; and (5) underlying diseases or other drugs taken.

Physical Examination

The first steps in treating a patient with poisoning are to *assess the vital signs, secure the airway, and assure adequate perfusion.* The airway of the overdosed patient may be obstructed, particularly if narcotics or sedative drugs have been ingested. Intubation and artificial ventilation are required when the central drive to breathe is severely depressed. Hypoventilation is a clue to narcotic or sedative OD. A patient sedate enough to allow unresisted endotracheal intubation almost certainly requires the airway protection and ventilatory support intubation provides.

Blood pressure and perfusion should be rapidly assessed and corrected if inadequate. Anticholinergic or tricyclic poisoning should be suspected in patients with marked *tachycardia.* Sinus *bradycardia* or conduction system block may result from overdoses of digitalis, cyanide, beta blockers, calcium channel blockers, or cholinergic drugs.

Core temperature may give valuable clues as well. Hyperthermia suggests anticholinergic poisoning, whereas hypothermia frequently accompanies alcohol or sedative-hypnotic overdose (see p. 233).

In the assessment of the poisoned patient, *it is important not to overlook concurrent trauma or serious medical illness.* For example, up to 40% of all motor vehicle accident patients with head injury are also intoxicated with alcohol or other substances.

The *head should receive particularly close attention,* both to exclude other causes of coma (e.g., head trauma, subarachnoid hemorrhage) and to provide data relevant to OD. Inspection of the *oral cavity* may yield unswallowed tablets or evidence of caustic injury. *Breath odor* may suggest a particular toxin. Ketones give a sweet odor, whereas cyanide presents an almond scent. The characteristic smell of hydrocarbons is easily distinguished, as is the "garlic" odor of organophosphate ingestion.

Narcotics commonly produce *miosis* whereas drugs with anticholinergic properties cause *mydriasis. Nystagmus* is often seen with phencyclidine (PCP) or phenytoin ingestion. Apparently fixed and dilated pupils can result from profound sedative overdose but are characteristic of glutethamide or mushroom poisoning. Pupils that are dilated but reactive suggest anticholinergic or sympathomimetic poisoning. Because *any* response to light (even if barely detectable) has prognostic implication, the pupillary response should be tested with a bright light in a darkened room. An ophthalmoscope focused on the plane of the iris serves the twin function of magnification and illumination.

Laboratory Testing

The *electrocardiogram (ECG)* can provide valuable clues in drug OD and should be reviewed at the earliest appropriate time. Ectopy is common in sympathomimetic and tricyclic poisoning. High-grade atrioventricular (AV) block may be due to digoxin, beta blockers, calcium channel blockers, cyanide, phenytoin, or cholinergic substances. A wide QRS complex or prolonged QT interval suggests quinidine, procainamide, or tricyclic antidepressant OD.

Arterial blood gases are always required to assess acid-base status and gas exchange and may yield a specific clue to salicylate intoxication if they reveal a *mixed respiratory alkalosis and metabolic acidosis*. Severe metabolic acidosis with hyperventilation is common with cyanide or carbon monoxide poisoning.

Six relatively common poisonings elevate the *anion gap*: (1) salicylates; (2) methanol; (3) ethanol; (4) ethylene glycol; (5) paraldehyde; and (6) carbon monoxide. In the presence of a coexisting osmolar gap (the difference between calculated and measured serum osmolarity), ethanol and ethylene glycol become the most likely candidates. Ketoacidosis suggests ethanol, paraldehyde, or diabetes as potential culprits. If ketones are present without systemic acidosis, isopropyl alcohol is the likely etiology.

In addition to routine arterial blood gases, measurement of *hemoglobin saturation and oxygen content* may be helpful. Both methemoglobin and carboxyhemoglobin lead to a disparity between the *measured* oxygen content or hemoglobin saturation and that *predicted* from the arterial oxygen tension (PaO_2). Carboxyhemoglobin is elevated in carbon monoxide poisoning, and a number of ingested drugs can oxidize hemoglobin to methemoglobin. Profound methemoglobinemia may be recognized at the bedside by the chocolate brown color it gives to blood.

Hypocalcemia is produced by the ingestion of ethylene glycol, oxalate, fluoride compounds, and by certain metals: manganese, phosphorus, and barium.

Chest and abdominal radiographs may help to identify radiopaque tablets of iron, phenothiazines, tricyclic agents, or chloral hydrate. When these drugs are involved, the abdominal radiograph may help to assure that the gut has been emptied following emesis or gastric lavage. With hydrocarbon poisoning upright abdominal radiography may show a 3-layered *fluid/fluid/air* level in the stomach (see Fig. 27.1).

Use of the Drug Screen

Most qualitative drug screens assay blood or urine using thin layer chromatography. Urine and gastric juice are the most reliable samples for toxin assay because many drugs may be detected as unabsorbed drug or excreted metabolites despite rapid clearance from the serum. Unfortunately, the drug screen has limited usefulness because significant delays invariably occur before the results are available, and the results seldom change empirical therapy. If a particular toxin is suspected, *specific* assay techniques may provide more rapid and quantitative results. *A negative drug screen alone does not exclude OD because of problems with sensitivity and timing of the test* in relation to ingestion. Whenever there is doubt regarding drug screen results, clinical judgment should prevail. Specific therapy is available for certain toxins (listed in Table 27.1) for which *quantitative* levels should be obtained to guide management.

TREATMENT OF DRUG OVERDOSE

Physiologic support is key to all OD management. Three basic precepts help minimize the toxic effects of drug ingestion: (1) *prevent toxin absorption*; (2) *enhance drug excretion*; and (3) *prevent formation of toxic metabolities*. Depending on the drug ingested, appropriate therapy may also include antidote administration or active removal.

Prevention of Toxin Absorption

After cardiopulmonary stabilization, the first step in the treatment of poisoning is to *stop absorption*. This may be accomplished by emptying the stomach using lavage or emesis, or by using absorbants (charcoal). If the patient is alert, retains an intact gag reflex, and is not subject to seizure, emesis may be induced by syrup of *ipecac*. Given orally, a 30-ml dose is promptly effective (< 20 min) in almost all patients. Emesis is not appropriate in

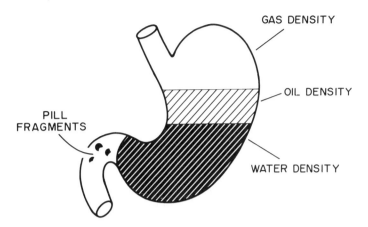

Figure 27.1 Composite diagram of radiographic features seen on an upright film of the stomach region after ingestion of radiopaque tablets and/or selected liquid hydrocarbons.

Table 27.1
Drugs for Which Quantitative Assay is Helpful

1. Acetaminophen	5. Ethanol
2. Theophylline	6. Ethylene Glycol
3. Digoxin	7. Methanol
4. Salicylates	8. Carbon Monoxide

ingestion of corrosive chemicals or petroleum distillates. Although equally effective as an emetic, *apomorphine* frequently produces significant respiratory depression and should probably not be used.

If emesis is contraindicated, a catheter can be used to empty the stomach. In patients with altered consciousness, the airway should be protected with a cuffed endotracheal tube before attempting *gastric evacuation and lavage.* Lavage should be performed in the left lateral decubitus position *using a large orogastric (Ewald) tube.* (Smaller nasogastric tubes fail to adequately remove pill fragments.) Vomitus or aspirated gastric contents should be sent for toxicological analysis. Gastric lavage is probably more effective than emesis at eliminating unabsorbed drug, removing most toxins in the stomach if performed within 4 hours of ingestion. Some poisons may be recovered even after 12 hours, particularly if they form concretions or impair gastric emptying (e.g., anticholinergic or tricyclic drugs, salicylates, meprobamate).

In most ingestions *activated charcoal* (AC) should be given following emesis or lavage. AC effectively absorbs orally ingested drugs and is safer than lavage or emesis. (Even when aspirated, charcoal does not produce pneumonitis.) One gram of charcoal has enormous absorptive area (> 1000 m^2) and completes toxin absorption within minutes of administration. Although AC tends to constipate, carthartics may deplete fluids and electrolytes and are not routinely needed unless large volumes or multiple doses of AC are given. If necessary, sorbitol is the preferred cathartic because it works faster than magnesium citrate and avoids the magnesium toxicity that could result if renal function is impaired. The only *relative* contraindication to the use of charcoal is in acetaminophen OD, in which AC *may* interfere with the absorption of acetylcysteine.

For cutaneously absorbed toxins (e.g., organophosphates), washing the skin and removing contaminated clothing is particularly important.

Enhancement of Drug Removal

Four therapeutic techniques enhance removal of circulating toxins: (1) "gut dialysis"; (2) ion trapping; (3) hemodialysis; and (4) hemoperfusion. Drugs undergoing enterohepatic circulation such as theophylline, digoxin, phenobarbital, phenylbutazone, and carbamazepine may be eliminated by "*gut dialysis,*" a process using repeated doses of oral charcoal to bind drug excreted into the bile.

Charged molecules do not cross lipid membranes easily; therefore, ionized drugs are not readily absorbed from the stomach and fail to cross the blood-brain barrier (BBB). Furthermore, once inside the renal tubule such molecules have a limited tendency to back-diffuse into the circulation. Altering the pH of body fluids to "*ion-trap*" drugs in the desired compartment (serum, gut, urine, etc.) is effective for only a small number of compounds. Alkalinization of the serum and urine impedes transfer of *weak acids* (salicylates, tricyclics, phenobarbital, and isoniazid) across the BBB and promotes their excretion. Conversely, acidification by ammonium chloride accelerates excretion of such *weak bases* as amphetamine, strychnine, PCP, and quinidine. Urinary acidification is questionably effective and potentially dangerous in patients with renal or hepatic dysfunction.

Dialysis may eliminate small, nonpolar compounds such as methanol and ethylene glycol. Salicylates and lithium are also effectively dialyzed.

Charcoal hemoperfusion removes theophylline and other lipid-soluble drugs from the blood but may initiate complement activation or coagulopathy.

Inhibition of Toxic Metabolite Formation

Some drugs (notably acetaminophen, methanol, and ethylene glycol) are relatively inert when ingested but form highly toxic compounds during metabolism. Inhibition of toxin formation will be discussed under specific therapy for these poisons.

SPECIFIC POISONS

Acetaminophen

Acetaminophen is very safe when taken in usual doses, but ingestion of as little as 6 gm may be fatal. (The usual fatal dose exceeds 140 mg/kg.) Acetaminophen is rapidly absorbed, especially when taken in the liquid form. The usual serum half-life approximates 2½ hours but lengthens with declining liver function. Normally the drug is hepatically metabolized to non-toxic compounds by linkage with sulphates and glucaronide. The hepatic cytochrome P-450 system converts < 5% of an ingested dose to reactive metabolites which are then detoxified by conjugation with glutathione. However, during massive OD, toxic metabolites overwhelm the supply of glutathione and accumulate to cause liver damage. Conditions that induce the hepatic cytochrome P-450 system such as chronic alcoholism and use of oral contraceptives or phenobarbital, predispose to acetaminophen toxicity.

With the exception of nausea and vomiting, adverse symptoms are minimal for the first 24 hours after ingestion. One to 2 days after ingestion deteriorating liver function tests, right upper quadrant pain, and oliguria (due to the antidiuretic hormone (ADH)-like effects of acetaminophen) become evident. Hepatic necrosis and hepatic failure evolve 3 to 5 days after massive ingestion.

As for all other drug ingestions, initial treatment should include evacuation of the stomach. A specific antedote, N-acetylcysteine (NAC, Mucomyst) is the drug of choice. Charcoal administration is controversial because charcoal *may* bind NAC, decreasing its effectiveness. Not all patients require therapy with NAC; the likelihood of hepatic toxicity may be predicted from the serum level using standard nomograms (Ref. 5). NAC probably acts by binding the toxic metabolities of acetaminophen. To be effective, NAC should be given as early as possible—certainly within 16 hours of ingestion. An oral loading dose of 140 mg/kg is followed by 17 additional doses of 70 mg/kg at 4-hour intervals.

Salicylates

Most salicylate OD occurring in adults results from therapeutic misadventure, not intentional ingestion. In high doses, salicylates inhibit cellular enzymes and uncouple oxidative phosphorylation.

The clinical presentation of salicylate OD includes: altered mental status, acidosis, hypoxemia, and (more rarely) hyperosmolarity and hyperthermia.

Initially, direct CNS stimulation causes a respiratory alkalosis and compensatory renal wasting of bicarbonate. Later, superimposed metabolic acidosis may produce a complex acid-base disturbance. Tachypnea may be absent if the patient has ingested a sedative or hypnotic concurrently. Large doses of aspirin may induce pulmonary edema, causing the adult respiratory distress syndrome (ARDS).

Salicylate intoxication should always be considered in the differential of an *anion gap acidosis*. The anion gap elevation results primarily from lactate and pyruvate generated during anaerobic glycolysis. (Ketones are also formed in response to decreased glucose and accelerated lipolysis.) However, very high serum levels of salicylate (> 80 mg/dl) may directly contribute to the anion gap. Furthermore, large insensible fluid losses deplete intravascular volume, thereby stimulating aldosterone secretion that depletes bicarbonate and potassium. Salicylate levels > 50 mg/dl commonly induce nausea and vomiting and may produce a metabolic alkalosis, leading to a triple acid base disorder.

Salicylates inhibit the formation of prothrombin, impair platelet function, and irritate the gastric mucosa—all contributing to the risk of *hemorrhage*. Patients with salicylate-induced coagulopathy or bleeding should receive vitamin K and, if immediate reversal is necessary, fresh frozen plasma and platelets.

If therapy is to prevent morbidity, salicylate intoxication must be suspected on clinical grounds. Although serum levels correlate poorly with toxicity, most patients do not experience toxic effects at levels below 30 mg/dl. If salicylate levels are not immediately available, "Phenistix" test strips can demonstrate a purple color when serum levels exceed 70 mg/dl. Although purely qualitative, the ferric chloride urine test is helpful if negative.

Gastric lavage followed by charcoal and cathartics increases stool excretion. Salicylates are normally absorbed rapidly, but in massive overdoses serum levels may continue to rise for up to 24 hours after ingestion due to delayed gastric absorption. As weak acids, salicylates remain nonionized at low serum pH and readily cross cell membranes; therefore, "ion trapping" may be used to lower toxicity and promote excretion. Apart from decreasing urinary excretion, an acidic pH favors movement of salicylates into cells and across the blood brain barrier. Therefore, serum and urine pH should be monitored and kept alkaline with bicarbonate titration or dialysis.

Alcohols

Many suicide attempts involve ethanol (ETOH), either alone or in combination with other drugs. Physiologic effects do not relate closely to serum concentrations, but blood levels > 150 mg/dl are inebriating. Death often supervenes when concentrations exceed 600 mg/dl. The therapy of acute alcohol intoxication is largely supportive. Ethanol may be removed by hemodialysis but is rarely necessary. One in 5 patients will transiently awaken in response to large doses of naloxone. There is no role for direct CNS stimulants in ETOH intoxication.

ETOH Withdrawal Syndrome

The ICU deprives the habituated patient of ETOH access. Deprivation may precipitate withdrawal (WD), a condition fully as dangerous as intoxication. Symptoms of WD usually start within 36 hours of the last drink (but may be delayed 5–7 days). Measurable serum levels of ETOH do not exclude the diagnosis of WD. Patients experiencing severe WD (hallucinosis, delerium tremens, DTs) are unpredictable, both in behavior and disease course. Therefore, most patients with DTs should be managed in an ICU to avert such fatal complications as seizures, aspiration, arrhythmias, and suicide attempts. Symptoms of WD (specifi-

cally, DTs) often mimic infection or primary neurological processes. It is important to emphasize, however, that *50% of febrile DT patients also have a concomitant infection, most frequently pneumonia or meningitis.*

The agitated WD patient should be *restrained in a lateral or prone position*, (not supine because of the risk of aspiration). Patients should be given nothing by mouth (NPO), with all fluids, electrolytes, and vitamins (B_{12}, thiamine, folate) administered intravenously. WD may be prevented or aborted in its early stages through the use of oral chlordiazepoxide, but if WD is fully manifest, intravenous diazepam becomes the sedative of choice. In this situation (intravenous diazepam (5 mg every 5 minutes) should be given until the patient is *calm but not obtunded*. After initial control with diazepam is achieved, chlordiazepoxide maintenance therapy should be instituted. Diazepam reduces hyperactivity and the risk of seizures. Recently, lorazepam has become popular because it has no active metabolites (a particularly useful property in patients with liver disease). Phenothiazines should not be used because they lower the seizure threshold.

Methanol and Ethylene Glycol Toxicity

The toxicity of methanol and ethylene glycol (M/EG) results from the formation of organic acids from parent compounds. Toxic metabolites of EG include: oxalic, glycolic, and glyoxylic acids. Formic acid and formaldehyde are responsible for methanol toxicity.

In their early phase, the clinical picture of M/EG ingestion resembles ETOH-related intoxication. However, as symptoms progress, almost any global CNS finding may be seen—coma, hyporeflexia, nystagmus, or seizures. Whereas the presentations of EG and M are often indistinguishable, cardiovascular symptomatology (tachycardia, hypertension, pulmonary edema, and renal failure resulting from oxalate crystalluria) more frequently complement EG. On the other hand, optic neuritis and blindness are hallmarks of M poisoning.

M/EG ingestion should be suspected in any patient with acidosis and coexistent anion and osmolar gaps. However, lethal levels of EG > 20 mg/dl may be present with minimal elevations in the osmolar gap.

The treatment of M/EG poisoning is 4-fold: (1) Remove any drug remaining in the stomach. (2) Prevent the formation of toxic metabolites. (3) Remove the parent drug from the circulation. (4) Treat metabolic acidosis. Emergency dialysis should be performed in all patients with toxic serum levels. Formation of toxins is attenuated by using ethanol to compete with EG or M for metabolism by alcohol dehydrogenase. To effectively inhibit toxic metabolite formation, an ethanol level > 100 mg/dl should be sustained by giving a loading dose of 600 mg/kg (about 4 ounces of whiskey) followed by a maintenance regimen (about 100 ml of 10% ethanol intravenously per hour, or 25 ml of 40% alcohol orally at the same rate). Ethanol doses must be increased during dialysis. Calcium replacement may be required in EG poisoning (see p. 123).

Sedative Hypnotic Drugs

Six major drugs comprise this group: barbiturates, benzodiazepines, meprobamate, methaqualone, chloral hydrate, and glutethimide. Although barbiturates historically were popular drugs with which to OD, now perhaps benzodiazepines are seen with a higher frequency. All sedative drugs depress consciousness and in large doses act as negative inotropes—occasionally causing cardiovascular collapse. The benzodiazepines however, have a wide therapeutic range, and when taken alone, doses of 50–100 times the usual therapeutic dose may be tolerated. In very large doses, benzodiazepines may produce neuromuscular blockade. Although clinical testing of a benzodiazepine antagonist is underway, there is currently no specific antidote available. Supportive therapy remains the cornerstone of management.

Barbiturates are hepatically metabolized before excretion. Delayed gastric emptying makes evacuation of the stomach a key therapeutic maneuver. However, the airway must be protected prior to lavage. The treatment of barbiturate OD is supportive. Forced alkaline diuresis has little effect on total drug excretion and is potentially dangerous. After all drug has been cleared, patients chronically habituated to barbiturates (and selected other sedatives) may enter a withdrawal phase. Tremor and convulsions may require temporary reinstitution of phenobarbital in theraputic doses, with gradual tapering. The anticholinergic effects of glutethimide may warrant gastric lavage long after ingestion of the drug. Installation of activated charcoal may bind unabsorbed drug or drug metabolites undergoing enterohepatic circulation.

Organophosphates

Organophosphates (OPs) and carbamates (related insecticides) inhibit the action of acetylcholinesterase, thereby causing accumulation of acetylcholine at neuromuscular junctions. Early specific treatment is important because binding of the toxin to acetylcholinesterase may become irreversible after 24 hours. OP initially stimulates but later blocks acetylcholine receptors. OPs penetrate the CNS, but carbamates do not. Toxic manifestations usually appear within 5 minutes but may be delayed for 24 hours after exposure. (Toxicity evolves rapidly after inhalation but more slowly during cutaneous absorption.)

The clinical presentation may be remembered by the mnemonic "STUMBLED": Salivation, Tremor, Urination, Miosis, Bradycardia, Lacrimation, Emesis, Diarrhea—all expressions of cholinergic excess. In some patients, nicotinic effects (fasciculation, skeletal cramping, hypertension, and tachycardia) predominate.

A *garlic odor* on the patient's breath suggests the diagnosis. Laboratory confirmation requires measurement of plasma pseudocholinesterase or erythrocyte cholinesterase. Acute reductions of enzyme activity by more than 90% correlate with severe toxicity. (With chronic exposures, enzyme levels may be dramatically reduced with few symptoms.) Alternatively, the diagnosis can be established by direct analysis of OP in serum, gastric, or urinary samples. Laboratory findings may also include hemolytic anemia (seen with carbamates) and an anion gap metabolic acidosis. Bradycardia and heart block frequently result from cholinergic stimulation.

Skin decontamination is an essential component of initial treatment. High doses of anticholinergics may block muscarinic CNS effects but do not reverse nicotinic manifestations. (Atropine, 2–4 mg, is usually given intravenously until muscarinic symptoms are reversed.) Therapy should continue for at least 24 hours following exposure. Pralidoxime (2-PAM) reverses the nicotinic (muscular) effects of OPs by uncoupling bound OP from the esterases. However, treatment retains efficacy for only ≃ 24 hours. Therefore, it should be given as soon as possible in a dose of 1 gm, repeated once if necessary. 2-PAM is ineffective in carbamate poisoning.

Theophylline Toxicity

Impaired theophylline clearance occurs commonly in patients with obstructive lung disease and heart and liver failure. The potential for impaired clearance due to drug interaction is frequently overlooked, particularly in patients who have had erythromycin or cimetidine added to chronic theophylline therapy. Smoking modestly improves the clearance of theophylline in patients without liver disease.

Toxic symptoms (tremors, arrhythmias, gastrointestinal upset) may occur at serum levels well within the therapeutic range (10–20 mcg/ml), particularly in patients predisposed by advanced age or underlying CNS or cardiac disease (Table 27.2).

A minority of hospitalized patients experience gastrointestinal (GI) warning symptoms before having refractory seizures—the most life-threatening toxic manifestation. (The *mortality* of theophylline-induced seizures exceeds 40% and a large percentage of survivors have persistent neurological deficits.) Leukocytosis may result from catecholamine-induced demargination of leukocytes. Cardiac arrhythmias of all varieties occur but serious arrhythmias do not generally emerge at therapeutic concentrations. Hyperglycemia can be effectively treated with beta blockers.

The treatment of theophylline intoxication initially includes correction of hypoxemia, acidosis, and electrolyte abnormalities. Oral charcoal should be administered following gastric lavage if ingestion is recent. When given in doses of 30–50 gm every 2–4 hours (up to a total dose of 120 gm), charcoal may double theophylline clearance. Lidocaine is the drug of choice for theophylline-induced ventricular arrhythmias, whereas phenobarbital is the preferred anticonvulsant. Charcoal hemoperfusion is probably indicated for theophylline levels > 60 mg/l and for refractory arrhythmias or seizures.

Tricyclic Antidepressants

It is not surprising that tricyclic antidepressants (TCA) are the single most common cause of drug overdose since they are widely used in depressed patients, have a long half-life, and accumulate in tissue. Despite the frequency of TCA OD, mortality remains below 1%. Signs and symptoms of TCA overdose are predominately anticholinergic. The phrase *"hot as a hare, blind as a bat, dry as a bone, red as a beet, mad as a hatter"* accurately describes these patients who often demonstrate hyperthermia, fixed and dilated pupils, dry red skin, and CNS hyperactivity (hallucinations and psychosis). The differential diagnosis of TCA OD includes other compounds having anticholinergic effects (e.g., atropine, phenothiazines, scolopamine, anti-Parkinson drugs, Jimson weed, and mushroom poisoning).

Due to their tendency to produce ileus, TCAs may remain in the gut long after ingestion; therefore, *gastric evacuation is a key therapeutic maneuver*. Oral charcoal binds TCAs during their enterohepatic circulation. Because TCAs are highly tissue bound, toxicity correlates poorly with ingested dose or serum level. The ECG warns of cardiac (and CNS) toxicity when the QRS complex widens to more than 0.12 seconds.

Both supraventricular and ventricular arrhythmias complicate TCA OD. Sinus tachycardia, conduction disturbances, and ventricular arrhythmias may persist long after serum levels normalize, because of avid tissue binding. Return of the ECG to normal is the best indication that the risk of significant arrhythmias has passed. Arrhythmias frequently respond to systemic alkalinization (pH > 7.50), which reduces the serum concentration of unbound drug. Lidocaine and phenytoin are the most helpful antiarrhythmics, but arrhythmias may be refractory to all standard therapy. Type Ia drugs (quinidine and procainamide) should be avoided because of their tendency to further impede conduction. TCA-related hypotension is usually due to volume depletion. If fluid administration fails to restore blood pressure, alpha agonists (e.g., norepinephrine) are the most effective vasopressors. Mixed-adrenergic agonists (e.g., dopamine, epinephrine) may paradoxically worsen the hypotension by increasing beta stimulation.

Interestingly, the tendency for seizures may be predicted by a QRS complex width exceeding 0.12 seconds. Diazepam or phenytoin are effective anticonvulsants in most cases, but physostigmine, a rapidly acting anticholinesterase inhibitor that penetrates the blood-brain barrier, may be necessary for refractory cases. Although physostigmine is occasionally helpful in *refractory* seizures or ventricular arrhythmias, its use is controversial. There is no evidence that physostigmine decreases mortality, and its own impressive spectrum of toxicity includes AV block, asystole, seizures, bronchospasm, and hypotension. Its short half-life necessitates hourly administration. Neither hemodialysis nor hemoperfusion are effective at TCA removal.

Table 27.2
Side Effects from Toxic Levels of Theophylline

Theophylline Level	Side Effects
> 20 mg/l	Nausea, vomiting, confusion
20–40 mg/l	Cardiac arrhythmias
> 40 mg/l	Refractory seizures

SUGGESTED READINGS

1. Jay JS, Johanson WG, Pierce AK: Respiratory complications of overdose with sedative drugs. *Am Rev Respir Dis* 112:591–598, 1975.
2. Marshall JB, Forker AD: Cardiovascular effects of tricyclic antidepressant drugs: therapeutic usage, overdose and management of complications. *Am Heart J* 103:401–414, 1982.
3. Milne MD, Scribner BH, Crawford MA: Non-ionic diffusion and the excretion of weak acids and bases. *Am J Med* 24:709–729, 1958.
4. Namba T, Nolte CT, Jackrel J, et al: Poisoning due to organophosphate insecticides. *Am J Med* 50:475–492, 1971.
5. Rumack BK, Peterson RC, Koch GG, et al: Acetominophen overdose: 662 cases with evaluation of oral acetylcysteine treatment. *Arch Intern Med* 141:380–385, 1981.
6. Steinhart CM, Pearson-Shaver AL: Poisoning. *Crit Care Clin* 4(4):845–872, 1988.

28

Coma, Seizures, and Brain Death

COMA

Definitions

Coma is unconsciousness from which the patient cannot be awakened. Although reflex movements (spinal reflexes and decorticate or decerebrate posturing) may occur, there is no speech or purposeful eye or limb movements. Less profound stages of suppressed consciousness are termed obtundation, stupor and lethargy. Such imprecise terms as "semicoma" or "light coma" may confuse subsequent examiners and should be abandoned in favor of a less ambiguous description of the highest level of neurological function.

Etiology

Unconsciousness results from *reticular activating system* dysfunction or from *diffuse bilateral hemispheric* dysfunction. Continuous stimulation by the brainstem's reticular activating system, (RAS), is required for the appearance of wakefulness. Conversely, *awareness*, a cognitive function, requires coordinated function of the cerebral cortex. From its origin in the mid-pons, the RAS radiates diffusely outward to the cerebral cortex. It is this wide distribution that prevents coma, unless a diffuse process impairs *both* cerebral cortices or the RAS is interrupted near its mid-pontine origin.

Coma may arise from a wide variety of diffuse or focal conditions affecting the central nervous system (CNS). The neurological impact of any potential cause of coma is modified by the patient's age and underlying cerebral and cardiovascular status. Only four basic pathophysiologic mechanisms incite coma: (1) *metabolic or drug encephalopathy*; (2) *generalized seizures*; (3) compression of the pons or cerebral cortices by *structural lesions or increased intracranial pressure (ICP)*; and (4) *inadequate cerebral perfusion*.

Metabolic Disorders

Outside the neurosurgical setting (e.g., head trauma, brain tumors), metabolic encephalopathy (ME) is the most common cause of coma. Because ME affects the cortex and brainstem diffusely, *abrupt* premonitory *focal defects* and *progressive rostro-caudal dysfunction* seen with supratentorial mass lesions do not usually occur. Rather, patients exhibit slowly evolving symmetric deficits, often preceded by progressive somnolence or confusion.

A variety of common disorders (including hypotension, dehydration, sepsis, hepatic encephalopathy, and uremia) contribute to impaired consciousness, but no absolute guidelines can be given as to the magnitude of an isolated abnormality that is necessary to cause coma, especially since multiple derangements often coexist. Furthermore, the age of the patient and the rapidity with which such disorders develop help determine their impact. It is difficult to state with certainty threshold values for critical metabolites. Yet, as a general rule it is uncommon for a glucose > 50 or < 500 mg/dl, a $Na^+ > 120$ or < 150 mEq/l, a $Ca^{2+} < 12$ mg/dl, or a $Mg^{2+} < 10$ mg/dl to produce coma without other cause. Only rarely do disorders of other electrolytes cause unconsciousness. Blood alcohol levels usually must exceed 300 mg/dl to cause frank coma. Uremia rarely causes coma until the BUN exceeds 100 mg/dl.

Cerebral perfusion pressure (mean arterial pressure (MAP) minus intracranial pressure (ICP)) must exceed 50 mmHg to perfuse the brain adequately (see p. 251). Otherwise healthy patients may maintain consciousness despite severe reductions in MAP. On the other hand, patients with cerebrovascular disease or elevated ICP may be underperfused at much higher pressures. Unconsciousness is rare when the oxygen saturation of hemoglobin is maintained at $\geq 90\%$ in otherwise healthy patients. For unclear reasons, a variety of systemic illnesses (especially sepsis) may impair consciousness, particularly in the elderly.

Seizures

Generalized seizures may induce coma during the ictal phase or as a post-ictal phenomenon. Distinguishing a seizure from other metabolic or structural causes of coma is seldom difficult. Consciousness usually returns rapidly after the termination of a brief seizure in otherwise healthy patients. Conversely, patients with underlying cerebral infarctions, metabolic encephalopathy, or prolonged seizures (status epilepticus) may undergo a prolonged post-ictal period. Therefore, delayed return of consciousness following a seizure suggests a precipitating structural lesion (e.g., tumors, stroke, subarachnoid hemorrhage, subdural hematoma), or an underlying metabolic disorder (e.g., hypoglycemia, toxin ingestion, or electrolyte disturbance). As with metabolic encephalopathy, seizures that cause loss of unconsciousness tend to produce *symmetric* neurological defects unless there is an underlying structural abnormality.

Structural Lesions

Although *supratentorial* mass lesions are generally confined to one hemisphere, they can cause coma by increasing ICP or by impairing RAS function through direct pressure on the brainstem. Unless located exactly in the midline, supratentorial mass lesions usually produce *hemispheric (unilateral) findings that precede loss of consciousness*. Because cerebral function is progressively affected in a rostro-caudal manner, there is a relatively *predictable progression* of signs. Supratentorial mass lesions, if unchecked, often cause uncal herniation across the cerebellar tentorium, manifested by a fixed dilated pupil, third cranial nerve palsy, and hemiplegia. In contrast, when *infratentorial* (brainstem) lesions cause coma, rapid or immediate loss of consciousness may be the initial manifestation. Such lesions (e.g., brainstem strokes, cerebellar hemorrhage) are often not associated with rostro-caudal progression and may be rapidly fatal.

Initial Approach to the Comatose Patient

History

Because pathophysiology and treatment differ radically, the metabolic versus structural origin of coma must be distinguished at the earliest possible time. The *history* may be helpful in making this separation if it reveals *trauma* or documents *drug or toxin ingestion*. History of an evolving *focal deficit* preceding loss of consciousness suggests a structural lesion, whereas a gradual progression to coma favors a metabolic cause. The circumstances under which coma evolved may suggest trauma, hyperthermia, hypothermia, or toxin exposure (e.g., organophosphates, carbon monoxide). *Medications or poisons* found near the comatose patient may be helpful. For example, medication containers may bear the name of the patient's physician, allowing further history to be obtained. In patients with known alcoholism, *intoxication with alcohol, ethylene glycol, methanol, or isopropyl alcohol* should be suspected. In patients with diabetes, *hypoglycemia* and diabetic *ketoacidosis* are common. Underlying medical problems such as hypothyroidism, renal failure, cirrhosis, or psychiatric illness suggest a metabolic etiology, whereas a clear history of falling, previous stroke, brain tumor, or chronic atrial fibrillation suggests a structural problem. Patients with *malignant tumors* are subject to both structural (metastasis) and metabolic (hyponatremia, hypercalcemia) coma. Similarly, uncontrolled hypertension can induce metabolic (e.g., hypertensive encephalopathy) or structural (e.g., intracerebral hemorrhage) coma.

Physical Examination

The physical examination is most helpful in differentiating structural from metabolic causes of coma when it reveals focal (lateralizing) signs. In such patients a metabolic etiology is uncommon. (The most frequent exceptions to this rule occur in *hepatic failure* and *hypoglycemia*.) Comatose patients should always be fully disrobed and examined for evidence of occult trauma. Physical evidence of head trauma suggests a structural cause. However, many trauma patients also suffer from intoxication.

Boggy areas of the skull suggest depressed skull fracture, while *Battle's sign*, "*raccoon eyes*", and *bloody nasal or aural discharge* suggest basilar skull fracture. Diffuse mucosal bleeding may implicate coagulopathy as the cause of intracranial bleeding. Incontinence of stool or urine or tongue lacerations strongly suggest a recent seizure. Atrial fibrillation, a large heart, and recent myocardial infarction are associated with cerebral embolic disease. Cardiac murmurs should raise suspicion of endocarditis-induced septic embolism or brain abscess. Arrhythmias only result in coma when they cause hypotension or cerebral emboli. Carotid bruits are of little significance. Nuccal rigidity suggests meningitis or subarachnoid hemorrhage. In traumatized patients it is critical to exclude cervical spine instability before the neck is manipulated.

Vital signs may provide valuable clues to diagnosis. Although hypertension may accompany any cause of increased ICP, severe hypertension suggests intracerebral or subarachnoid hemorrhage, particularly if accompanied by nuccal rigidity and focal neurological signs. Although hypertensive encephalopathy may produce coma, it is usually seen with systolic blood pressures > 240 mmHg or diastolic blood pressures > 130 mmHg. Although patients without underlying vascular or cerebral disease may remain awake with very low mean arterial pressures, the elderly, patients with chronic hypertension, and those with concurrent metabolic encephalopathy or structural lesions tolerate hypotension less well.

Aberrations of body temperature rarely cause coma until core temperatures exceed 105°F or fall below 80°F (see Thermal Disorders, Chapter 22). Heat stroke, neuroleptic malignant syndrome, malignant hyperthermia, and a variety of infections may cause fever sufficient to impair consciousness. Patients with both hyperthermia and hypothermia frequently have accompanying infection that may disturb consciousness (e.g., pneumonia, brain abscess, or meningitis).

In the setting of coma, *bradypnea/hypoventilation* commonly results from hypothyroidism, the sedative effects of drugs, alcohol, endogenous toxins, or far advanced brainstem compression. *Tachypnea* is a nonspecific finding but usually arises from one of three basic causes: (1) inappropriate ventilatory control; (2) hypoxemia or compensation for metabolic acidosis; and (3) reduced lung or chest wall compliance. Contrary to popular teaching, specific "pathognomonic" respiratory patterns have little localizing or prognostic value, with one notable exception—discoordinated, irregular (ataxic) respirations usually indicate severe medullary impairment and impending respiratory collapse.

Detailed Neurological Examination

After the vital signs are obtained and ventilation and perfusion are stabilized, neurological function should be examined in a stepwise fashion. The five key features of the neurological examination may be remembered by the mnemonic "SPERM": (1) State of consciousness; (2) Pupillary response; (3) Eye movements; (4) Respiratory rate and pattern; and (5) Motor function.

State of Consciousness

Only four terms should be used to describe the level of consciousness: (1) alert; (2) lethargic (aroused with simple commands); (3) stuporous (aroused only with vigorous stimulation—usually pain); and (4) comatose (unarousable).

Pupillary Response

Size, congruency, and response to light and accommodation should be described. Pupillary responses remain intact in *metabolic* causes of coma. (Exceptions to this rule include atropine and glutethimide intoxication in which "fixed and dilated" pupils may occur.) Pupillary function is controlled by the midbrain. Therefore, if the pupils function normally, the cause of coma either is a structural one located *above* the midbrain *or* is *metabolic*. Small "pinpoint" pupils usually result from pontine hemorrhage or from ingestion of narcotics or organophosphates. (Meperidine often fails to produce the miotic pupils typical of other narcotics.)

Eye Movements

The resting position of the gaze, the presence of nystagmus (horizontal/vertical/rotatory), and the response to head movements (oculocephalic) or to cold tympanic membrane stimulation ("caloric") testing should be recorded. Stability of the cervical spine *must* be assured before oculocephalic maneuvers are performed. Likewise, tympanic membrane integrity should be confirmed before caloric testing, to prevent introduction of water into the cerebrospinal fluid through a basilar skull fracture. Although pupillary function is usually retained in metabolic coma, coordinated eye movements can be disrupted by accumulations of endogenous (hepatic or renal) toxins. However, *exogenous toxins almost always spare eye movements*. In pontine disorders, the medial longitudinal fasciculus often becomes nonfunctional, but 6th cranial nerve function is preserved. Therefore, *ipsilateral ab*duction is intact, but *contralateral ad*duction is impaired. Quite simply, if rotation of the head (oculocephalic) and vestibular stimulation (calorics) produce no change in eye position, the pons is nonfunctional. If only the eye ipsilateral to the stimulus abducts, a lesion of the medial longitudinal fasciculus (encapsulated by the pons) should be suspected.

Respiratory Rate and Pattern

Description of the respiratory pattern is probably less helpful than has been suggested previously.

However, ataxic breathing is a marker of severe brainstem dysfunction. Despite the nonspecificity of most breathing patterns, the respiratory rate can provide valuable clues to the etiology of coma (as noted above).

Motor Function

The highest observed level of motor function should be noted (e.g., "spontaneously moves all extremities", "withdraws right arm and leg from noxious stimulus", or "no response to pain"). Motor function in pontine compression consists of extensor (decerebrate) posturing. If a structural lesion compresses the centers for respiration and heart rate control on the dorsal medullary surface, the patient will be flaccid, without eye movements, and will have mid-position, unreactive pupils.

Localizing the Level of Dysfunction

If examination reveals a sequential, rostrocaudal loss of function, either a *supratentorial mass lesion* or *increased ICP* should be suspected as the etiology of coma. A funduscopic examination that demonstrates papilledema is virtually diagnostic of increased ICP or hypertensive encephalopathy. Although the *thalamus-diencephalon* cannot be directly examined, injury to this area usually causes lethargy but spares motor function. (Because pupillary and ocular movements are controlled by the mid-brain and pons, respectively, they remain unaffected.) The respiratory pattern in thalamic dysfunction is unpredictable.

Injury extending to the *mid-brain* level usually results in loss of motor function and decorticate (flexor) posturing. Although pupillary diameter is usually midposition ($\simeq$ 3 mm), mid-brain injury tends to spare pupillary reactivity and ocular movements.

When damage extends to the *pontine* level, pupillary function is routinely impaired. Motor responses are often limited to extensor or decerebrate posturing.

If compression progresses to involve the medulla, all motor function is usually absent, as are pupillary responses and eye movements. It is only at this medullary level that respiratory rhythm is predictably affected. The physicial examination will usually reveal ataxic breathing.

Laboratory Evaluation

Appropriate body fluid samples should be collected to evaluate the patient for metabolic coma. Such testing may be indicated, even in patients with obvious head trauma, because of the possi-

bility that a metabolic cause may coexist or may have precipitated the trauma (e.g., alcohol). Such determinations should include indices of renal and hepatic function, serum glucose and electrolyte determinations, hematocrit and arterial blood gases, and, in suspicious circumstances, carboxyhemoglobin determinations.

Causes of Coma Not to Miss

Although many forms of critical illness are associated with coma that parallels disease severity (e.g., sepsis, renal failure), selected conditions present primarily with coma and must be recognized and reversed to prevent disastrous consequences (Table 28.1). Each of these is discussed in more detail elsewhere in this volume.

Treatment

An airway should be secured, perfusion stabilized, and oxygen administered. Immediately after obtaining appropriate laboratory specimens, an *intravenous line* should be established for the administration of fluids and medications. *Glucose* levels should be screened at the bedside. If testing is not immediately available or if the measured glucose value is low, 50% dextrose in water (D50W) and thiamine should be given (see p. 224). *Naloxone*, a narcotic antagonist, can reverse narcotic-induced coma and hypoventilation. In the setting of ventilatory failure, however, naloxone, a useful adjunct, is not a reliable substitute for intubation and mechanical ventilation. The duration of action of naloxone is less than that of most narcotics that produce unconsciousness. Therefore, relapse into coma often follows a single dose of naloxone in patients who are not closely monitored.

After initial stabilization and evaluation, specific diagnostic measures can be undertaken. In febrile comatose patients, immediate lumbar puncture and institution of antibiotics are indicated (see p. 190). However, if lateralizing neurological signs are present or there is a history of trauma, a head computed tomography (CT) scan should be the next diagnostic intervention.

Table 28.1
Reversible Causes of Coma

Hypoperfusion	Carbon monoxide
Hypoxemia/hypercapnia	Occult status epilepticus
Hypoglycemia	CNS infections
Wernicke's encephalopathy	CNS hemorrhage
Hypercalcemia	Expanding mass lesions
Myxedema	Temperature disorders

SEIZURES

Pathophysiology

A seizure results from paroxysmal neuronal discharge that causes generalized or focal neurological signs. Although seizure disorders have been classified in different ways, it is probably most useful to think of them in terms of their *duration* and *scope* (generalized versus focal). Duration is important because prolonged seizures may irreversibly injure neuronal tissue. Focality is also noteworthy because focal seizures suggest a discrete structural abnormality. Although seizures usually present as localized or generalized phasic muscle spasms, they occasionally masquerade as unexplained coma or puzzling sensory or psychiatric disturbances.

Etiology

Seizures arise from *intrinsic electrical instability* (idiopathic seizures), *metabolic disturbances* (e.g., hypoxia, electrolyte imbalance, or drug effects), or *structural damage* (e.g., trauma, CNS infections, or mass lesions). High fever (especially in children), drug withdrawal (particularly anticonvulsants, alcohol, or sedatives), and iatrogenic overdoses of isoniazid, penicillin, tricyclics, theophylline, or lidocaine are other common metabolic causes. Many electrolyte disturbances responsible for *coma* may also induce *seizures*, especially when such changes occur abruptly (e.g., acute hyponatremia, disequilibrium following dialysis).

Although most seizure disorders that occur in outpatients are idiopathic, this is true less often in the intensive care unit, where such treatable conditions as drug or alcohol withdrawal, metabolic imbalances and acute structural lesions must be excluded. Most important among the metabolic precipitants are uremia, hypoglycemia, hypocalcemia, hypomagnesemia, and hyponatremia. CNS infections (meningitis, encephalitis, and brain abscess) are frequent causes of ictus; $\simeq$ ⅓ of adults with bacterial meningitis will experience a seizure.

Diagnosis

The diagnosis of seizures is usually made from the history and from the observation of an attack. Occasionally, historical features and/or the clinical appearance are so atypical as to require confirmatory testing by electroencephalography. In such cases, an intra-ictal electroencephalogram (EEG) recording may be diagnostic. Rarely, an EEG recording may reveal unsuspected seizure activity in a patient with unexplained coma. EEG localization

of seizure discharge to the base of the temporal lobes (or intense uptake of radioisotope in the temporal lobes) suggests *herpes encephalitis*. A head CT scan is indicated in patients with *new seizures* (especially following trauma), in those accompanied by a preceding or persistent *focal neurological deficit*, and in those *refractory* to simple medical therapy. In such patients, a computed tomogram often reveals a structural cause (e.g., vascular malformation, subdural or subarachnoid hemorrhage, primary or metastatic tumor, or hemispheric bleed).

Why Are Seizures Bad?

Brief ictal episodes are of little consequence if they do not occur while the patient is involved in a dangerous activity, if oxygenation and ventilation are maintained, and if the episode does not cause musculoskeletal injury. However, continuous electrical firing during prolonged seizures depletes cellular reserves of oxygen and adenosine triphosphate (ATP), a process that may culminate in neuronal death. Thus, the long-lasting adverse effects of seizures are usually associated with *status epilepticus*, a condition in which uninterrupted seizure activity occurs or the patient fails to regain consciousness between intermittent but closely spaced ictal episodes. Prolonged seizures may also induce intracranial hypertension and intracerebral hypoglycemia. Fever resulting from sustained muscular activity may rise to dangerous levels (> 105° F). Furthermore, thermoregulation may be disturbed for days, even after cessation of seizure activity. Increased free water losses from sweating and hyperventilation may increase serum osmolarity and sodium concentration. Hypotension and (rarely) seizure-induced cardiovascular collapse, can further aggravate neurological damage. Seizure-induced neuronal damage does not require loss of consciousness or convulsive muscular contraction.

Treatment

Protection of the airway and *maintenance of perfusion* are primary considerations. Aspiration must be guarded against by prompt termination of the seizure and by proper positioning (lateral decubitus). As with all causes of altered consciousness, electrolytes and glucose should be tested and normalized. When hypoglycemia is noted and treated, thiamine should be administered concurrently.

In patients who experience a solitary seizure or a small number of brief seizures with known precipitant, long-term anticonvulsants are not always necessary. Although phenytoin (Dilantin) has received "bad press" because of its potential for adverse cardiovascular effects (arrhythmias, hypotension, conduction disturbances), it is probably the drug of choice in acute status epilepticus when it is given with appropriate caution. (No anticonvulsant is entirely free of side effects.) Loading doses should not exceed 1 gm (15–18 mg/kg), and the infusion rate should not exceed 50 mg/min. More rapid infusion may cause heart block, hypotension, arrhythmias, and death. Phenytoin must be administered only in saline; it is not compatible with glucose-containing solutions. Although the adult daily maintenance dose averages 300 mg intravenously or orally, therapy should be guided by serum drug levels. Phenytoin toxicity may produce diplopia, horizontal and vertical nystagmus, slurred speech, ataxia, clumsiness, and somnolence. Paradoxically phenytoin may even increase the frequency of seizures.

Diazepam (5–10 mg intravenously) and *phenobarbital* (150–400 mg intravenously, given slowly) are also used commonly to terminate seizures. Unfortunately, respiratory depression and hypotension often limit their use. Additionally, a very short duration of anticonvulsant activity makes diazepam impractical for prolonged use. Seizures refractory to combinations of benzodiazepines, barbiturates, and phenytoin frequently require unusual methods for control (e.g., paraldehyde and general anesthesia).

BRAIN DEATH

Because the brain is the organ most sensitive to deprivation of oxygen and perfusion, its function may be irretrievably lost despite preservation of other bodily functions. Firm criteria for diagnosing brain death (BD) are important to establish in order to prevent the wastage of valuable medical resources and, conversely, to avoid premature abandonment of hope for potentially salvageable patients.

To diagnose BD, the etiology of coma must be known with reasonable certainty. *Hypothermia, drug overdose, neuromuscular blockade,* and *shock must be excluded. No sedative or narcotic drugs may remain in the circulation.* Furthermore, the patient must be observed over a prolonged period ($\simeq$ 24 hours) to document the stability of the clinical picture. Seizure activity and decerebrate or decorticate posturing are inconsistent with the diagnosis. However, reflexes of purely spinal cord origin are compatible.

To confirm BD, cerebral function must be ab-

sent at hemispheric, mid-brain, pontine, and medullary levels. Lack of cortical function is evidenced by a totally *unreceptive* and *unresponsive* state. Patients in a *persistently vegetative state* lack awareness and responsiveness but appear awake because RAS arousal pathways remain intact. Such patients do not meet BD criteria. Patients with destructive lesions of the brainstem that give rise to the *"locked in"* syndrome also appear unresponsive. Detailed testing, however, reveals that these patients are aware but unable to respond, except for eye movements.

Absent *pupillary activity* indicates loss of midbrain function. Inability to evoke *eye movements* confirms lost pontine function. *Medullary dysfunction* is assured by demonstrating *apnea* when the patient is challenged by a profound hypercarbic stimulus. Apnea testing is performed by interrupting positive pressure ventilation, while continuing oxygenation. After pre-oxygenation with an F_iO_2 of 1.0, an O_2 catheter is introduced into the endotracheal tube. The patient is then observed for respiratory effort. Such precautions assure that the patient remains adequately oxygenated, even though unventilated. A $PaCO_2 > 60$ mmHg must be attained to assure adequate ventilatory stimulation. In apneic patients with a functioning circulation, the $PaCO_2$ normally rises 3–5 mmHg/min. Therefore, knowledge of the baseline $PaCO_2$ can be used to predict the apneic time necessary to assure a $PaCO_2 > 60$ mmHg. (In general, 4–6 minutes of apnea are required if the baseline $PaCO_2$ is normal.)

In some localities, a confirmatory EEG must be performed to document absence of cerebral electrical activity. An isoelectric EEG carries a dismal prognosis unless coma is drug induced. (Isoelectric EEGs have been recorded as long as 4 days after the initial presentation of patients with drug-induced coma.) Isoelectric tracings may also occur in patients who have lost cortical function but who retain brainstem activity (neo-cortical death). Such patients usually demonstrate a vegetative state in which arousal is intact but awareness is lacking. Brain death may also be confirmed by using contrast or radioisotope angiography to demonstrate absence of cerebral flow.

SUGGESTED READINGS

1. Aminoff MJ, Simon RP: Status epilepticus. Causes, clinical features and consequences in 98 patients. *Am J Med* 69:657–666, 1980.
2. Cloyd JC, Gumnit RJ, McLain W: Status epilepticus. The role of intravenous phenytoin. *JAMA* 244(13):1479–1481, 1980.

3. Engel J, Troupin AS, Crandall PH, et al: Recent developments in the diagnosis and therapy of epilepsy. *Ann Intern Med* 97:584–598, 1982.

4. Fisher CM: The neurological examination of the comatose patient. *Acta Neurol Scand* 45 (Suppl 36):4–56, 1969.

5. Guidelines for the determination of death: report of the medical consultants on the diagnosis of death to the President's Commission for the study of ethical problems in medicine and biomedical and behavioral research. *Neurology* 32:395–399, 1982.

6. Levy DE, Coronna JJ, Singer BH, et al: Predicting outcome from hypoxic—ischemic coma. *JAMA* 253:1420–1426, 1985.

7. Penry JK, Newmark ME: The use of antiepileptic drugs. *Ann Intern Med* 90:207–218, 1979.

8. Plum F, Posner JB: *The Diagnosis of Stupor and Coma*, ed 3. Philadelphia, FA Davis, 1980.

9. Ropper AH, Kennedy SK, Russel L: Apnea testing in the diagnosis of brain death. *J Neurosurg* 55:942–46, 1981.

Section 3

Surgical Crises

29 Head and Spine Trauma

SPINAL CORD TRAUMA

Mechanisms

The spinal cord can be injured by flexion-rotation, compression, or hyperextension. Cord *contusion* is the feature common to all three mechanisms. A minority of cord injuries result from primary *vascular disruption*. Spinal cord injury (SCI) should be suspected in every trauma patient with back or neck pain and sensory or motor deficits. Because SCI often occurs in conjunction with head injury, *all head trauma patients should be initially treated as if they have sustained cord injury*.

Flexion-rotation injury of the neck usually occurs when the neck is hyperflexed onto the trunk out of the midline axis, disrupting the posterior spinal ligament. Motor vehicle accidents are the most common cause. At a minimum, patients with flexion-rotation injury require closed reduction and traction. If radiographs demonstrate displacement of a vertebral body by more than ½ its width, instability and *bilateral* facet dislocation are likely. Displacement < ½ the width of the vertebral body suggests *unilateral* dislocation, a less serious problem. Such injuries are potentially unstable after reduction, but fewer than 10% require surgery for fixation. If facets in the lumbar region become "locked", surgery is usually necessary.

Compression injuries most commonly result from diving accidents. In this setting bone fragments may lead to neural damage by protruding into the spinal cord. However, these injuries are inherently stable because spinal ligaments remain intact. The usual treatment is bed rest with skeletal traction.

Hyperextension ("whip lash") injuries in the cervical region are usually stable. These injuries occur in older patients with cervical arthritis and are frequently associated with bleeding into the spinal gray matter, producing a "central cord" syndrome.

Physical Examination

Complete spinal cord disruption produces loss of all sensory and motor function below the level of the injury, initially resulting in flaccid paralysis that lasts for 2–7 days—the "spinal shock" phase. Incomplete cord injuries carry a better prognosis because some function is retained distal to the level of the injury. In a cooperative patient, many clinically important injuries may be diagnosed at the bedside. If the patient is able to take a spontaneous *deep breath*, cervical roots C2-C5 are probably intact and diaphragm function preserved. If the patient can *raise and extend the arms*, C5-C7 are intact. The ability to *open and close the hand* assures function of C7-T1, whereas the ability to *elevate the legs* confirms the integrity of L2-L4. *Wiggling the toes* indicates that L5-S1 roots are functional. Normal *anal sphincter* function implies preserved function of roots S3-S5.

Initial Management

All passive and active motion of the spine should be prevented in patients with suspected cord injury. Adequate ventilation and circulation should be assured and oxygen administered if indicated. Autonomic instability often occurs in the early phase, so that relative hypotension is not uncommon. Judicious filling of the intravascular compartment is indicated, but because of disordered vasoregulation it is important not to administer excessive volumes. Other measures key to the resuscitation of the trauma victim, such as chest tube insertion, should be performed immediately.

Following spinal immobilization and stabilization of the airway and circulation, a detailed neurological examination should be conducted and radiographs of the spine obtained. More than ⅔ of all spinal fractures may be seen on a single lateral view of the spine if proper technique is used. It is important to visualize all 7 cervical vertebrae because *C7 is the vertebra most commonly injured but least commonly seen on portable radiographs.* A "swimmers view" or traction on the patient's arms may aid visualization of C7.

The alignment of the anterior and posterior aspects of each vertebral body, the alignment of the spinolaminal lines, and the contour of the spinous processes and vertebral bodies should be reviewed. The prevertebral space should be examined for evidence of widening due to hemorrhage. Open mouth views should be obtained to look for odontoid fractures. Radiographs should visualize the entire spine if a fracture is found. (Up to 20% of patients have multiple levels of injury.) Myelography (plain film or computed tomography) should be reserved for cases in which the extent of injury is unclear after clinical evaluation and review of plain spine radiographs.

Neurosurgical consultation should be sought at the earliest possible time. Although the indications for immediate surgery in spinal cord trauma are controversial, commonly accepted criteria include: (1) progressive loss of neurological function due to suspected epidural or subdural bleeding; (2) a foreign body in the spinal canal; (3) cerebrospinal fluid (CSF) leak; and (4) bony instability requiring immobilization.

Complications

Progressive neurological impairment is only one of the many complications of SCI. The most significant of these are iatrogenically induced by spinal manipulation or inappropriate administration of fluids or vasopressors for the manipulation of blood pressure. In the first 48 hours following SCI the level of neurological impairment often ascends by 1–2 vertebral levels.

Cardiovascular

Cord lesions above the T6 level may cause hemodynamic instability by interrupting *sympathetic outflow.* Even in young, healthy persons the loss of sympathetic tone usually produces a stable supine blood pressure in the range of 100/60 mmHg. Hypovolemia, infection, or placement in the upright position often precipitates profound hypotension. The level of blood pressure is acceptable if urine output remains good and cerebration is clear.

However, if mean arterial pressure falls below 70 mmHg, a fluid challenge may be needed; invasive monitoring helps dictate proper therapy. Measures to reduce venous capacitance, including abdominal binding, Trendelenburg positioning, and compression stockings may help avoid postural hypotension.

Bradycardia often accompanies hypotension due to cord injury and does not require treatment unless symptomatic. Accommodation of the sympathetic and parasympathetic responses usually produce normal heart rates within 3–5 days following injury. However, *unopposed vagal stimulation* from pain, hollow viscus distention, hypoxemia, or endotracheal suctioning may produce profound bradycardia. If symptomatic bradycardia unrelated to hypoxemia occurs, atropine, isoproterenol, or temporary pacing is useful. It is the loss of compensatory tachycardia early in the course of SCI that makes *iatrogenic pulmonary edema* common following even modest fluid administration. If unequivocal *tachycardia* is present in a hypotensive patient with SCI, suspect another condition—sepsis, internal hemorrhage, or hypovolemia. Because autonomic paresis eliminates crucial vasoconstrictive reflexes, these patients have very limited stress reserves.

Respiratory

Respiratory impairment, the most common complication of SCI, results from respiratory muscle weakness, rib fractures, hemopneumothorax, lung contusion, and aspiration. Cervical roots 3, 4, and 5 innervate the diaphragm. Therefore, interruption of the cord above this level in an unsupported patient rapidly leads to apnea and death. Cervical spine injuries also cause problems when expiratory muscle weakness impairs cough and secretion clearance. The forced vital capacity (FVC) should be monitored several times daily in the acute phase of SCI. As a rule of thumb, such problems are unusual if FVC exceeds 1.5–2.0 liters. If the FVC is less than this value in patients with injuries below the C5 level, direct injury to the phrenic nerve(s) should be suspected.

Because quadriplegics have little ventilatory reserve, any condition that further impairs ventilation or increases minute ventilation may lead rapidly to fatigue and ventilatory failure. Lesions above T10 most commonly cause respiratory difficulty by impairing cough, altering ventilation/perfusion distribution (causing hypoxemia), and decreasing inspiratory capacity. Low lung volumes and atelectasis occur not only because of intrinsic muscle weakness, but also because abdominal distention (often from ileus) limits inspiration. Ventilation may be further compromised by unopposed parasympathetic responses that cause bronchorrhea and present an increased risk of vomiting and aspiration. Patients with spinal cord injury are particularly sensitive to the effects of paralytic agents.

Although seemingly paradoxical, quadriplegic patients often ventilate best in the supine position. Their only muscle of respiration (the diaphragm) is "cocked" into optimal position by such a posture through the upward pressure of the abdominal contents. Conversely, patients with isolated diaphragmatic paralysis ventilate best when fully erect. Upright positioning minimizes the cephalad pressure of the abdominal contents against the flaccid diaphragm. This action increases lung volume and helps to stabilize the diaphragm during contraction of the accessory muscles of inspiration.

Genitourinary

Urinary tract complications (sepsis, renal failure) are the most common cause for *late* death in SCI patients. Micturition may be impaired for months following SCI. Continuous Foley catheterization is probably indicated early in the hospital course to monitor urine output. Later, intermittent catheterization is preferred because of its reduced risk of infection. Regular surveillance cultures of urine help to detect infection at an early stage. Prophylactic antibiotics may prevent bacteremia but are unlikely to maintain sterile urine in patients with indwelling catheters.

Gastrointestinal

Immediately following SCI, *ileus* may occur that typically lasts 3–4 days. Ileus is likely to be protracted if SCI is accompanied by retroperitoneal hemorrhage. In most patients, a nasogastric tube should be inserted until bowel sounds return. Daily measurements of abdominal girth may also help assess gastrointestinal (GI) motility and the possibility of colonic impaction. In cord-injured patients the combination of tachycardia, hypotension, and absent bowel sounds should prompt consideration of an acute abdomen (pain may be absent or atypical).

Often there is no certain way to rule out intra-abdominal catastrophe, short of laparotomy or paracentesis. Pains referred to the shoulder or scapula are particularly valuable signs of abdominal inflammation in SCI.

Nutrients may safely be withheld for $\simeq$ 5 days before caloric supplementation is begun. When ileus resolves, enteral feedings are preferred if feasible, because of improved gut function, reduced cost, and avoidance of catheter related infections. Peptic ulcer disease is common following SCI, and *enteral feeding, antacids, and/or histamine blockers* are useful preventative measures. Corticosteroids increase the risk of peptic and stress ulceration and should be avoided unless clearly indicated. As soon as bowel sounds return and enteral feeding begins, a program of *bowel care* with regular evacuation and stool softeners should be started to prevent constipation and impaction. The level of the spinal cord lesion will dictate whether evacuation is spontaneous, reflex, or manually induced.

Cutaneous

Skin breakdown is a costly complication of SCI that presents a central focus for nursing care. Padding, physical therapy, and the use of rotating or air cushioned beds may be helpful in prevention. Cord-injured patients (particularly quadriplegics) should *not* be placed in the prone position because of the possibility of hypoventilation, hypoxemia, and bradycardia.

Miscellaneous

After the return of spinal reflexes, patients with lesions above the T6 level may develop episodes characterized by hypertension, diaphoresis, piloerection, and flushing. This syndrome, *autonomic hyperreflexia*, must be recognized because it can prove fatal unless rapidly reversed by a simple expedient—decompressing an *overdistended viscus* (usually bowel or bladder). In patients with excessive sympathetic activity, a vagally mediated *compensatory bradycardia* often occurs.

Thromboembolism is extremely common in the first 90 days after cord injury. The hemodynamic impact of embolism is accentuated by altered autonomic reflexes. Prophylactic heparin may be preventative, but there are risks of provoking hemorrhage in the early phase. Compression stockings and pneumatic boots may be useful if anticoagulants are contraindicated.

HEAD TRAUMA

Mechanisms/Pathophysiology

Head trauma injures neural tissue by primary (direct injury) or secondary mechanisms (vascular disruption and increased intracranial pressure). The concussive forces produced by a blow to the head are usually *greatest at the point of application* and diametrically across the skull from the site of the blow (*contre-coup injury*). Bony prominences on the base of the skull also commonly cause injury, particularly to the inferior surfaces of the frontal and temporal lobes.

Secondary brain injury, characterized by increased intracranial pressure (ICP), results from tissue edema, hydrocephalus or mass lesions (fluid/blood accumulations, epidural or subdural hematomas, intracerebral hemorrhage, abscess or empyema). Ischemia, hypoxia, and vascular disruption increase the severity of cerebral injury.

Cranial Disruption

Linear skull fractures are of particular significance when they traverse the normal course of the middle meningeal artery, suggesting the possibility of epidural hematoma. *Depressed skull fractures* or *penetrating injuries* produce damage as the inner table of the skull drives inward, injuring the brain surface. Such injuries usually result from the impact of small, high-velocity objects and carry a high risk of bacterial infection.

Basilar skull fractures are markers for the severity of the overall head impact. CSF leakage into the sinuses is common. In such cases trans-nasal tubes must not be inserted because of the possibility of passage through the base of the skull into the brain. Nasal packing should not be used in patients with CSF leakage because of the increased risk of meningitis. Febrile patients with basilar skull fractures must be treated as if meningitis is present, with a lumbar puncture and the early institution of antibiotics. Although recurrent meningitis is a feared complication of basilar skull fracture, CSF leaks seldom need surgical closure (fewer than 1% of all cases).

Injury to Brain Tissue

Cerebral contusion due to rapid deceleration is the most common mechanism of brain injury. Subsequent cerebral edema and increased intracranial pressure may exacerbate damage. The *brainstem contusion* syndrome is characterized by intermittent agitation, disordered autonomic regulation, and episodic hyperthermia.

Mass lesions and cerebral edema produce secondary brain injury by displacing cerebral contents across anatomic boundaries (Fig. 29.1). Translocation may occur through bony defects or by subfalcial, transtentorial, or foraminal herniation.

Epidural hematoma (EH) usually presents as a rapidly expanding mass (blood) in a patient with a linear skull fracture. Vascular disruption usually occurs where the fracture crosses the course of the middle meningeal artery or crosses the dural sin-

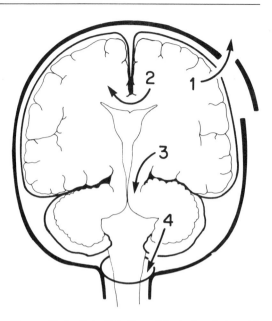

Figure 29.1 Potential sites of brain herniation: (1) transcranial; (2) subfalcial; (3) transtentorial; (4) foraminal.

uses or foramen magnum. Most EHs occur over the temporal lobes where the skull is thin and highly vascular. EH most commonly results in medial compression of the temporal lobe, causing contralateral hemiparesis and eventual death as the midbrain is compressed against the tentorium.

EH clinically presents as *loss of consciousness*, *contralateral hemiparesis*, and a *third nerve palsy* with *ipsilateral pupillary dilation*. Only ⅓ of patients have a classic "lucid interval". Because EH has an associated mortality approaching 50%, it usually requires urgent neurosurgical intervention. Therefore, any trauma patient who demonstrates a linear skull fracture or who loses consciousness (even transiently) for > 2 minutes probably should be admitted to the hospital for observation.

Acute subdural hematoma is an expanding mass that results from cortical contusion and laceration of a meningeal vessel. Like EH, this injury is associated with high mortality and usually requires immediate surgical intervention. *Subacute or chronic subdural hematoma* due to laceration of enlarged dural venous sinuses may occur as the result of even a trivial injury. Subdural hematoma most frequently occurs in the elderly because cortical atrophy stretches the subdural veins, predisposing them to injury. A typical presentation of a subacute or chronic subdural hematoma is slowly progressive confusion, somnolence, and headache leading eventually to hemiplegia. Anticoagulants greatly increase the risk of post-traumatic hematoma formation.

In severe brain injury an *intracerebral hematoma* may develop. The computed tomography (CT) scan is useful in delineating this mass, which appears initially as a dense intraparenchymal collection of blood. If an intracerebral hematoma produces mass effect, it should be surgically evacuated.

Intracranial Hypertension

Only 3 tissues occupy the intracranial cavity: *brain substance*, *cerebrospinal fluid*, and *blood*. None are readily compressible. Therefore, after head trauma, swelling of the brain substance, blockage of the normal circulation, or absorption of CSF leads to increased intracranial pressure (ICP), a process that may be mitigated by the movement of one of the ''liquid'' components (blood or CSF) out of the cranium. Clotting of *intraventricular blood* may obstruct the circulation of CSF, producing obstructive hydrocephalus. Blood products within the CSF can elevate the ICP by two other mechanisms: clogging CSF absorption at the subarachnoid villi and increasing CSF osmotic pressure during red cell lysis. Increased ICP reflects the severity of brain injury and in itself can be deleterious when it reduces tissue perfusion or encourages herniation of brain tissue. The swelling of injured tissue peaks within 72 hours of injury. ICP, however, can remain elevated for weeks if there has been significant intracerebral or intraventricular bleeding.

Cerebral Hemodynamics

ICP should be kept low enough to maintain cerebral perfusion and prevent cerebral herniation. The pressure perfusing the brain (the cerebral perfusion pressure, CPP) is the difference between mean arterial pressure and either the ICP or the pressure within the cerebral veins (whichever is higher). Whereas CPP normally exceeds 60 mmHg, the lowest acceptable level is $\simeq$ 40 mmHg. Neural dysfunction occurs when CPP < 40 mmHg. Neuronal death occurs at CPP < 20 mmHg.

In health, cerebral *autoregulatory mechanisms* sensitive to arterial oxygen tension (PaO_2), arterial carbon dioxide tension ($PaCO_2$), and blood pressure continuously adjust cerebral vascular resistance to maintain perfusion in proportion to metabolic need and changing perfusion pressure. Arterial blood gases, cerebral metabolism, and the components of perfusion pressure (blood pressure, ICP) must be watched cautiously in head injured

patients because the auto-regulatory mechanisms of injured tissue are impaired. In this setting *perfusion* of these tissues directly *parallels CPP* and perfusion adequacy is directly influenced by cerebral metabolism.

Complications of Head Trauma

In the acute phase, a number of metabolic and mechanical problems are common in the head injured patient. Direct neuronal injury causes *seizures* with sufficient frequency that prophylactic use of an anticonvulsant (e.g., phenytoin) may be prudent. Injury to the hypothalamus or pituitary may disrupt the normal secretion of hypophyseal hormones. Loss of *antidiuretic hormone* (ADH) may cause acute diabetes insipidus. Such patients can produce massive volumes (> 1 l/hr) of dilute urine despite increasing serum osmolality. Life-threatening hypovolemia and hyperosmolarity may result unless prompt treatment with hypotonic fluids and ADH are instituted. With the exception of ACTH deficiency, which may result in adrenal insufficiency, loss of other pituitary hormones (e.g., growth hormone, thyroid stimulating hormone) usually presents a less urgent problem.

Disruption of the dura by penetrating trauma or boney fracture (e.g., basilar skull fracture) may provide a pathway for the entry of microorganisms into the CSF, resulting in recurrent post-traumatic meningitis.

Finally, serious head injury may disrupt or cause blockage of normal channels of communication of CSF. Such disruptions may cause obstructive hydrocephalus with subsequent elevations in intracranial pressure.

Monitoring the Brain-Injured Patient

Careful monitoring of the neurological exam and use of objective ''coma scales'' may be helpful, especially in mild to moderate injury. Serial CT scans give invaluable information regarding the nature and evolution of the injury process. However, the only way to accurately assess intracranial pressure in the seriously injured, comatose patient is to monitor it directly.

Physical Examination

In addition to a careful neurological evaluation, the physical examination of patients sustaining head trauma should look for evidence of *penetrating wounds*, *spinal cord damage*, and *depressed or basilar skull fractures* (evidenced by blood behind the tympanic membrane, CSF rhinorrhea, ''raccoon eyes'', or discoloration behind the ears—

Battle's sign). Papilledema is a particularly useful finding in the head trauma patient, indicating an elevated ICP.

Intracranial Pressure Monitoring

There are four primary reasons to measure ICP: 1) to monitor patients at risk of developing life-threatening elevations of ICP, 2) to monitor for evidence of infection, 3) to monitor the progress of the underlying pathologic process, and 4) to assess the effects of therapy aimed at reducing ICP.

Mean ICP normally approximates 10–15 mmHg, and the ICP waveform normally undulates gently in time with the cardiac cycle. Extreme fluctuations of the ICP waveform (> 10 mmHg) suggest a position near the critical inflection point of the cranial pressure-volume curve, particularly when the contour shows a high "second peak" corresponding to the arterial pulse. Elevations in ICP to 15–20 mmHg compress capillary beds and compromise the microcirculation. At ICP levels of 30–35 mmHg venous drainage is impeded and edema develops in uninjured tissue. ICP elevations of this degree produce a viscious cycle in which impeded venous drainage leads to accumulating edema and elevated ICP. Even when auto-regulatory mechanisms are intact, cerebral perfusion cannot be maintained if ICP rises to within 40–50 mmHg of the mean arterial pressure. When the ICP approximates mean arterial pressure, perfusion stops and the brain dies. The urgency of reducing ICP may be assessed by following intracranial compliance, i.e., the response of ICP to a 1 ml challenge of sterile fluid injected through a ventricular catheter. This procedure is not risk free, however, and must be undertaken with extreme caution. Herniation can be precipitated unless the challenge is performed carefully.

In addition to sustained elevations of ICP, two specific transients have been described by Lundberg. "A waves", pressure elevations of 20–100 mmHg for periods of 2–15 minutes, are always pathologic. A waves are usually associated with abnormal eye movements, posturing, and abnormal neurological reflexes—physiologic responses resulting from inadequate cerebral perfusion during periods of extreme pressure elevation. Lundberg A waves indicate the likelihood of sudden deterioration and poor neurological outcome. Lundberg "B waves" are lower in amplitude, shorter in duration, and usually occur in relation to respiratory variation. B waves have no associated physicial findings at the time of occurrence

and unlike their A wave counterparts are not well correlated with neurological outcome.

Of the three fluid components contained within the fixed cranial volume, only the volumes of CSF and blood may be changed (unless brain tissue is removed or made less edematous). Starting from normal levels, ICP shows little response to volume change until a critical inflection point is reached. Thereafter, small increases in intracranial volume dramatically boost ICP, risking sudden neurological deterioration (Fig. 29.2). Direct ICP monitoring is important, because changes in other clinical indices—reflexes, blood pressure, and heart rate—usually occur too late to avert disaster. Bradycardia, a preterminal sign, is the least reliable of all clinical indicators of increased ICP. (Tachycardia is seen more frequently.)

Specific Indications for Monitoring ICP

Closed Head Injury. It is not practical to monitor all patients with head trauma, but several factors that correlate with elevations of ICP suggest benefit from intracranial monitoring. Patients who present with *hypotension or shock following head trauma*, particularly if elderly, are likely to have increased ICP. A normal CT scan of the head accurately predicts normal intracranial pressure in more than 80% of cases, whereas ICP is elevated in ≈ 50% of patients with *any specific lesion on head CT scan. Mid-line shift* of > 7 mm or blood in the lateral ventricles is especially worrisome. Head trauma patients with *Glascow coma scale (GCS) scores of < 7* frequently have an increased ICP, as do patients with decorticate/decerebrate *posturing or abnormal evoked potential testing.*

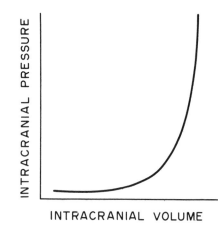

Figure 29.2   Relationship of intracranial pressure to intracranial volume. Intracranial pressure remains low until a critical volume is attained.

Abnormal eye or pupil movements are unreliable guides to increased ICP.

Reye's Syndrome. Increased ICP is a major cause of death in Reye's syndrome. Mortality approaches 100% without prompt diagnosis and treatment. Therapeutic reductions in ICP may reduce mortality to 20% or less, with survivors experiencing few sequelae. Therefore, ICP monitoring is indicated in patients with Reye's syndrome and GCS scores < 7.

Encephalopathy. As opposed to Reye's syndrome, the mechanism of increased ICP in acute hepatic failure of other etiologies and in other metabolic encephalopathies is largely unknown. At present there is little evidence to suggest that monitoring ICP reduces mortality in these disorders.

Brain Tumors. ICP monitoring is rarely necessary in patients with chronic supratentorial lesions. However, ventriculostomy may be useful preoperatively to allow reduction in the CSF volume of patients with large infratentorial lesions. In patients with large brain tumors or extensive edema on CT scanning, ICP monitoring may help guide therapy.

Contraindications to Monitoring

Coagulopathy (platelet count less than $100,000/mm^3$ or prothrombin time (PT) or partial thromboplastin time (PTT) > 2 × control) are strong contraindications to the placement of an ICP monitor. Isolated elevations of fibrin degradation products (FDPs) should not contraindicate catheter placement; FDP levels may be increased by brain trauma alone. Immunosuppressive therapy (particularly steroids) is a relative contraindication to ICP monitoring. If required, a subarachnoid bolt is preferred in such patients because of the lower risk of nosocomial infection.

Hardware and Devices

Ventricular Catheters. Ventricular catheters provide continuous, reliable data, enable compliance measurements to be performed, and allow therapeutic removal of CSF. Ventricular catheters may be inserted under local anesthesia at the bedside, through a burr hole in the skull.

Ventriculostomy presents several problems. Difficulty may be encountered in placing the catheter into a lateral ventricle compressed by extensive edema or mass lesion. In order to limit brain damage, no more than 3 passes should be attempted. After insertion, the CSF invariably shows evidence of catheter irritation (mild elevations of protein and leukocyte count). Infection is not uncommon (≈ 15%) after ventriculostomy, and relates to duration of monitoring and to sterility of catheter placement and maintenance. (To avoid adding to the infection risk, cranial compliance testing must be undertaken with close attention to sterility of technique.) Prophylactic antibiotics have shown no benefit in reducing infection rates, but tunneling the catheter through the skin may be helpful. Because bleeding commonly accompanies insertion of ventricular catheters, coagulopathy strongly contraindicates placement.

Epidural Transducers. Although epidural transducers present a lower risk of infection than ventricular catheters, they are technically more difficult to insert. For accuracy, the transducer membrane must be precisely juxtaposed to the dura. Once placed, these devices are difficult to keep calibrated. Another drawback to the use of epidural transducers is the inability to remove CSF.

Subarachnoid (Richmond) Screws. The subarachnoid screw is an open bolt inserted into the subarachnoid space through a burr hole (usually bored in the fronto-parietal suture). During placement the dura is opened and the screw is inserted onto the brain surface. Major problems with the subarachnoid screw include a relatively high risk of infection and the potential for seriously underestimating ICP if not placed on the side of an existing mass lesion. Problems with damping and clotting are sufficiently frequent that regular flushing is mandatory. Such flushing, however, exposes patients to an increased risk of herniation and infection. Finally, these devices are frequently dislodged, even with meticulous care.

Problems with Intracranial Pressure Monitoring

Metallic monitoring devices preclude magnetic resonance imaging (MRI) scans and produce artifacts on CT scans that can obscure important information. Infection occurs in 2–5% of patients who undergo ICP monitoring and is most common if the devices remain for more than 5 days or if open drainage systems are used. *Staphylococcus epidermidis* is the most common infecting organism. Volume-pressure testing of cranial compliance adds to the infection risk. Prophylactic antibiotics have not been demonstrated effective.

As with any monitoring technique, poor quality data may lead to inappropriate therapy. The intraventricular catheter gives the most consistent data. While the subarachnoid screw is less reliable, it carries the lowest infection risk.

Treatment of the Brain-injured Patient

The viability of injured brain depends on the critical balance of nutritional supply and demand. Because injured tissue cannot auto-regulate blood flow to metabolic need, a key component of the treatment strategy focuses on reducing the metabolic requirement while boosting CPP. Therefore, mean arterial and intracranial pressures must be maintained as close to their normal values as possible. (Very high elevations of ICP not only reduce CPP but also risk herniation.)

Therapy to Reduce Intracranial Pressure

Lowering Jugular Venous Pressure

The goal of reducing ICP is to *maintain cerebral blood flow by keeping cerebral perfusion pressure at or above 50 mmHg*. Patient positioning can be important; neck flexion, head turning, and tracheostomy ties impede venous drainage and may rapidly elevate ICP. Therefore, the head should be elevated to 45° and maintained in a midline position. Tracheostomy ties and bandages should be applied loosely. Increases of intrathoracic pressure related to straining and coughing should be minimized. Seizures should be prevented. Special caution should be taken during ventilation with positive end-expiratory pressure (PEEP). High levels of PEEP have the potential to reduce mean arterial pressure (MAP) and raise ICP simultaneously. However, judicious use of PEEP is not strictly contraindicated, especially since the ICP of trauma patients often exceeds the PEEP-affected pressure within the superior sagittal sinus.

Diuretics

Loop diuretics (furosemide and ethacrynic acid) have a twin therapeutic action—decreasing CSF production and producing a diuresis that reduces intravascular volume.

Osmotic Agents

When combined with loop diuretics, osmotic agents may produce marked but transient reductions in ICP. Diuretics help to oppose the volume-expanding effect of osmotic agents. *Glycerol and mannitol* establish an osmotic pressure gradient between the CSF and blood, promoting fluid transfer from brain cells to the circulation. In doses that produce a serum osmolarity greater than 320 mOsm/dl, osmotic agents slowly penetrate the blood brain barrier, gradually counterbalancing their own therapeutic effect. Furthermore, when given rapidly, large doses of osmotic agents may paradoxically expand the circulating volume and elevate ICP.

Rebound intracranial hypertension is a significant problem that may be seen after discontinuation of any osmotic agent. High osmolarity (greater than 340 mOsm/dl) may depress consciousness or impair renal tubular function. Acutely, volume expansion may induce metabolic acidosis and hemodilution. However, in the long term, excessive diuresis depletes intravascular and/or intracellular volume, delaying return to normal consciousness.

Hyperventilation

Hyperventilation is the *most rapid* method of *temporarily* lowering ICP. Acute reduction of $PaCO_2$ raises tissue pH, causing cerebral vasoconstriction in normally responsive cerebral vessels (Fig. 29.3). Within wide limits, reduced flow through normal brain tissue is well tolerated. As flow and vascular volume fall, ICP declines, thereby boosting CPP. Flow to injured, poorly auto-regulated brain actually improves because flow through injured brain is CPP dependent (Fig. 29.4).

Although moderate hyperventilation tends to reduce ICP, improve CPP, and improve nutrient flow to damaged tissue, extreme hyperventilation ($PaCO_2$ < 25 mmHg) offsets this beneficial action by causing excessive vasoconstriction and global reduction of perfusion. (Assuming a normal starting value, reducing $PaCO_2$ remains effective for $\simeq$ 48 hours; renal compensation restores acid-base status and eventually negates its effects.) Hyperventilation should be terminated in stages (over 24–48 hours) to avoid causing a rebound increase in ICP. Although the therapeutic benefits of deliberate *hyper*ventilation are uncertain, it is clear that *hypo*ventilation must be avoided at all costs; increased blood flow and vascular volume can drive ICP quickly to life-threatening levels. Associated hypoxemia accentuates the risk, as hypoxemia, like hypercapnia, is a cerebral vasodilator of auto-regulated brain tissue. Within the first 72 hours of injury special caution should be exercised not to interrupt hyperventilation for more than brief periods. (For example, prolonged disconnections to see whether the patient has spontaneous respirations may be ill advised during this period.)

Corticosteroids

Experimentally, corticosteroids appear to reduce CSF production and exert direct anti-edema effects. The ''anti-edema'' effect appears to increase linearly with the logarithm of the steroid dose, and therefore on this basis ''megadose'' therapy with 100–200 mg of dexamethasone may be

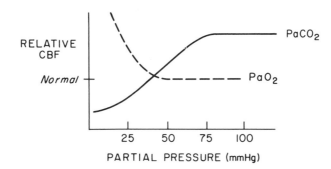

Figure 29.3 Effect of arterial gas tensions on cerebral blood flow (CBF) in normal brain tissue (auto-regulation intact). Whereas reductions of $PaCO_2$ lower CBF (and cerebral volume) in more or less linear fashion over the physiologic range, reductions in PaO_2 have an opposite effect that manifests only when the O_2 content of hemoglobin falls ($PaO_2 < 60$ mmHg). Injured tissue may lose this ability to auto-regulate flow in response to blood gas (or blood pressure) changes (see Fig. 29.4).

justifiable. However, steroids are much more effective at reducing *tumorogenic* edema than that of other causes. At present, there is no clear evidence that steroids are beneficial in head trauma.

Ventriculostomy Drainage

The removal of CSF may acutely lower ICP, especially when the system is poised on the steep portion of the intracranial pressure-volume curve. Because CSF production is a continuous process, the effects of intermittent CSF removal are usually transient (< 2 hours). Systems for continuously venting the CSF to maintain ICP at or below a given hydrostatic level are effective in reducing ICP but increase the risk of infection. Nonetheless,

CSF drainage makes consummate sense in the setting of aqueductal blockage (by clotted blood in the 4th ventricle, for example). Here, venting the CSF output until clot lysis occurs ($\simeq 5$–7 days) may prove life-saving. Withdrawal of spinal fluid from the lumbar region may precipitate brain herniation by increasing the pressure gradient across the tentorium.

Surgery

A direct attack on the cause of increased ICP may be indicated in such conditions as *obstructive hydrocephalus* (improved by shunting), *tumor*, or *large but focal hemorrhage* (particularly into the cerebellum). Prompt evacuation of a large *sub-*

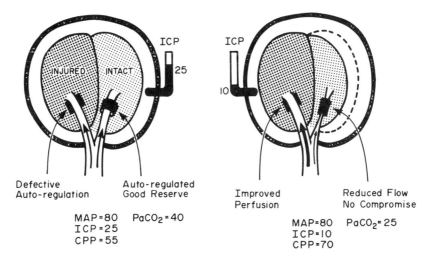

Figure 29.4 Effects of hyperventilation on cerebral blood flow and volume to injured and uninjured brain.

dural hematoma may be life-saving and, if necessary, can be performed at the bedside. Removal of a cranial flap may be an effective (if short-lived) temporizing maneuver.

Therapy to Minimize Cerebral Metabolism

Fever and agitation greatly increase cerebral metabolic requirements and should be prevented. However, it may be a serious mistake to use methods of temperature control (e.g., cooling blankets) that induce shivering. Semi-conscious patients are made more uncomfortable, thereby increasing cerebral metabolism and raising intrathoracic and intracerebral pressure. Antipyretics are preferable.

High dose barbiturates decrease cerebral metabolism and blood flow. Although such therapy may benefit head trauma patients, there is little evidence to support their usage in other settings. In any event, the decision to undertake high-dose barbiturate therapy should be carefully considered. These drugs depress cardiovascular function and obliterate both the electroencephalogram (EEG) signals and the clinical parameters used for neurological assessment. Barbiturate therapy mandates intracranial pressure monitoring.

The Recovery Phase

Recovery from cerebral trauma may be a prolonged process. However, once acute injury subsides, vigilance must be maintained to insure that reversible factors do not impede the return to normal function. All too often metabolic derangements (spontaneous or iatrogenic) are responsible for persistently depressed consciousness. Hyperosmolarity, hypovolemia, hyperglycemia, and hyponatremia are frequently induced by the therapies applied in the treatment of these disorders: diuretics, steroids, fluid restriction, osmotic agents, etc.

SUGGESTED READINGS

1. Bruce DA, Gennarelli TA, Langfitt TW: Resuscitation from coma due to head injury. *Crit Care Med* 6(4):254–269, 1978.
2. Cooper PR, Moody S, Clark WK, et al: Dexamethasone and severe head injury. *J Neurosurg* 51:307–316, 1979.
3. Gudeman SK, Miller JD, Becker DP: Failure of high-dose steroid therapy to influence intracranial pressure in patients with severe head injury. *J Neurosurg* 51:301–306, 1979.
4. Hooshmand H, Dove J, Houff S, et al: Effects of diuretics and steroids on CSF pressure. *Arch Neurol* 21:499–509, 1969.
5. Marsh ML, Marshall LF, Shapiro HM: Neurosurgical intensive care. *Anesthesiology* 47:149–163, 1977.
6. Ropper AH, Kennedy SK, Zervas NT: *Neurological and neurosurgical intensive care*. Baltimore, University Park Press, 1983.
7. Wilkinson HA: Intracranial pressure monitoring. In Cooper PR (ed): *Head Injury*, Baltimore, Williams & Wilkins, pp 147–184, 1982.

30 Chest Trauma

MECHANISMS OF CHEST TRAUMA

Blunt chest trauma may produce pneumothorax, neurological dysfunction, respiratory failure, or cardiovascular instability. Our approach to such problems, which are common to a wide spectrum of critical illness, is detailed elsewhere (see Chapters 31, 29, 20, and 3, respectively). The current discussion focuses on those mechanical problems unique to blunt (non-penetrating) chest injury. Rib fractures, increased intracavitary pressures, and shear forces are the major mechanisms producing intrathoracic injury in blunt chest trauma.

Rib Fractures

During chest trauma older patients frequently sustain bony fractures that injure the lung perimeter. In contrast, the increased chest wall flexibility of younger patients tends to allow direct energy transfer to the intrathoracic organs, without rib breakage.

Rib fractures, the most common form of thoracic injury, usually occur in the mid-chest along the posterior axillary line (the point of maximal stress). The uppermost ribs are infrequently damaged because of their intrinsic strength and protection by the shoulder girdle and clavicle. Therefore, fractures of the upper ribs imply a very forceful blow and should raise concern regarding injury of the major airways or great vessels. On the other hand, the flexibility of the lowermost ribs makes them less prone to injury. Hence, fracture of the lower ribs suggests an unusually powerful regional impact and the possibility of concurrent splenic, hepatic, or renal injury. Aligned fractures of multiple ribs, *"curbstone fractures"*, usually result from striking a sharp edge. *"Cough fractures"* most frequently involve ribs 6–9 in the posterior axillary line. Although cough fractures produce significant pain, they are non-displaced

and difficult to detect. A bone scan is occasionally required for diagnosis.

Rib fractures often injure adjacent tissues. Displaced rib ends or fragments may cause lung laceration or contusion, pneumothorax, and hemothorax. Large hemothoraces can occur when intercostal vessels are disrupted. Pain associated with rib fractures frequently causes splinting, hypoventilation, secretion retention, and atelectasis—complications minimized by adequate narcotic analgesia or intercostal nerve blocks. Fractures of multiple ribs at two or more sites may produce a free-floating, unstabilized section of the chest wall known as a flail segment (see p. 259). Forceful displacement may also disrupt chondral attachments, producing a flail sternum.

Increased Intracavitary Pressures

Abrupt elevation of intracavitary pressures may rupture any air-filled or fluid-filled structure unbraced for the impact. Leak of oral/gastric secretions following *esophageal* rupture may result in mediastinitis or empyema. *Alveolar* rupture may cause pneumothorax, pneumomediastinum, or pulmonary hemorrhage. Sudden increases of intraabdominal pressure can rupture the *diaphragm*, herniating the abdominal contents into the chest. Unprotected by the liver, the left hemidiaphragm is at greatest risk. By a similar mechanism, a distended stomach or urinary bladder may also rupture when struck forcefully.

Shear Forces

To varying degrees, all intrathoracic structures are tethered to adjacent tissues. Consequently, shear forces produced by differential organ motion may cause visceral or vascular tears. Aortic rupture is the most serious injury produced by this mechanism. Tracheobronchial disruption may also result from deceleration-induced shearing.

Direct blows or rapid deceleration may tear pulmonary micro-vessels, causing pulmonary contusion. If the leak from these vessels is sufficient to form a discrete fluid collection, a pulmonary hematoma may form.

SPECIFIC CONDITIONS

Bronchial and Tracheal Disruptions

Fracture of the first two ribs and clavicle are the most common bony injuries associated with airway disruption. Hemoptysis, lung collapse, subcutaneous emphysema, or pneumothorax that fails to improve with tube thoracostomy may signal major airway disruption. (The occurrence of bilateral pneumothoraces following blunt trauma strongly suggests this possibility.) Most disruptions occur within 2 cm of the carina in the form of a spiral tear of the main bronchi or a longitudinal tear in the posterior membranous portion of the trachea. If disruption of a major bronchus is complete, the amputated lung can fall away from its normal hilar position to rest on the diaphragm and posterior chest wall.

Immediate recognition of airway disruption is important to avert the atelectasis, infection, and bronchial stenosis associated with delayed repair. Fiberoptic bronchoscopy allows its detection and facilitates selective intubation with a dual-lumen tube. On the affected side the inflatable cuff is positioned distal to the site of disruption. Partial disruption is often not detected until bronchial stenosis and atelectasis occur several weeks later. Because complete disruption is generally recognized earlier than partial disruption, it is associated with fewer long-term complications.

Hemothorax

Hemothorax is diagnosed when the hematocrit of pleural fluid exceeds 1%. Thoracentesis should confirm the diagnosis prior to chest tube placement. Indications for drainage include the presence of > 500 ml of blood in the chest or brisk ongoing hemorrhage into the pleural space.

Aortic tears or laceration or avulsion of intercostal or internal mammary vessels produce massive bleeding. Rib fractures, esophageal tears, and avulsion of periesophageal vessels frequently accompany large hemothoraces. If more than 1000 ml of blood are evacuated from the chest on the first tap or if there is continued bleeding of > 100 ml/hr, exploratory thoracotomy should be strongly considered. Tube thoracostomy drainage is satisfactory in most cases, but the natural course of an undrained hemothorax is highly variable. Large effusions are less likely to reabsorb spontaneously and therefore require drainage. However, the late complications of hemothorax (fibrothorax, empyema, and trapped lung) are not clearly prevented by early evacuation of pleural blood.

Pericardial Tamponade

Traumatic tamponade may be the result of aortic root disruption, coronary artery laceration, or rupture of the free ventricular wall. The diagnosis should be suspected when muffled heart sounds, hypotension, tachycardia, and elevated jugular pressure are noted. Echocardiography may support the diagnosis by showing pericardial fluid and/or diastolic collapse of the right atrium or ventricle. QRS alternans is highly suggestive. Right-heart catheterization confirms the diagnosis by demonstrating diastolic equalization of pressures throughout the cardiac chambers. Although needle aspiration of pericardial fluid is a worthwhile initial approach, trauma-induced tamponade usually requires surgical decompression ("drainage window") or pericardiectomy.

Cardiac Contusion

Cardiac contusion should be considered whenever a displaced or fractured sternum, multiple rib fractures, or a convincing history indicates a significant blow to the chest (e.g., high speed steering wheel injury). Common consequences of cardiac contusion include myocardial ischemia, arrhythmias, and conduction system defects (particularly heart block). Contusion may transiently produce output-impairing "stunned myocardium".

Elevated cardiac isoenzymes of creatinine phosphokinase (CPK) confirm the diagnosis. Although the electrocardiogram may demonstrate ST segment elevations that simulate myocardial infarction, reciprocal changes and Q waves are characteristically absent. Technetium pyrophosphate infarct scanning may reveal "hot" areas of myocardium in the contused region. The treatment of cardiac contusion is the same as that for acute myocardial infarction and includes close monitoring for arrhythmias, pump failure, and pericardial disease.

Aortic Disruption and Dissection

The aorta can withstand massive uniform elevations in transmural pressure (up to 2000 mmHg) but tolerates the shear forces of impact injuries much less well. Most aortic ruptures occur just distal to the ligamentum arteriosum. (In a minority of cases, disruption occurs at the aortic root just above the aortic valve.) When rupture of the ascending aorta occurs, damage to the aortic valve or coronary arteries is also possible.

Aortic disruption, a result of abrupt deceleration, is frequently fatal at the accident scene. Older patients are more likely to suffer aortic avulsion. No evidence of external trauma is present in many patients with fatal aortic rupture; rib or sternal fractures are not required for diagnosis. Clues to aortic disruption are similar to those for aortic aneurysm and include acute valvular insufficiency, hoarseness, dysphagia, carotid pulse differential, and arm-to-leg blood pressure differential. Typical chest pain penetrates to the intra-scapular region. Aortic disruption may present as a stroke syndrome if the carotid circulation is compromised.

Some radiographic clues to aortic aneurysm or disruption are illustrated in Figure 30.1. Angiography is more sensitive and specific than computed tomography (CT) scanning with contrast. Although possible, tears and disruptions of the pulmonary artery are rare without penetrating injury.

RADIOGRAPHIC SIGNS OF LEAKING AORTIC ANEURYSM

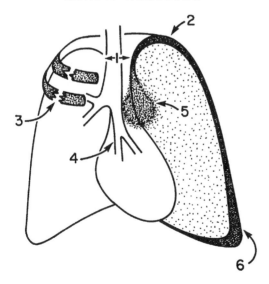

Figure 30.1 Radiographic clues to aortic disruption include: (1) mediastinal widening (best detected on upright films); (2) apical pleural capping; (3) fractures of the first two ribs or sternum; (4) depression of the left main bronchus; (5) indistinct aortic knob; and (6) pleural effusion (shown here for a supine exposure with "ground glass" appearance of left lung field).

Diaphragm Injuries

Blunt trauma may rupture the diaphragm, herniating the abdominal contents into the chest. Almost all such ruptures are left-sided, because the liver shields the right hemidiaphragm from direct injury. Major clues to diaphragmatic injury include a left-sided infiltrate or atelectasis, combined with signs and symptoms of bowel obstruction. Hearing bowel sounds above the diaphragm on physical examination or seeing air fluid levels above the diaphragm on radiograph are also suggestive. CT scanning or placement of contrast within the bowel may be confirmatory.

Flail Chest

Flail chest results from multiple contiguous fractures of bony ribs or cartilaginous attachments that dislodge a free-floating section of rib cage or sternum. Restrained by negative intrapleural forces, the floating segment lags during inspiration, producing an apparent "paradoxical motion" during forceful breathing. This instability may go unnoticed until vigorous efforts cause major swings in intrapleural pressure. Flail chest should be suspected in every patient with blunt chest trauma, particularly if rib fractures are evident. Whenever possible, a brief period of spontaneous breathing (5–10 breaths) should be observed to bring any flail segment to clinical attention.

A flail segment impairs normal coordinated action of the respiratory muscles and produces regional hypoventilation due to splinting and pain. Oxygen exchange is further impaired by underlying lung contusion and retained secretions. Although the work of breathing may be only modestly affected at low levels of ventilation, it rises dramatically during hyperpnea as breathing efficiency worsens. Because the sternum retains a relatively fixed position and is not located in a strategic position in relation to the ventilatory function of the rib cage, flail sternum is usually better tolerated than flail segments elsewhere.

In patients with extensive injury and ventilatory compromise, a high level of mechanical assistance may help to reduce fluctuations of intrapleural pressure for the 7–14 days needed to stabilize the chest wall. More than in most patients, it is important to minimize the minute ventilation requirement and ensure excellent bronchial hygiene to reduce the breathing workload before weaning is attempted. Taping, sandbagging, or other attempts at external chest wall stabilization do not significantly improve pain or ventilatory mechanics and may encourage atelectasis. Intercostal nerve blocks may reduce pain without impairing consciousness or ventilatory drive and thereby facilitate the weaning process.

Pulmonary Contusions

A forceful blow to the chest may contuse the lung at the site of impact or cause a contre-coup injury. In a sense, this condition may be thought of as localized tissue bleeding and edema, with the consequent ventilation/perfusion mismatching resulting in severe hypoxemia. Hemoptysis is common. Pulmonary contusion should be considered in all patients with ill-defined chest x-ray infiltrates and hypoxemia developing shortly after chest trauma, particularly when the radiographic abnormality is aligned with the known path of a forceful blow. Within 6 hours of trauma, pulmonary contusions are radiographically visible as localized nonsegmental infiltrates. Resolution begins within 24–48 hours of injury and is usually complete within 3–10 days. Pulmonary contusions tend to be less severe in the obese because of decreased energy transfer to the lung underlying the thickened chest wall.

Occasionally, pulmonary contusions coalesce to form a *pulmonary hematoma* that typically appears as a spherical 1–6 cm density. A pulmonary hematoma is a large pocket of blood located deep within the pulmonary parenchyma. Hematomas arise from significant vascular disruption and may require weeks or months to clear. Resolution is often incomplete, leaving a permanent scar deep within the lung.

Esophageal Rupture (Boerhaave's Syndrome)

Esophageal rupture (ER) should be suspected in patients with a history of major chest trauma and a pleural effusion, especially if it is left-sided or accompanied by pneumothorax. Empyema following blunt chest trauma should suggest the possibility of esophageal or diaphragmatic rupture with subsequent bacterial contamination of the pleural space. Although interscapular, substernal, or epigastric pains are common, fever, hypotension, a rapidly evolving pneumothorax, or a pleural effusion may be the only manifestation. Thoracentesis may be highly suggestive of ER. The diagnosis may be confirmed by aspirating food particles from the pleural space. A marked elevation of pleural fluid amylase is often present, a result of leakage of salivary amylase into the pleural space.

The mortality of untreated ER, a highly lethal problem, approaches 2% per hour. Mediastinitis is the most frequent cause of death, fatal in almost ½ of patients within the first day. Chest radiographs demonstrate mediastinal widening and gas in the mediastinum or pleural space. Extravasation of swallowed contrast material into the mediastinum or pleural space confirms the diagnosis. Surprisingly, endoscopy is frequently unrevealing, and CT scan may only suggest the problem by demonstrating fluid with or without gas in the pleural space and mediastinum.

Fat Embolism

The fat embolism syndrome (FES) may occur 1 hour to 3 days after trauma. Although FES is usually associated with multiple long bone or pelvic fractures, diabetes, fatty liver, pancreatitis, joint surgery, and sickle cell anemia are reported causes. It is theorized that injury is produced when lipases hydrolyze neutral triglycerides to liberate unsaturated fatty acids toxic to the lung parenchyma. Fat confined to the pulmonary circulation may precipitate diffuse coagulopathy and clinical disseminated intravascular coagulation (DIC). Fat microglobules may even pass through the pulmonary capillary bed to enter the systemic circuit and produce characteristic retinal, central nervous system, and skin lesions.

A triad of *confusion*, *pulmonary dysfunction*, and *skin abnormalities* characterize this disorder. Frequent symptoms include cough, dyspnea, and pleuritic chest pain. These are often accompanied by physical findings of fever, rales, tachypnea, and disorientation. Although a petechial rash over the upper torso may be present in the full-blown syndrome, it is unusual in less obvious cases. Serum and urine lipase levels may be elevated, and fat globules can sometimes be found in the urine, sputum, or bronchial lavage fluid. Retinal fat emboli may also be seen. Initially the chest x-ray is normal in a large percentage of patients, despite severely impaired gas exchange. Decreased lung compliance, impaired diffusing capacity, hypoxemia, and respiratory alkalosis are common respiratory manifestations. In cases of FES-induced adult respiratory distress syndrome (ARDS) infiltrates may require 1–4 weeks to resolve.

Lung Torsion

Lung torsion is an uncommon result of severe chest trauma that forces the lung to rotate on its hilar axis. A radiographic clue is reversal of the normal pattern of bronchovascular markings, with the major pulmonary vessels coursing cephalad rather than caudad. "Ground glass" opacification of the affected hemithorax may accompany this pattern, due to vascular congestion, edema and atelectasis in the affected lung. Torsion must be surgically reversed to avoid infarction or gangrene.

SUGGESTED READINGS

1. Kirsh MM, Sloan H: *Blunt Chest Trauma: General Principles of Management*. Boston, Little, Brown, 1977.
2. Majeski JA: Management of flail chest after blunt trauma. *South Med J* 74(7):848–849, 1981.
3. Rothstein RJ: Myocardial contusion. *JAMA* 250(16):2189–2191, 1983.

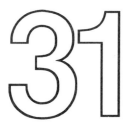

Pneumothorax and Barotrauma

ETIOLOGY OF BAROTRAUMA

The varied forms of pulmonary barotrauma—interstitial emphysema, pneumomediastinum, pneumoperitoneum, subcutaneous emphysema, cyst formation, and pneumothorax (PTX)—are prominent among the iatrogenic causes of critical illness. Although PTX may arise from such diverse medical problems as pulmonary infarction, eosinophilic granuloma, or spontaneous rupture, a confined set of etiologies causes most problems in the intensive care unit: *pleural puncture*, *lung necrosis*, and *ventilator barotrauma*.

Missiles, sharp instruments, and displaced rib fractures cause PTX by direct puncture of the visceral pleura. Pneumothorax may complicate any medical procedure in which a needle enters the thorax, especially thoracentesis, pleural biopsy, transthoracic aspiration of a pulmonary mass, and central line placement. Precise single punctures of the lung are less likely to cause problems than multiple punctures or slashing actions of the bevel of the needle. Disruption of the visceral pleura and PTX may follow necrotizing pulmonary infection.

Although direct rupture of the visceral pleura undoubtedly occurs in some patients, the barotrauma that complicates mechanical ventilation frequently develops by a more circuitous mechanism. Rupture of weakened alveolar tissues is particularly likely to occur in "non-partitional" or "marginal" alveoli which have bases that abut on vessels, bronchioles, or fibrous septae. During positive pressure ventilation (or severe blunt chest injury that occurs with the glottis closed), alveolar pressures rise more than interstitial pressures, allowing pressure gradients to develop between marginal alveoli and the contiguous perivascular connective tissue. If rupture occurs, extravasated gas follows a pressure gradient down the path of least resistance, tracking along the perivascular sheaths toward the hilum. The *interstitial emphysema* produced en route may be detected against the radiopaque background of infiltrated lung as lucent streaks and small cysts that do not correspond to the bronchial anatomy. The gas continues to track centrally, forming a *pneumomediastinum* which may or may not be radiographically evident. In the absence of pre-existing mediastinal pathology, gas freely dissects along fascial planes, usually decompressing into the soft tissues of the neck (*subcutaneous emphysema*) or retroperitoneum (*pneumoperitoneum*). *PTX* occurs in a minority of such cases (perhaps 20–30%) when soft tissue gas ruptures into the pleural space via an interrupted or weakened mediastinal pleural membrane. Interstitial emphysema, pneumomediastinum and subcutaneous emphysema have little hemodynamic significance and seldom affect gas exchange in adult patients. However, because their presence signals alveolar rupture and the potential for PTX, these signs are important to detect in the ventilated patient.

Pressure gradients usually favor decompression of interstitial gas into the mediastinum. However, when normal bronchovascular channels are blocked, gas accumulates locally or migrates distally to produce *subpleural air cysts* that compress parenchymal vessels, create deadspace, increase the ventilatory requirement, and cause major problems for ventilation-perfusion matching. The development of *cystic barotrauma* is a common and omnious finding that usually presages tension PTX occurring a short time afterward. Two other forms of barotrauma, bronchopulmonary dysplasia and systemic gas embolism, have been described as complications of mechanical ventilation in infants, but not in adults.

PATHOPHYSIOLOGIC CONSIDERATIONS

Parenchymal Injury and Cystic Barotrauma

Widespread cystic barotrauma (CB) is most likely to develop in young patients with necrotizing pneumonitis, small airway narrowing, and retained secretions. Alveolar rupture and focal gas trapping are key to its pathogenesis. As predicted by the Law of Laplace ($P = 2T/R$) the pressure (P) required to maintain a fixed tension (T) in the wall of a spherical structure falls as its radius (R) increases. Therefore, it is not uncommon for a cyst created by positive pressure to grow quickly to a large dimension (> 10 cm diameter).

Once underway, CB tends to be pernicious and self re-inforcing. As cysts develop, they compress normal lung tissue, stiffening the lung and increasing the airway pressure needed for effective ventilation. Furthermore, blood flow diverts away from areas of cyst expansion, creating deadspace that increases the ventilatory requirement and mean alveolar pressure. Increased peak and mean ventilatory pressures accentuate the tendency for further lung damage, while higher requirements for alveolar ventilation tend to keep the patient ventilator-dependent. Secretion management, treatment of infection, and, most importantly, reduction of airway pressure are fundamental to effective management.

Uncomplicated PTX

Ordinarily, the visceral and parietal pleurae are closely approximated during all phases of the respiratory cycle. The negative pressure between them is maintained by the joint tendencies of the chest wall to expand and the lung to recoil to their natural resting volumes. At equilibrium, these opposing forces create a small negative pleural pressure. *PTX disrupts the normal relationship of the lung to chest wall.* The lung collapses toward its resting volume, which occurs below residual volume at ambient surface pressure. Simultaneously, PTX allows the chest wall to expand toward its unstressed volume, which occurs at approximately 60% of the normal vital capacity. The natural tendency of the chest wall to expand—"the counter-springing effect"—is diminished or lost when thoracic volume increases. *Coupling between the lung and chest wall is impaired* by the gas buffer separating them. Outward migration of the chest wall places the bellows at a *mechanical disadvantage.* Expansion of the chest wall shortens the resting length of the inspiratory muscles, placing them on a less advantageous portion of their length-tension relationship. Less obviously, the total force developed by the muscles of the chest wall normally distributes over a larger surface area than that offered by the collapsed lung. Therefore, even if the inspiratory muscles generate the same intrapleural pressure, the total force applied to the lung is reduced, in proportion to the degree of lung collapse.

As tidal excursions of the unaffected lung increase to maintain ventilation, elastic and flow resistive work increase. This increase is well tolerated by healthy patients with adequate ventilatory reserve. However, those with significant airflow obstruction, neuromuscular weakness, or parenchymal restriction may experience dyspnea, progressive hypoventilation, and respiratory acidosis.

Tension Pneumothorax

The term "tension PTX" implies sustained positivity of pleural pressure. A tension component occasionally develops when a ball valve mechanism pumps air into the pleural cavity during spontaneous breathing, but *it is much more common when positive pressure provides the ventilatory power.* Positive intrapleural pressure expands the ipsilateral chest cage, rendering the muscles less efficient generators of pleural pressure. Contralateral pleural pressure tends to be maintained near normal levels until late in the process. However, a shifting mediastinum may encroach on the contralateral hemithorax, compromising lung expansion. Eventually, rising pleural and central venous pressures impede venous return sufficiently to cause *cardiovascular deterioration.*

Vigorous inspiratory efforts tend to maintain intrapleural pressure (averaged for both lungs over the entire respiratory cycle) at near normal levels until the patient fatigues or receives increased machine assistance. Then, abrupt cardiovascular deterioration may occur as mean pleural pressure rises sharply. Such considerations explain why so many patients who develop pneumothoraces while *mechanically ventilated show a tension component* and why ventilated patients with PTX who receive sedating or paralytic drugs frequently experience abrupt hemodynamic deterioration. In the non-intubated patient, muscle fatigue and *respiratory arrest may precede the cardiovascular collapse* classically described with the tension PTX syndrome. It should be emphasized that tension can develop without major volume loss.

RISK FACTORS FOR BAROTRAUMA

Although the peak airway cycling pressure has frequently been cited as the most important risk factor for ventilator-related barotrauma (VB), it is clearly not the only one (Table 31.1). A necrotizing parenchymal process, non-homogeneity of lung pathology, young age, excessive airway secretions, and duration of positive pressure ventilation

Table 31.1
Predispositions to Barotrauma

Necrotizing lung pathology	Peak cycling pressure
	Mean alveolar pressure
Secretion retention	Minute ventilation
Young age	requirement
Duration of ventilation	Non-homogeneous parenchymal disease

are major predispositions. The process of alveolar rupture is one that appears to require sustained hyperexpansion of fragile alveoli. Therefore, the *mean alveolar pressure*, averaged over an entire respiratory cycle, may be an important factor. As major determinants of mean alveolar pressure, *minute ventilation requirement and positive end-expiratory pressure (PEEP)* contribute greatly to the PTX hazard.

Notwithstanding these considerations, *peak dynamic (P_D) and static (P_S) airway pressures* appear to contribute most significantly to VB. P_D can be reduced by improving lung compliance, reducing tidal volume (V_T) or PEEP, lowering airflow resistance, or slowing peak inspiratory flow rate. On first consideration it might seem that P_S (the pressure that in conjunction with thoracic compliance determines overall lung volume and alveolar stretch) should correlate even more closely with PTX than P_D. However, although P_S does bear a strong relationship to PTX, it should be kept in mind that airway resistance varies greatly among the bronchial channels of a non-homogeneously affected lung, so that increasing the dynamic pressure within the central airway may encourage regional over-distention and alveolar rupture in channels with open pathways to weakened alveoli. Therefore, raising the peak flow rate is not risk free. On the other hand, slowing the rate of inspiratory flow prolongs alveolar distention, increasing mean alveolar pressure. This is especially true in patients with critical airflow obstruction. Improving airway resistance or lung compliance and reducing V_T and PEEP are preferable methods for lowering P_D.

As a general rule, high peak pressures applied to a stiff lung cause less alveolar stretch than the same pressures applied to a compliant lung. Yet, the inherent susceptibility of lung tissue to rupture and the degree of regional inhomogeneity play crucial roles. Largely for these reasons, there does not seem to be a sharp threshold value of peak ventilator cycling pressure below which VB does not occur. Nevertheless, as a rough rule of thumb,

PTX becomes much more likely at peak ventilator cycling pressures > 40 cmH_2O.

Secretion accumulation, blood clots, or foreign objects can increase the degree of non-homogeneity or create ball-valve phenomena that exacerbate the risk of VB. The crucial role of inhomogeneity of lung injury in producing VB may explain why *PTX tends to develop 1–3 weeks after diffuse lung injury*, a time when some regions are healing while others remain intensely inflamed.

DIAGNOSIS OF PNEUMOTHORAX

Clinical Features

Early recognition of PTX is of paramount importance in patients ventilated with positive pressure because of their proclivity to develop tension. During episodes of acute clinical deterioration compatible with PTX the risk of mortality rises when physicians delay intervention, awaiting roentgenographic confirmation. Pleuritic chest pain, dyspnea, and anxiety comprise the most common symptoms of uncomplicated PTX. Symptoms indicative of other forms of extra-alveolar air that may precede PTX include transient precordial chest discomfort, neck pain, dysphagia, and abdominal pain. These nonspecific symptoms are often transient. *Tension PTX frequently presents with tachypnea, respiratory distress, tachycardia, diaphoresis, cyanosis, or agitation.*

In mechanically ventilated patients the airway manometer usually (but not always) shows increased peak inspiratory airway pressures, especially if tension is present, and the calculated compliance of the respiratory system usually falls from previous values. Volume cycled ventilators may "pressure-limit" or "pop-off", resulting in ineffective ventilation. Close examination of the affected hemithorax often reveals signs of hyperexpansion, with unilateral hyperresonance, diminished ventilatory excursion, and reduced breath sounds on the affected side. The examination must be performed carefully; *massive atelectasis can present a similar clinical picture, simulating PTX on the contralateral side.* Palpation of the pericervical tissues and suprasternal notch is important to detect subcutaneous emphysema or a *trachea deviated away from the side of tension.* Tension is reflected in elevations of central venous, right atrial, and pulmonary arterial pressures. Such hemodynamic changes do not generally occur during atelectasis.

Radiographic Signs of Barotrauma

Extra-alveolar Gas

Extra-alveolar air in the lung parenchyma can manifest as interstitial emphysema or as subpleural air cysts. Both are easiest to detect when the parenchyma is densely infiltrated. Sharp black lines that outline the heart, great vessels, trachea, inferior pulmonary ligament, or diaphragm suggest mediastinal emphysema, even when the pleural membrane itself cannot be visualized (Fig. 31.1).

The *"complete diaphragm"* sign indicates that the heart is separated from the diaphragm by a cushion of air. Subcutaneous emphysema, subdiaphragmatic air, and pneumoperitoneum are other manifestations of barotrauma that may precede or coexist with PTX. *Subpleural air cysts are commonly seen in basilar regions.*

Pneumothorax

The radiographic signs of PTX are detailed elsewhere in this volume (see Chapter 10, Radiology in the Intensive Care Unit). A number of points deserve emphasis here, however. A smooth, two-sided visceral pleural line is roentgenographically diagnostic but must be distinguished from skin folds and other artifacts at the skin surface. A pleural line may be particularly difficult to detect on a standard supine view if pleural air loculates anteriorly or if ribs or mediastinal vessels obscure the pleural margin. Two useful markers of occult PTX visible on supine films are the *"deep sulcus"*

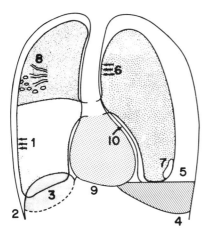

Figure 31.1 Radiographic signs of barotrauma: 1) visible visceral pleural line; 2) deep sulcus sign; 3) hyperlucency localized to the upper abdomen; 4) inverted hemidiaphragm; 5) air-fluid level; 6) mediastinal shift; 7) subpleural air cyst; 8) interstitial emphysema; 9) complete diaphragm; and 10) pneumomediastinum.

sign and *hyperlucency centered over the ipsilateral abdominal upper quadrant*. A lateral *decubitus view* allows air to collect along the upper margin of the hemithorax, facilitating visualization. An *expiratory chest film* may also prove revealing. (Although the volume of intrapleural air remains constant, it occupies a greater percentage of the available space as the volume of the thoracic cage decreases.)

PTX under tension can be strongly suspected from a single film when *diaphragmatic inversion* or *extreme mediastinal shift* occur. A sequence of films demonstrating progressive migration of the mediastinal contents into the contralateral hemithorax secures the diagnosis. It should be emphasized that *life-threatening tension can exist without complete lung collapse or mediastinal displacement* if the lung adheres to the pleura, the lung is densely infiltrated, the airway is obstructed, or the mediastinum is immobilized by infection, fibrosis, or previous surgery. It should be emphasized that the mere presence of a *chest tube may not prevent tension* if the tube is nonfunctional, the space drained is loculated, or intraparenchymal tension cysts coexist.

MANAGEMENT OF PNEUMOTHORAX

General Principles

Recent studies indicate that pulmonary barotrauma developing in the setting of acute lung injury is a self-perpetuating, auto-amplifying, and highly lethal process that must be prevented. Once extra-alveolar air begins to manifest in its cystic form, impaired gas exchange often forces an increase in minute ventilation requirement and therefore in mean airway pressure. In time, higher mean airway pressure worsens the tendency for alveolar rupture. The key interventions aimed at avoiding barotrauma are:

1. *Treat the underlying disease*, especially suppurative processes.
2. *Maintain excellent bronchial hygiene* but minimize unnecessary coughing.
3. *Reduce the minute ventilation requirement* by treating agitation, fever, metabolic acidosis, and bronchospasm. Some physicians advocate deliberate hypoventilation achieved by sedation (or paralysis). If necessary, respiratory acidemia can be counterbalanced by an infusion of bicarbonate.
4. *Reduce peak and mean airway pressures* by limiting PEEP and tidal volume and by increasing the percentage of spontaneous versus ma-

chine-aided breaths (i.e., reduce the number of ventilator breaths given during synchronized intermittent mandatory ventilation, SIMV). Ventilator settings for tidal volume should be varied, peak pressures measured, and thoracic compliance calculated. During volume-cycled ventilation reducing tidal volume by 100–500 ml may greatly reduce P_D and P_S. Peak flow should be set to the lowest value that satisfies inspiratory demand without incurring additional patient work, thus lowering peak dynamic (but not peak static or mean alveolar) pressure. Although several new modes of ventilation have been advocated to reduce peak airway pressure (high frequency, pressure-supported and pressure-controlled ventilation), these forms of positive pressure ventilation do little to alter *mean airway pressure*, and their therapeutic efficacy in preventing VB is currently unknown.

Preventing Ventilator-Related Barotrauma

Minimize minute ventilation ($\dot{V}_E$)	Normalize lung compliance
Minimize PEEP	Improve chest wall compliance
Use lower V_T	Encourage spontaneous breathing
Decrease I:E	
Decrease bronchial obstruction	
Use newer modes of ventilation (?)	

Chest Tube Drainage

Indications for Thoracostomy

Vigilant observation and conservative management are appropriate options in the spontaneously breathing, uncompromised patient with a *small* PTX. Simple observation is frequently a useful strategy for well-compensated patients who experience PTX after thoracentesis, aspiration needle biopsy, or central line placement. A substantial fraction of such patients will not require more aggressive management. Serial radiographs must demonstrate gradual improvement. An air collection that fails to show convincing improvement over several days may indicate an unresolved process, with equilibration between the rates of leakage and absorption. However, spontaneous resolution of PTX is a slow process. Once leakage stops, the absorption of intrapleural air occurs at a variable rate, averaging approximately 1.5% of the hemithorax volume each day. Even a moderate PTX may take weeks to resolve. During this period the partially

collapsed lung clears secretions poorly. *Large collections of undrained pleural air predispose to infection* of the lung or pleural space, to fibrosis, and to the formation of a restrictive outer shell.

PTX is particularly dangerous in the mechanically ventilated patient. The high risk of tension mandates early decompression. Other patients to consider for early intervention are those with ipsilateral lung infection or secretion retention, ventilatory insufficiency, or high ventilatory requirements.

Tube Options

The ideal chest tube system provides a reliable, low impedance conduit that ensures unidirectional flow of gas and liquid from the chest. It should restore the normal sub-atmospheric intrapleural pressure and reapproximate pleural surfaces. To be in *best position for drainage of unloculated air*, the tube should be directed *superiorly and anteriorly*. Small tubes can be introduced anteriorly in the second intercostal space. Larger tubes are best introduced laterally and directed upward. *When the pneumothorax is evenly distributed and suction is used, actual position of the tube tip makes little difference*. However, if loculations develop, a poorly placed chest tube, especially one not connected to suction, may fail to evacuate the appropriate area.

Although large tubes are usually needed to drain substantial collections of fluid, chest tubes placed for simple air drainage are usually 28 F in caliber, or smaller. Iatrogenic pneumothoraces without major airleak can often be managed in stable patients with short flexible tubes of very small diameter. One example, the McSwain Dart, can be attached to a lightweight flutter valve (Heimlich valve) to facilitate the mobility of ambulatory patients. Such small catheters can be introduced with minimal patient discomfort. Larger tubes are selected if liquid drainage is needed. Tube radius is a major determinant of the evacuation capability of the system. However, unless the tube caliber is very small, or the leak very large, system resistance does not usually limit evacuation. (*Tube placement and patency are much more important.*)

Drainage Apparatus

One-way drainage is usually provided by a water seal (Fig. 31.2). A collection column (or bottle) may be inserted in tandem and proximal to the water seal column, or one ''bottle'' may serve both functions. In the traditional ''one bottle'' system, accumulated liquid drainage makes air leakage difficult to visualize and, more importantly, may cre-

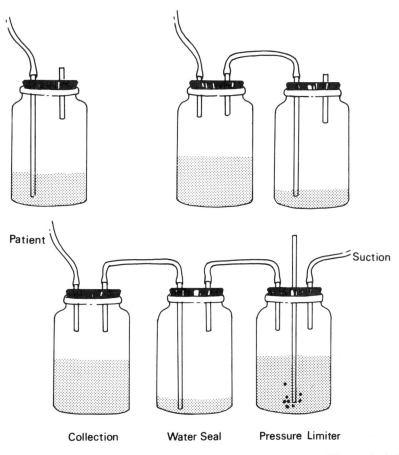

Patient

Suction

Collection   Water Seal   Pressure Limiter

Figure 31.2 Schematic diagram of one-, two-, and three-bottle drainage systems. When a single bottle is used both to collect fluid drainage and to provide the "water seal", compensation must be made for the rising liquid level. Otherwise, there will be increasing back pressure as the tube submerges. Furthermore, foaming will occur as air bubbles through proteinaceous liquid. Separation of collection and water seal functions obviate these problems. The addition of a third "pressure-limiting" bottle enables the application of a safe, constant level of suction from any vacuum source. (A controlled pressure pump fulfills this function in a two-bottle system.)

ate sufficent back-pressure to hinder lung expansion. Adjustment of applied suction or periodic liquid removal can obviate this problem. The vertical distance separating the thoracostomy incision and the liquid level must be sufficient to prevent suction of liquid into the pleural space during vigorous inspiratory efforts. Because maximal static inspiratory forces may approach -100 cmH$_2$O within the pleural space, a 1-meter vertical separation is appropriate when suction is not applied, as during transport. To avoid back pressure, the end of the water seal tube should be placed no deeper than 2 cm beneath the fluid surface.

Monitoring Tube Function

Fluid movements in the water seal tube reflect tidal variations in *regional* intrapleural pressure.

In the spontaneously breathing patient fluid rises in inspiration and falls during exhalation. The reverse is true during passive inflation with intermittent positive pressure. The direction of tidal fluctuations during triggered machine cycles varies with the vigor of the respiratory effort. The degree of fluctuation of the water seal without suction applied *("tidaling")* can provide useful clinical information. (Tidal fluctuations are generally smaller during suction.) An abrupt increase in tidaling suggests undrained air, lobar atelectasis, upper airway obstruction, impaired secretion clearance, or hyperpnea. Decreased fluctuation can reflect resolution of any of these problems, partial outflow obstruction (e.g., by fluid in a dependent loop of tubing), or decreased air leakage through a bronchopleural fistula. Absent fluctuations may be due to tube obstruction by fibrin, blood clots, or extrinsic compression.

Because of the risks of infection the chest tube should be removed as soon as it no longer fulfills a useful function. Because 25–50 ml of liquid will drain each day from the normal pleural space, drainage of this amount is expected through a functioning tube. There should be noticeable fluctuations during respiratory efforts. A "dead tube" (< 50 ml/24 hr of drainage, no gas leak, and no respiratory fluctuation) should be pulled. Another tube should then be placed if the need for drainage is still apparent radiographically. If the water seal level rises and ceases to fluctuate with respiration after several days of declining drainage, pleural re-apposition has likely occurred, and the tube should be removed after x-ray confirmation. The rising level reflects sealing of the air leak and subsequent reabsorption of the air contained within the chest tube. If the liquid column remains patent, fluid will rise until negative pressure within the gas filled lumen offsets the hydrostatic column.

Persistent bubbling at the water seal signals an airleak within the lung or tubing connections. If the leak is within the lung, its magnitude can be quantified during mechanical ventilation by comparing the inspiratory volume delivered by a machine cycle to the exhaled tidal volume. (Some drainage systems also provide crude flow detectors.) If the inspired and expired volumes are equivalent, air leakage is likely to originate external to the lung. Cessation of the air leak when the tube is clamped near the chest wall indicates a *bronchopleural fistula* or air entry at the incision site. The latter can be excluded by careful approximation of the skin edges and the application of airtight occlusive dressings. If the leak does not stop after occlusion near the chest wall, there has been a breach of system integrity. Migratory (transient) clamping of the tubing (moving away from the patient) will then allow localization. All connection sites should be inspected with special care.

Indications for Suction

In certain clinical situations natural pressure gradients (fluid siphon effects, expiratory contractions) may be adequate to empty the pleural space of gas and liquid. However, *suction may be needed for large air leaks or for drainage of viscous or clotting fluids.* When the lung is surrounded by gas, pressure applied to one portion of the pleural surface distributes equally throughout the hemithorax. However, when normal pleural surfaces are approximated, the negative pressure applied to

one area transmits poorly to other regions. The explanation is that lung tissues adjacent to the tube effectively isolate a pocket of negative pressure. In addition, tissue may be drawn into the "eyes" of the tube, preventing generalization of applied pressure. When this happens increasing suction only increases the risk for local tissue injury. Adhesion-related loculation may also impede pressure transmission. In this instance multiple tubes in different locations may be required. Suction can usually be discontinued (but water seal continued) when bubbling stops. The tube itself can be safely removed after 24–48 hours of additional observation, provided that no air leakage occurs during coughing and a PTX is not visible radiographically. *Some physicians advise keeping a functioning chest tube in place as long as the patient receives positive pressure ventilation.*

Suction Systems

Two common mechanisms regulate safe levels of suction pressure. The Emerson suction generator links a servomechanism to a fan. A high-capacity, low-impedance system, it is capable of maintaining essentially constant negative pressure at flow rates up to 40 l/min. If power is interrupted, air escaping from a bronchopleural fistula can vent between the fan blades, preventing tension. If increased gas leakage develops in the system, the servomechanism increases the evacuation rate in an attempt to maintain constant pressure. It is important to recognize, however, that *pressure is sensed within the apparatus itself*, and the manometer will continue to register a substantial level of negative pressure, even if the pump becomes completely disconnected from the patient. As recommended by the manufacturer, the collection and water seal functions are combined—a setup that protects the motor but causes problems when there is substantial liquid drainage.

Several commercially available units incorporate a pressure regulated "three bottle" system in a single molded plastic container. A third chamber added in series to the fluid collection and water seal columns serves as a pressure governor, modulating excessive wall suction pressures (− 80 to − 200 cmH$_2$O) to the desired level (typically < 30 cmH$_2$O). The filling level of the vacuum control tube determines and limits the degree of applied suction. Suction is increased until continuous bubbling occurs in the control chamber, indicating that sufficient negative pressure has been applied to the water surface to offset the hydrostatic column. *Continuous bubbling in the control chamber must be maintained* throughout the respiratory cycle to ensure the desired level of suction. Increasing the applied vacuum then serves only to increase fluid perturbations in the suction control bottle, leaving unaffected the suction applied to the pleural space. The *magnitude of bronchopleural air leakage must be gauged from the water seal column.* If the delivered wall suction abruptly increases, air will rush from the atmosphere through the suction control straw, preventing transmission of the increase to the pleural space. A fail-safe mechanism (a positive pressure pop-off valve, ≃ 2 cmH₂O) must be provided to open the pressure control chamber to atmosphere when suction is disconnected. Otherwise, the water column developed within the control tube would impede egress of air from the pleural space.

Three easily remediable problems commonly cause failure to deliver the desired level of negative pressure: fluid accumulation in the water seal chamber (common with Emerson pump), evaporation from the pressure-limiting tube of a three-bottle system, and the development of a fluid-filled dependent loop (Figure 31.3).

SPECIAL PROBLEMS OF BAROTRAUMA

Extensive Subcutaneous Emphysema

A small amount of subcutaneous emphysema is frequently palpable about the chest tube entrance site. However, extensive unilateral emphysema suggests focal accumulation of air under pressure near the thoracostomy wound. Forced exhalation, straining, and coughing tend to drive gas into soft tissues. Extensive subcutaneous emphysema usually indicates inadequate evacuation of a large airleak and should prompt careful examination for problems that might decrease system efficiency. In the absence of these, management options include increasing suction pressure, changing to an evacuation system with greater capability (e.g., Emerson suction generator), readjusting tube position, or placing a second chest tube to diminish the impedance to pleural emptying.

Persistent Bronchopleural Fistula

Unresolving airleaks commonly occur after rupture of emphysematous blebs, after subtotal pulmonary resection, and during ventilator treatment of adult respiratory distress syndrome (ARDS). In the latter setting, the development of a bronchopleural fistula (BPF) portends a very poor prognosis for survival, largely because BPF is a marker of underlying disease severity. Adequate gas exchange can usually be maintained by conventional ventilator adjustments or by one of the techniques outlined below. Interestingly, *the effluent from BPF contains CO₂.* Although the ''flow-through'' ventilation provided by the fistula is less efficient than tidal breathing, the gas that exits the fistula has participated in gas exchange and is not entirely ''wasted''. For this reason effective tidal volume is somewhat greater than that measured from the exhalation line of the ventilator circuit.

Routine Management

A large body of clinical data suggests that approximating the visceral and parietal pleura facil-

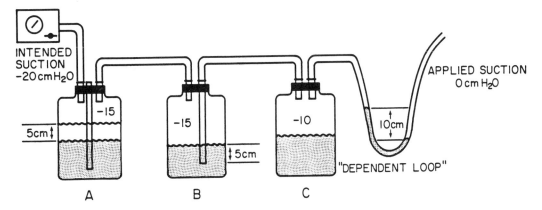

Figure 31.3 Factors contributing to failure of applied suction. An intended suction pressure of −20 cmH₂O applied in a three-bottle system can be attenuated by evaporation of water from the pressure-limiter bottle, by submersion of the water seal tube below the appropriate level of 1–2 cm, and by the presence of liquid in a dependent loop of connecting tubing.

itates healing of pleural rents. The initial approach to management may include tube re-positioning and/or a trial of increased suction in an attempt to appose the pleural surfaces more tightly. However, in certain situations excess suction may perpetuate flow through the fistula by increasing the pressure gradient between the airway and pleural space. If increasing suction fails, lowering or removing the suction may in rare instances promote healing by relieving tension on the margins of the tear. Increased lung collapse may compromise gas exchange, however.

Specialized Techniques

Management of a life-threatening air leak in the mechanically ventilated patient can prove very difficult. Several techniques have been described for modifying the apparatus, either to prevent flow through the chest tube during inspiration or to maintain a common level of PEEP in the airway and the affected pleural space. In some instances independent lung ventilation may be necessary. A few studies conducted primarily in children suggest that high-frequency ventilation (HFV) is associated with a lower incidence of barotrauma. However, although *HFV is occasionally helpful in adults*, it is not generally an attractive or effective option for management of severe lung injury.

After several weeks of observation and manipulation of the drainage system, surgical intervention may be considered, especially in less critically ill patients with cystic or bullous lung disease. Primary suturing or stapling of the injured area and pleural abrasion usually suffice. In the case of large fistulas, direct tamponade by a pedicle flap or tissue resection may be needed. Chemical pleurodesis with tetracycline has been successfully used as an alternative to surgical intervention, but this treatment must be considered hazardous until more information is available. Attempts at chemical sclerosis are seldom successful unless performed

with meticulous technique. Closure is unlikely to be achieved in the presence of multiple adhesions, large air leaks, or inability to appose the pleural surfaces.

SUGGESTED READINGS

1. Albelda SM, Gefter WB, Kelley MA, et al: Ventilator-induced subpleural air cysts: clinical, radiographic, and pathologic significance. *Am Rev Respir Dis* 127:360–365, 1983.
2. Batchelder TL, Morris KA: Critical factors in determining adequate pleural drainage in both the operated and non-operated chest. *Am Surgeon* 28:296–302, 1962.
3. Christman BW, Marini JJ: Pneumothorax and barotrauma: diagnosis and management. *Pulm Clin Update* 1(4):1–8, 1985.
4. Duncan C, Erickson R: Pressures associated with chest tube stripping. *Heart Lung* 11:166, 1982.
5. Macklin MT, Macklin CC: Malignant interstitial emphysema of the lungs and mediastinum as an important occult complication in many respiratory diseases and other conditions: an interpretation of the clinical literature in the light of laboratory experiment. *Medicine* 23:281–358, 1944.
6. Marini JJ: Chest tubes. In *Respiratory Medicine for the House Officer*, Baltimore, Williams & Wilkins, ed. 2, pp 62–70, 1987.
7. Petersen GW, Baier H: Incidence of pulmonary barotrauma in a medical ICU. *Crit Care Med* 11(2):67–69, 1983.
8. Pierson DJ, Horton CA, Bates PW: Persistent bronchopleural air leak during mechanical ventilation. *Chest* 90(3):321–323, 1986.
9. Powner DJ, Grenvik A: Ventilatory management of life-threatening bronchopleural fistulae—a summary. *Crit Care Med* 9:54–58, 1981.
10. Rohlfing BM, Webb WR, Schlobohm RM: Ventilator-related extra alveolar air in adults. *Radiology* 121:25–31, 1976.
11. Rothberg AD, Marks KH, Maisels MJ: Understanding the pleurevac. *Pediatrics* 67:482–484, 1981.
12. Steier M, Chung N, Roberts EB, Nealon TF: Pneumothorax complicating continuous ventilatory support. *J Thorac Cardiovasc Surgery* 67:17–23, 1974.
13. Woodring JH: Pulmonary interstitial emphysema in the adult respiratory distress syndrome. *Crit Care Med* 13(10):786–791, 1985.

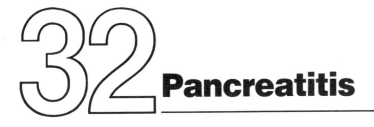

32 Pancreatitis

CAUSES AND PATHOPHYSIOLOGY

Cytotoxic effects of alcohol and gallstone-induced reflux of bile into the pancreatic duct account for 80% of all cases of acute pancreatitis (APT). Other causes include trauma, tumors, medications, electrolyte disturbances, toxins, infections, and surgery.

Gallstones causing APT usually impact at the ampulla of Vater. About ½ of all patients with gallstone pancreatitis have concurrent biliary tract infection (cholangitis), a complication that heightens mortality. Two-thirds of patients with gallstone pancreatitis who do not undergo stone removal experience recurrence. Tumors of the pancreas and common bile duct or ampullary stenosis following biliary tract surgery may also obstruct the free flow of bile.

Visualization of the pancreatic duct by endoscopic retrograde cholangio-pancreatography (ERCP) reveals structural abnormalities in many cases of recurrent APT of obscure etiology. The ERCP procedure itself may elevate serum amylase in as many as 60% of patients; however, the majority of these are asymptomatic.

Ethanol leads the list of toxins and medications that commonly cause APT. Other direct pancreatic toxins include methanol, carbon tetrachloride, and organophosphate insecticides. Medications known to cause APT include antihypertensives, diuretics, selected antimicrobials, corticosteroids, and cancer chemotherapeutic agents.

In lipid-induced APT, triglyceride levels usually exceed 1000 mg/dl. The diagnosis is often difficult to make because triglycerides interfere with assays of serum amylase and are frequently elevated even when APT has another cause. Hypercalcemia-induced APT usually occurs in association with untreated hyperparathyroidism. Cholesterol emboli following arteriographic procedures may incite APT, particularly in the anticoagulated patient.

For uncertain reasons, pancreatitis is also common in patients undergoing heart-lung transplantation.

Regardless of the inciting stimulus, all pancreatitis results from in situ activation of autodigesting pro-enzymes (e.g., trypsin, chymotrypsin). Such inflammation results in disruption of pancreatic ducts, breakdown of vessel walls, and death of both exocrine and endocrine pancreatic cells.

DIAGNOSIS

Symptomatology

Patients with pancreatitis usually present with abdominal and/or back pain, nausea, and vomiting; however, alternative presentations (chest pain, shock, respiratory distress) are commonly encountered.

Chemical Analysis

Many conditions unassociated with symptomatic APT elevate the *amylase* level, making this test much less specific than is commonly perceived. For example, up to ⅓ of all patients undergoing laparotomy and ⅕ of those having major *extra-abdominal* surgery have elevated amylase levels without pancreatic manipulation or clinical evidence of APT. Non-pancreatic causes of amylase elevation are listed in Table 32.1.

Amylase determinations also lack sensitivity. As many as ⅓ of patients with clinical and radiographic features of APT do not have elevated serum amylase values. In patients with APT, peak

Table 32.1
Non-Pancreatic Causes of Amylase Elevation

Macroamylasemia	Peptic ulcer disease
Small bowel obstruction	Morphine administration
Ectopic pregnancy	Lung cancer
Gallbladder disease	Surgery
Hepatic failure	Ovarian tumors

amylase elevations occur within 24 hours and then gradually decline. High rates of false positive and false negative results limit the clinical utility of amylase clearance tests. Renal failure is one of many conditions that increase the ratio of amylase clearance to creatinine clearance.

Lipase is another pancreatic enzyme assayed to confirm the diagnosis of APT. Lipase peaks later and clears more slowly than amylase, remaining elevated for up to 14 days. It can therefore be helpful in making a diagnosis in a patient who presents late in the course of disease. Unfortunately, lipase determinations require up to 24 hours to perform, and therefore, "stat" results cannot be obtained. Unlike amylase, lipase is not elevated in patients with burns, diabetic ketoacidosis, pelvic infection, salivary gland dysfunction, or macroamylasemia. Assays of both *trypsin* and *methemalbumin* are ancillary but nonspecific tests used to support the diagnosis.

Radiographic Studies

The *chest x-ray* commonly demonstrates bibasilar atelectasis, diaphragmatic elevation, or pleural effusion. Diffuse infiltrates suggest adult respiratory distress syndrome (ARDS). *Abdominal films* may reveal signs of localized ileus, such as "the colon cut off sign" or the "sentinal loop". Free air may enter the abdomen in cases of pancreatitis resulting from ulcer perforation. A "soap bubble" appearance of the pancreatic bed, calcifications suggestive of chronic pancreatitis, ascites, and widening of the duodenal sweep on upper gastrointestinal (GI) series offer other clues. Retroperitoneal inflammation may obscure the psoas margins.

Computed tomographic (CT) scanning and *ultrasound* (US) are neither sensitive nor specific. Although CT scanning demonstrates some abnormality in 2/3 all patients, it requires transport of the patient from the intensive care unit. Furthermore, CT is inferior to US in identifying pancreatic edema or gallstones. Although US may be performed at the bedside, obesity and excessive abdominal gas limit its usefulness. Although *magnetic resonance imaging* is time consuming and not universally available, it appears promising in its ability to detect tissue edema.

Because *ERCP* can exacerbate acute inflammation and cause infection, it should probably be reserved for instances of APT in which stone extraction is anticipated. Stones must be extracted within 24–48 hours of symptom onset to abort a full-blown attack.

PROGNOSTIC FEATURES

Certain features associated with APT predict an adverse outcome (Table 32.2). Patients with fewer than three of the tabulated factors fare well. Conversely, few patients survive if more than six of these are present. *Hemorrhagic* pancreatitis (a disorder usually caused by a non-alcoholic precipitant) is much more serious than the edematous variety. Death from *alcohol-induced* pancreatitis usually occurs early in the hospital course, often as a result of hypovolemia, whereas death from *gallstone-induced* pancreatitis usually occurs later, as a result of sepsis.

MEDICAL THERAPY

Because marked reductions in circulating volume are common, adequate *fluid resuscitation* remains key to the initial management of APT. Causes of hypovolemia include: extravascular ("third space") losses into the pancreas and retroperitoneum, vomiting, and intraluminal gut sequestration (due to ileus).

Withholding oral feeding reduces pancreatic enzyme synthesis and release, speeding resolution of inflammation. Continuous *nasogastric suction* has been used to decrease acid delivery to the duodenum and thereby decrease pancreatic stimulation, but this has not been shown to speed resolution. Nonetheless, nasogastric suction may help relieve ileus-related discomfort or intractable vomiting.

Total parenteral nutrition should be considered in symptomatic patients from whom food is withheld for longer than 3–5 days. Although intravenous amino acids stimulate gastric acid production, there is no evidence that amino acid or lipid preparations aggravate APT.

Few other interventions improve the course of APT. Inhibition of gastric acid secretion by *antacids or histamine blockers* reduces the incidence

Table 32.2
Adverse Prognostic Features of Acute Pancreatitis*

Age > 55 yr	Calcium < 8 mg/dl
Glucose > 200 mg/dl	ARDS
WBC > 16,000/mm^3	Rise in BUN > 5 mg/dl
SGOT or LDH > 350 units/dl	Base deficit > 4 mEq/l
	Repletion volume > 6
Falling hematocrit	liters

*WBC, white blood cells; SGOT, serum glutamic oxaloacetic transaminase; LDH, lactic dehydrogenase; BUN, blood urea nitrogen.

of stress ulceration and upper GI bleeding but does not shorten the course of APT. *Corticosteroids* predispose to both infectious and metabolic complications and do not appear to benefit APT. Convincing evidence is also lacking that the use of *anticholinergic agents*, *somatostatin*, or *glucagon* is worthwhile.

If *narcotics* are used to relieve pain, meperidine is preferred to morphine, which can evoke ampullary spasm.

Prophylactic antibiotics directed against enteric gram-negative rods, anaerobes, and enterococci are indicated in gallstone pancreatitis because of the high associated incidence of biliary tract infection.

SURGICAL THERAPY

In a recent randomized prospective study, no clear advantage of *peritoneal lavage* in reducing mortality or morbidity of APT was demonstrated (Ref. 7). It remains possible, however, that the subgroup of patients with severe or hemorrhagic disease may benefit.

There are four major indications for laparotomy in critically ill patients with APT—"the four D's": (1) **D**iagnostic uncertainty; (2) **D**ecompression of biliary obstruction; (3) **D**rainage of pancreatic abscess; and (4) **D**eterioration in the face of conservative therapy.

In APT, the clearest indication for surgery is obstructive choledocholithiasis. Without surgery, the mortality from gallstone pancreatitis approaches 50% but is dramatically improved by early surgical intervention. Endoscopic stone removal appears to be as successful as surgery in aborting pancreatitis if the removal is performed early. In APT, pancreatectomy carries a high mortality and does not reduce the incidence of complications. Nonetheless, surgery may be appropriate in the treatment of the *late complications* of APT: pseudocyst, lesser sac abscess, and pancreatic ascites.

COMPLICATIONS OF APT

Pulmonary

Hydrostatic pulmonary edema frequently complicates unmonitored fluid replacement for the treatment of APT. Although exudative pleural effusions are usually left sided, bilateral or right sided effusions are possible. Most pleural effusions should be tapped to exclude the possibility of empyema, particularly if fluid appears suddenly or late in the course. Pneumonia and fat embolism are not uncommon. ARDS, the most dreaded complication of APT, is more common in patients with severe disease and is possibly related to the circulatory release of activated enzymes.

Coagulation

Pancreatic inflammation commonly activates the coagulation cascade, providing laboratory evidence of disordered clotting: elevated levels of thromboplastin, factor VIII, and fibrin split products. Clinical evidence of coagulopathy, however, is unusual. Although bleeding disorders are more common, splenic or portal vein thrombosis may also complicate APT.

Infectious

Although low-grade fever may be observed in uncomplicated APT, infection accounts for up to $\frac{1}{4}$ of all deaths in this disorder. Common infections include pancreatic or subdiaphragmatic abscess, cholangitis, urinary tract infection, and peritonitis. Whenever possible, antibiotic therapy in established infections should be guided by Gram stain and culture of appropriate body fluids. However, when uncertainty exists as to the site of origin or infecting organism, antibiotic coverage should include drugs directed against gram-negative aerobes, anaerobes, and staphylococci.

Electrolytes

A variety of fluid and electrolyte disorders are common in acute pancreatitis (see Chapter 12, Fluid and Electrolyte Management). Hypocalcemia may persist for weeks after the onset of APT. Calcium levels usually reach a nadir at $\simeq 5$ days after pain begins. Mechanisms include: the formation of intra-abdominal calcium complexes, hypoalbuminemia, and increased release of glucagon or thyrocalcitonin. Treatment parallels that of any case of *symptomatic* hypocalcemia. Serum magnesium may be reduced by vomiting, diarrhea, poor oral intake, or deposition in necrotic fat. Hypomagnesemia, especially common in alcohol-induced APT, may precipitate refractory hypokalemia and hypocalcemia.

Hemorrhage

Pseudocysts can erode into major vessels, resulting in massive GI hemorrhage. Although only 10% of patients bleed directly into the pancreatic parenchyma, this condition (hemorrhagic pancreatitis) carries a very high mortality, related largely to subsequent infection in devitalized pancreatic tissue. Hemorrhagic pancreatitis has no distinctive clinical features. Although the diagnosis is suggested by methemoglobin in peritoneal fluid, virtually any source of intraperitoneal blood can produce this finding. Coagulation disorders that accompany APT worsen the hemorrhagic tendency, regardless of bleeding source. Attempts at specific treatment of hemorrhagic APT, including pancreatectomy and peritoneal lavage, have limited effectiveness.

Renal

Acute renal failure resulting from hypovolemia, hypotension, or drug-induced renal damage is frequent and often fatal.

Ascites

APT can produce ascites when transudative fluid crosses the retroperitoneal boundary or when ductal disruption causes spillage into the peritoneum. When pancreatic secretions leak into the peritoneal cavity, intense inflammation of the lining membrane causes massive exudation ("pancreatic ascites"). Overt disruption of the pancreatic duct commonly accompanies traumatic or hemorrhagic APT. When ductal disruption occurs, amylase levels in ascitic fluid typically exceed the corresponding serum levels, often rising to > 1000 IU. Three to six weeks of bedrest and nutritional support may be required for spontaneous healing of the pancreatic leak and resolution of the ascites. Surgical repair is indicated in refractory cases and should be guided by preoperative ERCP.

Chronic Inflammation

Pseudocysts form in about ½ of all cases of APT within the first 3 weeks of illness. However, ½ of this subgroup show prompt spontaneous resolution. In the remainder, 6 months or longer may be required for spontaneous resolution. Although pseudocyst drainage or excision often proves difficult, operative intervention should be considered for those with acute complications or persistent, incapacitating symptoms. A drop in hematocrit with signs of shock and abdominal distention are reasons for immediate operation.

Abscesses or phlegmons may also form in the pancreatic bed, usually *after 3 weeks* of illness. Abscess is suggested radiographically by air-fluid levels in the lesser sac or gas bubbles in the pancreatic bed. Surgical or catheter drainage and culture-directed antibiotics are indicated in such cases. External drainage often is sufficient for early suppuration, but later complications usually require internal drainage. Repeated bouts of APT may incite *chronic pancreatitis*, a disease characterized by pain and deficiency of endocrine and exocrine pancreatic function (diabetes, malabsorption, etc.).

SUGGESTED READINGS

1. Acosta JM, Pellegrini CA, Skinner DB: Etiology and pathogenesis of acute biliary pancreatitis. *Surgery* 88(1):118–125, 1980.
2. Balart LA, Ferrante WA: Pathophysiology of acute and chronic pancreatitis. *Arch Intern Med* 142:113–117, 1982.
3. Frey CF: Hemorrhagic pancreatitis. *Am J Surg* 137:616–623, 1979.
4. Geokas MC, Baltaxe HA, Banks PA, et al.: Acute pancreatitis. *Ann Intern Med* 103:86–100, 1985.
5. Levant JA, Secrist DM, Resin H, et al: Nasogastric suction in the treatment of alcoholic pancreatitis. A controlled study. *JAMA* 229(1):51–52, 1974.
6. Martin JK, van Heerden JA, Bess MA: Surgical management of acute pancreatitis. *Mayo Clin Proc* 59:259–267, 1984.
7. Mayer AD, McMahon MJ, Corfield AP, et al: Controlled clinical trial of peritoneal lavage for the treatment of severe acute pancreatitis. *N Engl J Med* 312(7):399–404, 1985.
8. Moossa AR: Diagnostic tests and procedures in acute pancreatitis. *N Engl J Med* 311(10):639–643, 1984.
9. Ranson JHC: Etiological and prognostic factions in human acute pancreatitis: a review. *Am J Gastroenterol* 77:633–638, 1982.
10. Ranson JHC, Turner JW, Rose DH, et al: Respiratory complications in acute pancreatitis. *Ann Surg* 179:557–566, 1974.

33 Gastrointestinal Bleeding

Burns, coagulation disorders, respiratory failure, renal failure, central nervous system disease, and advanced age predispose to gastrointestinal (GI) bleeding in the critically ill. Because diagnostic and therapeutic strategies are site specific, it is important to distinguish upper from lower GI bleeding early in the hospital course. Diagnostic or therapeutic maneuvers should be undertaken only after resuscitation and stabilization have been accomplished.

UPPER GASTROINTESTINAL BLEEDING

Stress Ulcers

Erosive gastritis or gastric stress ulceration (GSU) is particularly common in critically ill patients with sepsis, hypotension, or burns. Although superficial, GSU may result in severe bleeding, particularly in patients with coagulopathy. GSU results from the combined actions of acid, ulcerogenic drugs, and ischemia and typically develops 5–7 days after intensive care unit (ICU) admission. Antacids and histamine blockers can prevent GSU, provided gastric pH is maintained above 4.0. Sucralfate may also be helpful.

Gastric and Peptic Duodenal Ulcers

Bleeding is an uncommon initial manifestation of peptic ulcer disease. Most patients with peptic ulcers relate a history of epigastric pain (particularly nocturnal) relieved by food or antacids. Esophago-Gastro-Duodenoscopy (EGD) is the most rapidly performed diagnostic test and may enable control of bleeding with laser therapy or electrocoagulation. Angiography may also be used to confirm the diagnosis and allow embolization or vasoconstrictor infusion to control severe bleeding. However, as with GSU, most gastric and duodenal peptic ulcers stop bleeding spontaneously with supportive care and control of gastric pH.

Mallory-Weiss Tears

Forceful vomiting may disrupt the mucosa of the gastroesophageal (GE) junction, resulting in a Mallory-Weiss tear. Precipitating or contributing factors include: (1) alcohol usage; (2) intractable vomiting; and (3) food impaction within the esophagus. No precipitating cause is determined in ≃ 20% of cases. Mallory-Weiss tears account for at least 10% of all upper GI bleeding. Even though these lesions commonly lead to massive hemorrhage, bleeding almost always stops spontaneously. The diagnosis is suggested by a history of forceful, painless hematemesis and is confirmed by EGD demonstrating linear tears at the GE junction. (An upper GI series is usually unrevealing.) Supportive treatment includes antiemetics, control of gastric pH, and expectant observation. (Attempts at balloon tamponade may splay the mucosa, extend the laceration, and aggravate the bleeding.)

Esophageal Varices

Varices are venous channels that shunt portal blood to the systemic circuit in response to portal hypertension. The largest collateral channels form at the GE junction; however, hemorrhoidal and retroperitoneal veins may also dilate and bleed. As many as 40% of all cirrhotic patients eventually develop variceal hemorrhage characterized by abrupt, painless, massive upper GI bleeding. The acute mortality of variceal bleeding approaches 50%. Approximately ⅔ of patients die within 12 months of the first episode.

Because *half* of all bleeding episodes in patients with known esophageal varices originate in *nonvariceal sources* (e.g., ulcers, Mallory-Weiss tears, etc.), it is important to determine the bleeding site before instituting definitive therapy. Hemodynamic stabilization and stomach evacuation must be achieved before diagnostic procedures are attempted. Once stability has been accomplished, *confirmation* of variceal bleeding by endoscopic observation should be undertaken.

Aortoenteric Fistulas

Prosthetic aortic grafts may erode into the GI tract, causing massive hemorrhage. Exsanguination often follows a moderate to large "herald" bleed that spontaneously stops. Aortoenteric fistulas usually occur in the distal duodenum and occasionally cause pulsatile bleeding from the mouth or nasogastric tube. Endoscopy and aortography are the only methods currently available to establish this diagnosis. Immediate laparotomy should be undertaken in patients with a confirmed diagnosis or intractable bleeding.

Angiodysplasia

Angiodysplasia occurs most commonly in the large bowel. It is, however, a common cause of *upper* GI bleeding in patients with renal failure (second only to erosive gastritis). Microvascular malformations involving the upper GI tract are usually located in the duodenum. The diagnosis must be made by angiography or EGD.

Miscellaneous Causes of Upper GI Bleeding

Hemobilia, a rare cause of upper GI bleeding, occurs when hepatic blood drains via the bile ducts into the duodenum. Hemobilia may be due to tumor involvement of the bile ducts or liver but most commonly follows blunt chest or abdominal trauma. The triad of abdominal pain, jaundice, and upper GI bleeding should prompt consideration of this condition. Hemobilia is seldom massive and spontaneously resolves in most cases.

Although *pancreatic disease* is an unusual primary cause of upper GI bleeding, hemorrhage may occur when pseudocysts or pancreatic tumors erode the posterior duodenal wall. Patients with acute pancreatitis frequently bleed from gastritis, ulcers, Mallory-Weiss tears, or esophageal varices unrelated to their pancreatitis. Coagulation disorders that accompany pancreatitis worsen the bleeding tendency.

LOWER GI BLEEDING

Two major disorders, *diverticulosis* and *colonic angiodysplasia*, account for approximately 80% of all lower GI bleeding (LGB), in more or less equal proportion.

Diverticulosis

Diverticulosis is responsible for $\simeq$ 40% of all LGB. Although diverticular bleeding is often severe, it usually stops spontaneously but often recurs. Although most diverticuli arise in the left colon, more than 70% of *diverticular bleeding* originates from the *right side*. Interestingly, diverticular bleeding does not usually occur in patients with acute diverticulitis (characterized by fever and lower abdominal pain).

Angiography demonstrates the site of active bleeding in ½–¾ of cases and offers the therapeutic option of intra-arterial pitressin infusion. The barium enema is not often helpful, and the value of colonoscopy is usually compromised by large amounts of colonic blood and stool in the unprepared patient.

Angiodysplasia

There are no unique historical features that distinguish angiodysplastic bleeding from diverticular bleeding. However, the *venous bleeding of angiodysplasia* is usually less severe than the *arterial bleeding of diverticulosis*. Aortic stenosis murmurs have been associated with some cases of angiodysplasia. Angiodysplastic bleeding recurs even more commonly than diverticular bleeding.

Like diverticular bleeding, angiodysplastic hemorrhage most frequently originates in the right colon and terminal ileum. Angiography reliably displays the vascular malformations but, unfortunately, confirms hemorrhage much less often—only about 10% of the time. Because of the high incidence of rebleeding, the involved portion of colon should be removed if hemorrhaging angiodysplastic vessels are demonstrated.

Colon Carcinoma

Colon carcinoma more commonly produces slow, continuous blood loss than massive GI hemorrhage. Premonitory symptoms include a change in bowel habits, melena, and crampy abdominal pain, with or without weight loss. Sequential rectal examination, colonoscopy, and barium enema are likely to reveal the cancerous site of blood loss.

Other Causes of Lower GI Bleeding

Ischemic colitis and bowel infarction due to mesenteric thrombosis or embolism may produce mucosal sloughing, bowel necrosis, and LGB (see Chapter 34, Acute Abdomen, p. 282).

Inflammatory bowel disease may cause massive LGB in the young. Bloody diarrhea is usually superimposed upon chronic, crampy abdominal pain.

Rectal ulcers are another rare but potentially fatal cause of massive LGB in patients with chronic renal failure.

DIAGNOSTIC TESTS

Localizing the Bleeding Site

Hematemesis or blood in the stomach are reliable signs of upper GI (UGI) bleeding. Even though *massive* UGI hemorrhage can produce bright red rectal bleeding, hematochezia originates from a lower site in > 90% of cases. As little as 15 ml of blood in the upper tract may produce guaiac positive stools, but melena (black, tarry stools formed by the digestion of blood by acid and bacteria) requires a loss of > 100 ml of blood over a relatively brief period. Because blood in the gut speeds transit time, melena seldom results from LGB unless it originates in the proximal colon and is delayed in passage.

The *nasogastric aspirate* helps to localize the site of bleeding in patients without a clear history of an UGI source and helps to assess activity of bleeding. An UGI bleeding site is unlikely if the aspirate does not reveal fresh blood or "coffee ground" material. However, 5–15% of patients with UGI bleeding have negative gastric aspirates. These "false negative" aspirates usually occur when a competent pylorus prevents the gastric reflux of blood originating in the distal duodenum. Testing gastric contents for occult blood is rarely necessary and may produce false-positive results in patients who have recently eaten meat or who have an alkaline stomach pH.

Once the general area of bleeding has been determined (upper versus lower), specific diagnostic tests are indicated to isolate the exact site. Plain *abdominal x-rays* may be helpful if they demonstrate free air (indicating perforation of a viscus) or "thumb printing" of the bowel (suggesting ischemic colitis).

A contrast *UGI series* is seldom helpful. It reveals only gross anatomical features, often failing to show more subtle features (varices, gastritis, and Mallory Weiss tears). Furthermore, even if the UGI series detects an abnormality, it never directly confirms it as the bleeding site. Finally, barium compromises subsequent tests, including CT scanning, angiography, and colonoscopy, and makes surgery technically more difficult. Barium studies also require transport of potentially unstable patients to the radiography suite.

Specialized Procedures

Upper GI Endoscopy

Upper GI endoscopy (EGD) performed within 24 hours of bleeding cessation improves diagnostic yield. However, there is not clear evidence that endoscopy in the early phase of active bleeding improves outcome, rebleeding, or mortality rate.

Uses of EGD
1. Demonstrating bleeding esophageal varices and allowing injection sclerotherapy
2. Predicting the need for surgery when a spurting vessel is visible in an ulcer crater
3. Reducing anesthesia time by allowing a planned approach before entering the operating room

Limitations of EGD
1. An optimal examination requires patients to take nothing by mouth (NPO) for 6 hours.
2. Sedation may compromise ventilation in patients with borderline respiratory status.
3. The procedure proves dangerous as well as unrewarding when a viscus perforates or the patient fails to cooperate.

Angiography

A diagnostic angiogram requires a skilled radiologist, a cooperative patient, and a rapidly bleeding lesion. To demonstrate extravasation of contrast, patients must be actively bleeding at a rate > 1 ml/min. Angiography reveals a site of active bleeding in most patients with GI hemorrhage but is of greatest use in LGB. This test is better at finding diverticular than angio-dysplasic lesions. Angiography offers the option of injecting emboli or vasoconstrictors into the parent vessel to stop bleeding. The combined incidence of allergic dye reactions, contrast-induced renal failure, vascular perforation, and cholesterol embolization is $\simeq 2\%$, even in experienced centers.

Barium Enema

The barium enema (BE) only defines structure. Therefore, BE may demonstrate inflammatory bowel disease, diverticulosis, or colonic carcinoma but does not prove any of these to be the source of bleeding. BE lacks resolution to define angiodysplasia or rectal ulceration.

Colonoscopy

Colonoscopy, a bedside procedure with high yield, reveals a bleeding site in about half of all cases of LGB and does not preclude subsequent diagnostic procedures. However, meticulous bowel preparation and hemodynamic stability are mandatory, and emergent colonoscopy risks perforation.

GI Bleeding Scans

Nuclear scans are more helpful than endoscopy or arteriography in detecting *intermittent* bleeding. Three tests used to detect GI bleeding include the technetium-sulphur colloid (TSC) scan, the indium scan, and the Meckel's scan.

Meckel's diverticuli may be localized using a radioactive tracer secreted by ectopic gastric mucosa lining the diverticulum. Although highly sensitive and specific, false-positive Meckel's scans are seen in non-fasting patients and in those with large arteriovenous malformations.

TSC studies are accomplished by scanning the abdomen for "puddling" of labeled red blood cells at the site of bleeding. With a longer half-life than technetium, *indium* allows repeated scanning for up to 5 days, a feature that may be particularly useful in patients with intermittent bleeding.

Imprecision is the major problem with all radionuclide scanning. Some tracers concentrate in the liver and spleen, while others are secreted into the gut lumen obscuring underlying bleeding sites. Therefore, although the general region of GI bleeding may be confirmed, precise localization usually requires endoscopy or arteriography.

Nuclear scans can detect bleeding as slow as 0.1 ml/min. No bowel preparation is necessary. About half of all positive studies are diagnostic within minutes. Nonetheless, these tests may be time consuming, occasionally requiring 6–18 hours for definitive results. Delayed scanning (at 24 hours) improves sensitivity but decreases specificity because isotopes are normally excreted into the gut lumen. False positive studies may be minimized by using continuous nasogastric (NG) suction to rid the stomach of secreted radionuclide.

PREVENTION AND THERAPY

Prevention

Four major factors may be manipulated to prevent GI bleeding:

1. Enteral feeding helps restore mucosal integrity and inhibits GI bleeding. *Nutrition* should be maintained by this route whenever feasible.
2. *Drugs* that cause esophageal, gastric, and small bowel bleeding should be avoided. These include corticosteroids, slow-release potassium, and aspirin or other non-steroidal anti-inflammatory agent.
3. *Hypotension* is a reversible risk factor for stress ulceration and mesenteric ischemia.
4. Reducing *gastric acid* production decreases the incidence of bleeding in ulcer disease and stress gastritis. Numerous histamine blockers and antacids are now available. All have comparable effectiveness if gastric pH is maintained consistently > 4.0. Continuous enteral feeding also buffers gastric pH.

Treatment

General Measures

Circulatory Support

Blood, colloid, or crystalloid should be used to maintain adequate perfusion (see Chapter 3, Support of the Circulation). As a rule, hemoglobin concentration should be kept > 10 mg/dl and coagulation and platelet abnormalities should be corrected (see Chapter 24, Coagulation Disorders). Although patients with impaired liver function may benefit from removal of intestinal blood that may precipitate hepatic encephalopathy, gastric lavage does not decrease the rate of UGI bleeding, even when the solution is cooled or fortified with norepinephrine. Lavage with water may induce hyponatremia, whereas saline may cause fluid overload.

Acid Control

Antacids both prevent and decrease bleeding from stress ulcers. There is little evidence, however, that they stop bleeding from any other source, perhaps because blood itself is an excellent buffer. Continuous instillation of antacids may help ensure that gastric pH is maintained > 4.0 for optimal benefit. Potential side effects of antacid therapy include diarrhea, phosphate binding, and (in patients with renal insufficiency) magnesium toxicity. Because *sucralfate requires acid production* for dissolution and tissue binding, it may be ineffective if administered concurrently with antacids or histamine (H_2) blockers.

Histamine blockers (cimetidine, ranitidine) prevent and heal stress ulcers with effectiveness similar to antacids. Yet, whether H_2 blockers help control ongoing bleeding is open to question. H_2 blockers appear to reduce mortality, the incidence of rebleeding, and the need for surgery in peptic ulcer disease. When using H_2 blockers it is important to monitor gastric pH, because some patients fail to suppress acid secretion with commonly used doses. Continuous infusions inhibit gastric acid secretion more consistently than intermittent dosing. Side effects of H_2 blockers include *altered drug metabolism* and *central nervous system disturbances*. The latter have been reported most commonly with cimetidine in elderly patients.

Specific Measures

Treatment of Varices

As with all massive GI bleeding, fluid resuscitation, hemoglobin maintenance, and correction of coagulation abnormalities are key components of therapy. There is no evidence that gentle NG tube insertion aggravates variceal bleeding. However, NG tubes may induce esophagitis and gastric erosion if left in place for prolonged periods.

Vasopressin (VP), a splanchnic vasoconstrictor, often controls variceal bleeding by decreasing portal blood flow through hepatic and collateral vascular channels. It is not known whether VP lowers the incidence of rebleeding. VP is usually administered as a continuous infusion of 0.2 to 0.6 units/ minute, given in a peripheral vein and continued 24 hours after clinical bleeding has stopped. Intra-arterial administration is useful for patients with diverticular or peptic ulcer hemorrhage but offers no advantage for variceal bleeding. VP-associated complications include arrhythmias, myocardial or mesenteric ischemia, stroke, and renal insufficiency. Vasopressin routinely decreases cardiac output and may cause cardiac decompensation by increasing afterload. The concurrent use of nitroglycerin minimizes the tendency for cardiac ischemia. *Somatostatin*, another promising splanchnic vasoconstrictor, is not yet available for clinical use.

Propranolol has also been used chronically to decrease portal blood flow and reduce portal pressure. Although it may decrease rebleeding episodes in patients with varices, beta-blockade blunts compensatory cardiovascular responses and therefore should not be used in *acute* variceal bleeding.

Balloon tamponade may control esophageal bleeding in patients refractory to other modalities. Unfortunately, half of all patients so treated rebleed on decompression. Currently, a four lumen catheter with gastric and esophageal balloons (e.g., the Minnesota tube) is preferred over the three-lumen Sengstaken-Blakemore tube because it enables the evacuation of the proximal esophagus, reducing the risk of aspiration.

The Minnesota tube is inserted through the *mouth* into the stomach. Appropriate positioning of the gastric balloon *must be checked by x-ray before inflation* to prevent esophageal rupture. Following inflation, traction should be applied to secure the gastric balloon against the esophagogastric junction. If bleeding continues, the esophageal balloon should then be inflated. Upon completion of this inflation sequence, it is crucial to confirm the proper configuration by x-ray. The tube should be kept in place for at least 24 hours following cessation of bleeding.

Without meticulous technique and monitoring, complications occur in a high percentage of patients who undergo balloon tamponade. Aspiration remains the most frequent complication, although recent modifications of tube design have decreased the risk. Cephalad migration may produce *upper airway obstruction*, a catastrophic event for the patient whose airway is unsecured. (Scissors should be kept at bedside for immediate tube transection if airway obstruction occurs.) *Esophagogastric rupture*, another devastating complication, usually results from improper tube placement and inflation of the gastric balloon in the esophagus. *Pressure necrosis* of the nose, mouth, and gastroesophageal mucosa are common.

Surgical approaches to variceal bleeding include techniques that obliterate the varix by interrupting the esophagus or stomach and those that shunt blood around the high vascular resistance of the liver to decompress the portal system. Even though interruption of esophagus or stomach is transiently effective at controlling variceal bleeding, portal pressure remains elevated and bleeding elsewhere often becomes a problem.

Shunting procedures may be total (porto-caval, meso-caval) or selective. Selective procedures (Warren shunts) decompress portal circulation by joining the splenic and renal veins. Selective shunts preserve hepatic perfusion but decrease portal pressure and varix diameter. In experienced centers, selective shunts are the preferred operations for *elective* decompression but are time consuming and therefore not usually feasible in unstable patients. Selective shunts produce lower rates of encephalopathy than nonselective shunting procedures and prevent recurrent hemorrhage. Unfortunately, they do not improve long-term survival.

Endoscopy with variceal injection of a sclerosing agent (*injection sclerotherapy*, IS) usually controls variceal hemorrhage and offers improved short term survival when compared to balloon tamponade. Sclerotherapy reduces transfusion requirements and is less dangerous than emergent surgical shunting. (However, overall survival is similar in groups treated by IS or shunting.) After the control of acute bleeding, IS may obliterate the dilated vessels and reduce the incidence of rebleeding.

There is no significant difference in efficacy or complication rates among the various sclerosing agents currently available. Complications of IS include: (1) oversedation and aspiration; (2) pulmonary dysfunction (adult respiratory distress syndrome, ARDS) secondary to sclerosants; and (3) local esophageal problems including ulceration, perforation, stricture, dysmotility, and abscess formation. Perforation of the esophagus may produce empyema, mediastinitis, or mediastinal hematoma. Occasionally sclerotherapy incites bacteremia.

Endoscopy for Non-variceal Lesions

EGD may be used in conjunction with direct epinephrine injection or laser photocoagulation to reduce rebleeding and transfusion requirements in patients with ulcers and visible, spurting vessels. Unfortunately, laser therapy may perforate the mucosa or intensify bleeding. Thermal coagulation via the endoscope may be used to halt bleeding from duodenal or gastric ulcers and Mallory-Weiss tears.

The Role of Surgery in Control of GI Bleeding

Upper GI Bleeding.   Unfortunately, the worst candidates for surgery often are those most in need because of their limited tolerance of anemia and hypotension. In patients with ulcer-related UGI bleeding who are not good surgical candidates, consideration should be given to endoscopic injection of epinephrine and to laser or thermal coagulation. Angiography with embolization or selective pitressin infusion may also be helpful if general anesthesia must be avoided.

Several indications prompt surgical intervention in upper GI bleeding: (1) A *visible* or spurting *vessel* in the base of an ulcer crater rebleeds at least 50% of the time, even if initially controlled by non-surgical means. Because of this high risk of rebleeding, surgical repair is indicated. (2) Brisk hemorrhage from a lesion that perforates a GI vis-

cus warrants surgical intervention. (3) *Massive ongoing blood losses* from any source (more than 1500 ml or 6–10 units of blood in the first 24 hours) is also used as a criterion for surgery in upper GI bleeding.

Lower GI Bleeding.   Embolization via angiographic catheter or selective infusion of vasopressin may be helpful in patients with diverticular or angiodysplastic lesions. Because of the high incidence of rebleeding in angiodysplasia, however, resection is usually recommended. In patients with massive LGB of undetermined origin, exploratory laparotomy will identify the bleeding site in only 1/3 of cases. If the bleeding site cannot be found at the time of laparotomy, a right hemicolectomy is usually favored because both bleeding diverticuli and angiodysplastic lesions are more common there.

PROGNOSTIC FACTORS

Advanced age, massive transfusion requirement, rebleeding, multisystem illness, shock, ascites, and renal or hepatic failure are adverse prognostic factors. Patients requiring massive transfusion ($>$ 10 units of packed red blood cells) face a mortality exceeding 35%.

SUGGESTED READINGS

1. Athanasoulis CA, Wlatman AC, Novelline RA, et al: Angiography. Its contribution to the emergency management of gastrointestinal hemorrhage. *Radiol Clin N Am* 14:265–280, 1976.
2. Hastings PRK, Skillman JJ, Bushness LS, et al: Antacid titration in the prevention of acute gastrointestinal bleeding: a controlled, randomized trial in 100 critically ill patients. *N Engl J Med* 298(19):1041–1045, 1978.
3. Johnson WC, Widrich WC, Ansell JE, et al: Control of bleeding varices by vasopressin: a prospective randomized study. *Ann Surg* 186:369–376, 1977.
4. Larson DE, Farnell MB: Upper gastrointestinal hemorrhage. *Mayo Clin Proc* 58(6):371–386, 1983.
5. Miskowiak J, Nielsen ST, Munck O: Scintigraphic diagnosis of gastrointestinal bleeding with 99mTc-labeled blood-pool agents. *Radiology* 141:499–504, 1981.
6. Pingleton SK: Gastrointestinal hemorrhage. *Med Clin N Am* 67(6):1215–1231, 1983.
7. Waldram R, Davis M, Nunnerley H, et al: Emergency endoscopy after gastrointestinal haemorrhage in 50 patients with portal hypertension. *Br Med J* 4:94–96, 1974.

34 Acute Abdomen

PRINCIPLES OF MANAGEMENT

Diseases causing acute abdominal pain (AAP) rarely present in a typical fashion in the intensive care unit (ICU) population. Patients with spinal cord injuries, those in coma, and those receiving corticosteroids may experience an abdominal catastrophe with few signs or symptoms. Several principles should be kept in mind when critically ill patients with AAP are being treated: (1) Carefully exclude such emergent nonabdominal processes as myocardial infarction and pneumonitis. (2) Until a firm diagnosis is established, *consider the problem to be urgent and life threatening.* (3) *Make repeated observations.* A changing examination provides valuable clues to diagnosing abdominal disorders. (4) *Avoid potent analgesics* or narcotics in patients with undiagnosed AAP. (5) Withhold all enteral feedings and medications. (6) Involve a *surgeon and/or gynecologist early* in the evaluation. All consultants should follow the evolving course of the illness; furthermore, this strategy avoids unnecessary repetition of painful pelvic and rectal examinations.

DIAGNOSIS

History

An accurate history is key to the workup. Description of the *onset* and *character* of the pain as well as *exacerbating* or *relieving factors* is helpful in diagnosis. All conscious patients should be asked to localize the pain to a discreet site with one finger. AAP awakening patients from sleep or persisting longer than 6 hours is frequently a surgical problem. AAP arises from one of three mechanisms: (1) visceral ischemia; (2) serosal inflammation; or (3) distention of a hollow viscus.

Pain of *sudden onset* suggests a vascular catastrophe or perforation of a hollow viscus. Pain of *gradual onset* that builds to a crescendo is more typical of hollow viscus overdistention, as is *intermittent pain* in a "colicky" pattern. *Steady pain* suggests serosal inflammation, especially when it is markedly exacerbated by changes in position or local pressure (rebound tenderness). A *pleuritic component* raises the possibility that an "intra-abdominal process" either abuts the inferior surface of the diaphragm or actually extends into the chest. (Conversely, lower lobe pneumonias may be confused with acute AAP, because of diaphragmatic irritation.)

Physical Exam

The specific site of the pain may be helpful in diagnosis. The abdomen should first be *examined visually*, then *auscultated*, and finally *palpated*. Palpating the abdomen as the first part of the examination is likely to produce voluntary guarding or artifactual bowel sounds, even in patients with severe ileus. The most painful area of the abdomen should be examined last. The abdominal examination must answer the following specific questions:

1. Is there rebound tenderness?
2. Are the *bowel sounds absent*?
3. Are there *palpable masses*?
4. Is there evidence of *free air or fluid* in the abdomen?

A positive response to any of these questions strongly indicates surgical intervention. Peritoneal signs are the most reliable in predicting the need for urgent laparotomy.

Laboratory Tests

Routine laboratory tests are rarely diagnostic during acute AAP. Leukocyte count and temperature may be normal even with severe intra-abdominal disease. The serum amylase is helpful in the clinical setting of pancreatitis, but both false negatives and false positives occur (see Pancreatitis, Chapter 32). A triad of hyperkalemia, hyperphosphatemia, and metabolic acidosis (in the absence of renal failure) suggests well-advanced bowel infarction. The abdominal x-ray may give important clues to the etiology and urgency of AAP and is discussed separately (see Radiology in the Intensive Care Unit, page 103).

SPECIFIC CONDITIONS PRODUCING THE ACUTE ABDOMEN

The most rapidly lethal condition compatible with the presentation should be considered first, particularly in patients with overt abdominal signs and hypotension. The fulminant development of shock associated with AAP is usually attributable to vascular disruption and intra-abdominal hemorrhage. Two conditions of this type in most urgent need of surgical intervention are *ruptured abdominal aortic aneurysm (AAA)* and *ruptured ectopic pregnancy*.

Ruptured Aneurysm

Immediate diagnosis and surgical correction are needed to salvage patients with a ruptured AAA. AAA usually presents with *back and abdominal pain and shock*. An *expanding abdomen* or *pulsatile* abdominal *mass* with the *loss of one or both femoral pulses* completes the classic presentation. Unfortunately, hypotension often impedes comparison of pulse volumes, and examination of the abdomen and pulses may be difficult in obese patients.

When clear signs and symptoms of a ruptured AAA are present, the patient should be taken directly to the operating room after initiation of fluid resuscitation. If the patient is hemodynamically stable, intravenous lines should be inserted and blood ordered before diagnostic testing. A contrasted computed tomographic (CT) scan or aortic arteriogram may be helpful to confirm and delineate the aneurysm in the stable patient, but *ultrasonography is the quickest non-invasive bedside test* to confirm the aneurysm or free fluid (blood) in the belly.

Pelvic Disease in the Female

Ruptured ectopic pregnancy typically presents as *AAP, hypotension, vaginal bleeding*, and *a mass in the cul-de-sac*. (AAP occurs in almost all patients; $\simeq$ ¾ have vaginal bleeding, and $\simeq$ ½ have a pelvic mass.) A serum beta-human chorionic gonadotropin (HCG) should be performed on every fertile female with AAP, to screen for pregnancy. Urinary HCG testing, although immediately available, is less sensitive. Hematocrit determinations are usually not helpful because of the acute nature of the bleeding. Young women with unexplained AAP and shock should undergo immediate laparotomy for a presumed ruptured ectopic pregnancy. In patients with AAP, stable blood pressure, and no evidence of peritoneal signs, elective evaluation should be performed before operation.

Ovarian tumors or *cysts* may also produce pelvic pain if they undergo torsion or ischemia. Rupture of a normal ovarian follicle into the peritoneum may produce worrisome but otherwise benign peritoneal signs. *Pelvic inflammatory disease* (PID), the most common cause of pelvic pain in young women, is often difficult to differentiate from appendicitis or a ruptured ectopic pregnancy. PID usually starts within 7 days of the menstrual period, a helpful point in the differential with ectopic pregnancy. The pain of PID is gradual in onset and usually bilateral, whereas the pain of appendicitis tends to be of sudden onset and unilateral when fully developed. Diffuse bilateral tenderness elicited by moving the cervix during pelvic examination is key to detecting PID.

Mesenteric Ischemia

Mesenteric ischemia afflicts the *elderly*, particularly those with *underlying heart and vascular disease*. The mortality of bowel infarction approaches 70%, primarily because of *delayed diagnosis*. The differential diagnosis of mesenteric ischemia includes bowel obstruction, diverticulitis, and inflammatory bowel disease.

Pathophysiology

Bowel ischemia may result from *arterial or venous* occlusion of the superior or inferior mesenteric vessels. About 50% of patients with acute bowel ischemia have superior mesenteric artery disease. Superior mesenteric artery (SMA) occlusion usually presents as the sudden onset of AAP and a striking leukocytosis. Conversely, inferior mesenteric artery occlusion (accounting for about 25% of bowel ischemia) usually has a more subtle, chronic pattern.

Bowel infarction most often is the result of *thrombotic* occlusion near the aortic origin of mesenteric vessels in patients with extensive atherosclerotic vascular disease. In patients with slowly progressive occlusion, a history of "intestinal angina" may be elicited. *Embolism*, the second major mechanism producing bowel obstruction, is a likely etiology in patients with chronic atrial fibrillation or recent myocardial infarction complicated by mural thrombosis. *Vasculitis* (lupus, radiation, and polyarteritis) is occasionally responsible. It has recently been recognized that many critically ill patients have *non-occlusive bowel infarction* due to generalized hypotension and vasopressor drugs.

Initially, ischemia produces mucosal and submucosal injury and edema. Later, mucosal sloughing occurs. Unless corrected within 2–4 days, bowel necrosis and perforation occur, resulting in generalized peritonitis and death. After initial stabilization with fluid and electrolytes, early angiographic diagnosis and surgical correction are crucial for a good outcome. Therefore, unless there are clear signs of early resolution, patients should undergo surgical exploration if there is to be any chance of salvage. Prognosis is best when revascularization is performed on a "non-surgical" abdomen.

Signs and Symptoms

The signs and symptoms of mesenteric ischemia are often minimal or poorly localized. The most common symptom of mesenteric occlusion is constant, non-discrete back and abdominal pain. More than ½ of all patients have either occult blood in the stool or bloody diarrhea. Bowel sounds increase early in this process but decrease later. Shock may be the presenting symptom if perforation or infarction has already occurred. Atrial fibrillation or congestive heart failure are present in as many as ½ of all patients with bowel infarction.

Diagnostic Tests

Laboratory tests are seldom sufficiently specific or timely to aid in diagnosis. Although loss of circulating volume may cause hemoconcentration, more typically, the *hematocrit* remains normal as the leukocyte count rises. Refractory *metabolic acidosis* in conjunction with increased levels of *potassium and phosphate* is typical of infarction. Unfortunately, these abnormalities are often recognized too late to impact favorably on crucial therapeutic decisions.

Plain *abdominal radiographic findings* (seen in a minority of cases) include an ileus localized to the area of bowel ischemia with dilation of large and small bowel loops and loss of haustral markings. Occasionally, gas may be seen in the portal venous system, in the bowel wall, or free in the peritoneal cavity. Hemorrhage and bowel wall edema may result in a classic "thumb printing" pattern on the plain radiograph. *Angiography*, the procedure of choice for diagnosis, may aid in the

therapy but must be performed without delay. Angiography helps to distinguish thrombosis, embolism, and vasoconstriction and allows the local infusion of a vasodilator (papaverine). *Barium studies* should not be performed if ischemic bowel is suspected, because extraluminal barium may cause peritonitis.

Therapy

After angiographic diagnosis, infusion of papaverine or nitroglycerin may improve the perfusion of the ischemic gut. Thrombolytic agents are not yet of proven benefit. In patients with *peritoneal signs*, *immediate surgery* should follow confirmation of the diagnosis. At the time of surgery, non-viable segments of bowel should be removed. A "second look" operation 24–36 hours following revascularization has gained popularity to allow dying tissue time to demarcate before removal. Unfortunately, the diagnosis of ischemic bowel disease is often overlooked or delayed until the clinical condition is too poor to permit salvage.

Appendicitis

Again in appendicitis, early diagnosis is critical to prevent its major complications—perforation and abscess formation. The *classic features* of acute appendicitis—mid-epigastric pain migrating to the right lower quadrant accompanied by nausea and vomiting—are *seen in* < ½ of all patients. The site of pain is not predictable because of the variable location of the cecum and appendix. The pace and intensity of this surgical problem are highly variable. Appendicitis is often overlooked in the absence of fever, leukocytosis, a localizing physical examination, or a "classical" history.

Physical examination usually reveals a mildly elevated temperature with moderate AAP. Generalized peritoneal signs are usually absent unless perforation has occurred. Pelvic and rectal examinations are particularly helpful in localizing the pain.

Laboratory examination reveals an elevated white blood cell (WBC) count in most patients, but leukocyte counts may be normal in older patients or in those receiving steroids or cancer chemotherapy. Even when perforation is demonstrated surgically, free intra-abdominal air is only seen radiographically in ½ of all patients.

Cholecystitis and Cholangitis

Pathophysiology

A low threshold for surgical intervention must be maintained to prevent mortality in patients with cholecystitis and cholangitis. Many ICU patients with these disorders have coexisting problems. The increased mortality in elderly patients with biliary infection seems to be related to delays in diagnosis and institution of therapy. Cholangitis, a problem that arises primarily in elderly patients, occurs when bacteria reflux into a partially obstructed biliary duct, producing inflammation. Life-threatening bacteremia may result as infected bile, under pressure, seeds the bloodstream. Chronic or recurrent cholangitis may result in abscess or stricture formation.

Cholangitis and cholecystitis are most common among patients with gallstones, previous biliary surgery, pancreatic or biliary tumors, or other obstructions to bile flow. Instrumentation of the biliary tract, including endoscopic retrograde cholangio-pancreatography (ERCP), surgery, or T-tube cholangiography are major risk factors. When cholecystitis occurs among ambulatory patients, gallstones are found 85–95% of the time; however, *acalculous cholecystitis* (ACC) is much more common in hospitalized patients. Cholestasis may be key to the development of ACC. Thus, ACC tends to occur in patients deprived of the oral alimentation that produces the normal pattern of phasic gallbladder emptying.

Signs and Symptoms

The signs and symptoms of acute biliary inflammation are referred to as either a "classic" triad or pentad. The complete *triad of cholecystitis* (fever, chills, and right upper quadrant pain) is seen in 70% of patients. The addition of mental status changes and shock complete the *pentad of cholangitis* in another 10%. The diagnoses of cholecystitis or cholangitis are unlikely in the absence of fever.

Laboratory Findings

The *leukocyte count* is elevated in ≈ 2/3 of patients with cholecystitis. Even if the WBC count is normal, granulocytes usually predominate. The *bilirubin* is elevated in 80% of cases of acute cholecystitis, but in most it remains < 6 mg/dl. Only 25% of patients are overtly jaundiced. The *alkaline phosphatase* is usually modestly elevated (2–3 times normal) unless obstruction is severe or prolonged. Serum levels of other liver enzymes are usually only modestly elevated. A low-grade *coagulopathy* is common, manifest as a decreased platelet count and prolonged prothrombin time.

Radiographic Procedures

Although *plain x-rays* visualize only 20% of gallstones, gas demonstrated in the biliary tract is virtually diagnostic of cholangitis. Ultrasound (US) will visualize gallstones and dilated biliary ducts reliably if obesity and bowel gas are minimal, and sufficient time has elapsed for distention to occur. Patients with ACC do not have evidence of gallstones, but "sludge" may be detected. *US* does not demonstrate pancreatic detail as well as CT scanning, but it is a rapid bedside test that offers high resolution of structures in the right upper quadrant. *CT scanning* may be a superior method of demonstrating dilated intrahepatic channels and processes in the region of the common bile duct, but it is expensive and lacks portability. *Percutaneous cholangiography* is feasible and helpful if the biliary ducts are dilated, but otherwise has a low yield. Unfortunately, percutaneous cholangiography fails to outline the pancreatic duct and may result in liver laceration, bile leak, and sepsis. A postoperative T-tube in the biliary tract may provide a convenient channel for cholangiography.

Nuclear biliary scans may also be used to evaluate the function of the liver and biliary tract. A radioactive tracer is administered, taken up by the liver and secreted into the bile, where it outlines the major intrahepatic ducts, gallbladder, and common bile duct. Non-visualization of the gallbladder may occur with cystic or common duct obstruction. *Non-visualization in the absence of gallbladder disease may occur with starvation, total parenteral nutrition use, and severe hepatic dysfunction.* The specificity of biliary scans is high (> 90%) if gallstones are present, but in *acalculous* cholecystitis the specificity falls to ≈ 40%.

ERCP requires a skilled operator and transport of the patient to the radiology suite. This technique, however, allows direct visualization of the ampulla and radiographic visualization of the intrahepatic and pancreatic ducts—information that is helpful when malignancy is suspected. ERCP also offers the option of stone extraction or dilation of a stenotic ampulla.

Bacteriology

In most patients with cholecystitis, frank cholangitis is not seen until ≥ 48 hours following ductal obstruction. Intraoperative bile cultures are positive in 85% of patients; two or more organisms grow more than 50% of the time. Although the most common organisms are aerobic gram negative rods (*Escherichia coli*, *Klebsiella*, and *Streptococcus faecalis*), anaerobes (i.e., *Bacteroides fragilis* and *Clostridium perfringens*) are isolated in ≃ 40% of infected patients.

Treatment

Patients with cholangitis or cholecystitis should be stabilized hemodynamically, cultured, and given appropriate antiobiotics; however, *antibiotics are not an alternative to biliary drainage*. Drugs normally excreted into bile are unlikely to achieve effective concentrations in unrelieved biliary obstruction. Antibiotic selection should include broad coverage directed against anaerobes (clindamycin, chloramphenicol, metronidazole, or cefoxitin), gram-negative rods (aminoglycosides), and enterococci (ampicillin). Although achieving adequate serum concentrations is important, the renal toxicity of aminoglycosides increases with biliary obstruction; therefore, special care must be exercised in their use. Doses should be adjusted by serum levels to an appropriate therapeutic index. Ampicillin is effective against most biliary pathogens and provides coverage of enterococcus (*S. faecalis*) not obtained by using cephalosporins. (In the penicillin-allergic patient, vancomycin may be substituted for ampicillin.)

Most patients should undergo *semi-elective* drainage of the biliary tract after hemodynamic stabilization. Severity of illness in biliary tract obstruction should not preclude surgery because drainage offers the only chance for recovery. In the critically ill patient, it is generally best to do the simplest effective procedure and to reoperate at a later time, if necessary. T-tube drainage of the biliary tract (with or without cholecystectomy) is effective, but *cholecystostomy alone is unreliable*, even if the cystic duct is patent. Nonoperative drainage options include percutaneous drainage, a useful technique for biliary drainage in the high-risk ICU patient or in the terminally ill patient. Unfortunately, bile peritonitis, a potentially lethal problem, may complicate this procedure. For bedside drainage of the biliary tract, ERCP is another option that may be performed without general anesthesia. ERCP is most helpful for stones impacted in the ampullary region, but cannulation can be difficult because of ampullary edema and obstruction.

Small Bowel Obstruction

The triad of nausea, vomiting, and AAP should suggest small bowel obstruction (SBO). SBO can be classified as (1) simple, (2) strangulated (in which vascular compromise is the predominant manifestation), or (3) closed loop (in which vascular compromise and complete bowel obstruction rapidly escalate intraluminal pressure).

About ¾ of cases are due to adhesions; incarcerated hernias and malignancy comprise the majority of the remainder. Inflammatory bowel disease accounts for a small minority of cases.

On examination, occult blood in the stool signifies compromised bowel wall integrity. Incarcerated hernias or abdominal scars are suggestive physical findings. Bowel sounds are usually rushing and high pitched early in SBO, but later they become hypoactive.

Abdominal radiographs taken with the patient in the upright position demonstrate *multiple air-fluid levels* with distal *evacuation of the colon and rectum*. Treatment of SBO is usually less urgent than treatment of colonic obstruction. Strangulated bowel with perforation, a potentially disastrous problem, is often misdiagnosed as simple SBO. Unfortunately, there is no clinical way to distinguish between simple SBO and strangulated bowel. Good candidates for conservative management with nasogastric suction include patients who are hemodynamically stable, those with a partial SBO, those with recurrent obstruction following radiation therapy, and those with SBO occurring within 30 days of abdominal surgery.

Colonic Obstruction

Colonic obstruction, a disease of the elderly, presents with AAP, obstipation (50%), and vomiting (50%). The most common causes of obstruction include *colon cancer*, *diverticular disease*, and *volvulus*. Impaction may confuse or imitate this picture. About 20% of patients with colon cancer will have both perforation and obstruction and will demonstrate free air on abdominal x-rays. Preoperatively, the etiology of obstruction is often unknown, although the plain radiograph may be quite helpful. Plain radiographs are diagnostic of volvulus in > 50% of patients. When x-rays show an acute increase of cecal diameter to > 9 cm, perforation of the colon may be imminent.

Rarely, "*pseudo-obstruction*" (Ogilvie's syndrome) may occur in which signs and symptoms of bowel obstruction are present without a *mechanical* cause. Colonic pseudo-obstruction may be due to electrolyte imbalances (magnesium or potassium), anticholinergic drugs, myxedema, or ganglionic blockers. Pseudo-obstruction usually results from ileus of the right colon and is treatable by correction of the underlying disorder.

Diverticulitis

Diverticulitis accounts for up to 10% of all abdominal pain in the elderly. It is produced when a "pseduodiverticulum" of the colon becomes inflamed. Even though diverticulitis has been referred to as "left-sided appendicitis," the pain has no typical pattern. Nausea, fever, and constipation are common. Frankly *bloody* stools and vomiting are quite unusual.

The physical examination frequently demonstrates a *palpable mass* in the lower abdomen or pelvis. The stool, although often *guaiac positive*, is rarely bloody. Often, colonoscopy and other diagnostic tests are necessary to rule out cancer, because diverticulitis typically causes extrinsic compression of the bowel lumen, mimicking colon carcinoma. Steroid therapy may impair the "walling off" process and predispose to free perforation into the peritoneum.

Medical therapy is successful in 80–90% of cases. Withholding food and providing mild analgesics, nasogastric suction, and intravenous fluids are standard. Broad spectrum antibiotics (e.g., ampicillin plus clindamycin and an aminoglycoside) should be administered. Indications for operation in diverticulitis include: perforation, obstruction, abscess formation, fistula tract formation, malignancy, and failure to respond to several days of conservative management.

Perforated Viscus

Ulcer Disease

The perforated gastric or duodenal ulcer is often misdiagnosed as pancreatitis because of similar symptomatology (mid-abdominal pain radiating to the back, nausea, vomiting, and elevated serum amylase). Perforation more commonly complicates duodenal ulceration (5–10%) than gastric ulceration (< 1%). Anterior ulcer perforation produces a chemical peritonitis with diffuse AAP and ileus.

About 80% of all ulcer perforations release free air into the peritoneal cavity. To demonstrate free abdominal gas it may be necessary to position the patient upright or in the left lateral decubitus posture for 5–10 minutes before film exposure. Patients with perforated ulcers usually appear very ill with diffuse AAP, tenderness, and decreased bowel sounds. A minority of such patients have the abrupt onset of AAP or a rigid abdomen. Perforations of the gastrointestinal (GI) tract may be confirmed by demonstrating extravasation of Gastrografin (not barium) into the peritoneum.

Surgical intervention is indicated in ulcer disease for (1) intractable pain, (2) bleeding, (3) obstruction, and (4) free perforation. If the ulcer is located in the duodenum and the patient is stable, a definitive resection (vagotomy and drainage) should be performed. In unstable patients, however, the ulcer should be oversewn and the operation quickly terminated. Whenever possible, gastric ulcers should be resected because of the high potential for carcinoma.

Colonic Perforations

Perforation of the colon is frequently associated with colonic obstruction due to malignancy or diverticular disease. Diverticular perforation is frequently responsible for free intraperitoneal gas in the elderly, but many perforated diverticuli do not liberate intraperitoneal gas.

Pancreatitis

Pancreatitis, another condition causing AAP, is discussed in Chapter 32.

Unusual Causes of APP

Carcinoma is found in 5–10% of *elderly* patients with AAP. Although no one knows the cause, patients with *diabetic ketoacidosis* often present with AAP. (Diabetic ketoacidosis should be excluded in all patients before laparotomy.) *Sickle cell disease* may produce abdominal pain by infarcting the bowel or spleen. *Inferior myocardial infarction* and *pneumonia* in the basilar segments of the lung may both present predominately with abdominal discomfort. In these patients, nausea and vomiting are also common, mimicking acute cholecystitis.

Typhlitis, bacterial invasion of the bowel wall in immunosuppressed patients, may be confused with ischemic colitis, diverticulitis, or appendicitis. Several forms of *chemotherapy* may produce nausea, vomiting, and GI bleeding (particularly cytosine arabinoside). Up to ¼ of all leukemic patients have neoplastic infiltration of the bowel wall that may cause perforation either in the natural history of the disease or shortly after the initiation of chemotherapy.

RADIOLOGIC DIAGNOSIS OF SUSPECTED INTRAABDOMINAL CRISIS

Plain Films of the Abdomen

In patients with AAP, plain films of the abdomen are often helpful and occasionally diagnostic. Radiographic signs that should be sought include:

1. mass effect,
2. extraluminal gas,

Table 34.1
Merits of Radiological Diagnostic Methods for Acute Abdominal Pain

Characteristic	CT and US	Radionuclide Scans (Ga and In)
Operator dependence	Require directed study of a suspected area by skilled operator	Whole body scan
Specificity for inflammation	Failure to determine whether fluid collections contain leukocytes	More specific for the presence of WBCs
Rapidity	Rapidly accomplished	Usually requires 24–48 hours
Portability	Only US portable	Not portable
Body habitus	US best in thin patients; CT requires body fat to define tissue planes	Not as effective in obese patients

3. obliteration of normal soft tissue planes,
4. localized ileus,
5. thumbprinting of bowel,
6. evidence of gas in the biliary tree.

For a more extensive discussion of plain films in abdominal disorders, see Chapter 10, Radiology in the Intensive Care Unit. An upright chest x-ray should also be reviewed in all patients with AAP to look for subdiaphragmatic air or a lower lobe pneumonia.

Biliary Scans

Radionuclide scans (''-IDA'' scans) are sensitive but lack specificity for biliary tract inflammation, particularly in the absence of gallstones. The high sensitivity of these tests renders them useful for excluding the diagnosis of cholecystitis, provided that an adequate study is obtained. Failure to visualize the gallbladder may result from obstructive biliary tract disease, starvation, total parenteral nutrition use, or severe parenchymal liver failure.

Gallium and Indium Scans

The question of abdominal abscess arises frequently and is difficult to resolve noninvasively. Whole body or directed gallium and indium scans may be useful in the search for localized inflammation. Unfortunately, there are many problems. Indium[111]-labelled white blood cells are difficult to produce because the isotope is very expensive, short lived, and cyclotron generated. Indium scanning is likely not to work if WBCs are dysfunctional, as in patients with acquired immune deficiency syndrome, with malnutrition, or receiving dialysis. False positive scans may result in the presence of pneumonia, sinusitis, GI bleeding, or tumors of the bowel. Indium may be used to localize acute infections, but chronic infections may not have sufficiently numerous or active WBCs to enable visualization.

Gallium[67] concentrates in any site of inflammation (not just areas of infection) and may visualize tumors, hematomas, fractures, infections, sarcoidosis, or adult respiratory distress syndrome.

Table 34.2
Characteristics of CT, MRI, and US Examinations

Computed Tomography	Magnetic Resonance Imaging	Ultrasound
Not portable	Not portable	Portable
Expensive	Expensive	Less Expensive
Can evaluate through wounds and bandages	Can evaluate through wounds and bandages	Requires skin contact
Better in fat patients	Body habitus not critical	Better in thin patients
Cross-sectional views best	Infinite number of sectional views	Wide range of sectional views
Metal causes artifact	Impossible to perform with metallic implants	*Air* causes artifact
Static images	Static images	Dynamic images possible
Uniform resolution throughout field	Uniform resolution throughout field	Limited area of high resolution
Not operator dependent	Not operator dependent	Highly operator dependent
Requires contrast to distinguish vascular structures	Exquisite detail of flowing blood and soft tissues	Cystic and dilated structures provide best contrast; air interferes

Gallium is normally excreted into the colon and kidney, producing "physiological hot spots". Resolution is characteristically poor, and precise localization is difficult.

The CT scan and US are frequently used to diagnose intraabdominal conditions. Each has its own specific advantages and limitations as outlined in Tables 34.1 and 34.2.

SUGGESTED READINGS

1. Field S: Plain films: the acute abdomen. *Clin Gastroenterol* 13(1):3–40, 1984.
2. Jordan GL, Jr: The acute abdomen. *Adv Surg* 14:259–315, 1980.
3. Laing FC: Diagnostic evaluation of patients with suspected acute cholecystitis. *Radiol Clin N Am* 21(3):477–493, 1983.
4. Silen W (ed): *Cope's Early Diagnosis of the Acute Abdomen*, ed. 16. New York, Oxford University Press, 1983.

35 Burns

BURN EVALUATION

Mortality rates for burn patients vary widely, depending upon the *depth* and *size of the burn*, *underlying health*, and *age*. *Age* is a powerful predictor of mortality. A 20-year-old individual sustaining a 50% full thickness burn has a 75% chance of survival, whereas the same burn is nearly always fatal in a 70–year-old. Once the airway is secured and hemodynamics have stabilized, the patient should be carefully examined to determine the depth and extent of thermal injury and the burns should be gently washed.

Severity

Burns are classified by their depth (partial or full thickness) or by severity of injury (first to third degree) (Table 35.1).

Estimation of Burn Size

The percentage of body surface affected by burn injury can be estimated by the "rule of nines". This rule assigns percentages of the total body surface area (BSA) to the anterior and posterior surfaces of the head, limbs, and trunk (see Fig. 35.1). As another useful measure, the palm of the patient's hand, estimates 1% of total BSA.

Estimation of the total area involved by second and third degree burns is useful in determining fluid requirements and expected mortality. Adults

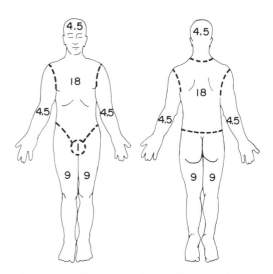

Figure 35.1 Burn wound diagram illustrating the surface area of selected body regions. Numbers correspond to percentages of total body surface area.

with extensive or severe burns and most burned children require admission.

Criteria for Hospital Admission (Adults)

1. Second-degree burn > 20% BSA
2. Third-degree burn > 5% BSA
3. Any second or third-degree burn in a patient ≥ 60 years
4. Inhalation injury
5. Circumferential burns of trunk or extremities
6. Burns of hand, face, feet, or perineum

INITIAL MANAGEMENT

Initial management of the patient with severe burns should include careful assessment of the *airway* and *vital signs* to assure adequate ventilation and perfusion. Inadequate ventilation or perfusion demand immediate intubation or fluid resuscitation.

Table 35.1
Classification of Burns by Severity

Severity	Skin Examination	Sensation
First*	Erythema	Painful
Second*	Erythema/blisters/ edema	Painful
Third**	White or charred Firmly indurated	Anesthetic

*Partial thickness; **Full thickness.

After securing the airway, *repletion of circulating volume* should be undertaken, guided by invasive monitoring if required by tenuous hemodynamic status. Hypovolemic shock is the most common cause of death in the first 24 hours following admission. Most adult patients with burns that require vigorous volume repletion should have urinary and central venous or pulmonary artery catheters inserted for the assessment of volume status. The goal of volume replacement is to establish adequate vital organ perfusion as judged by mental status and urine output (see Chapter 3, Support of the Circulation).

Fluid Management

Burns cause hypovolemia as a result of massive shifts of fluid from intravascular to extravascular compartments and exudation through injured skin.

Hemoconcentration (due to fluid losses from the intravascular space) or *anemia* (due to hemolysis induced by thermal effects and vascular damage) may also occur; therefore, the packed cell volume (PCV) should be checked frequently during resuscitation and kept greater than 30%. Hemoconcentration rarely presents a clinical problem.

Numerous strategies have been advocated for replacing circulating volume. A central feature of all plans is to administer *large volumes of salt-containing fluid* in the initial 24 hours. As a general rule, 3–4 ml of normal saline/kg/% body burn are given in the first day. Customarily, half of the fluid deficit is replaced in the first 8 hours, and the remainder in the next 16 hours. (In fluid replacement, calculated burn areas $\geq$ 50% are all considered 50% BSA). After 24 hours, sodium requirements decline. Free water and colloid are then administered to maintain circulating volume and electrolyte balance. Evaporative water losses after the first 24 hours may be estimated by the following formula: Hourly evaporative water loss (in milliliters) = (25 + % area of burn) × (total BSA in m^2). This formula predicts that a patient with a 25% burn and a 2 m^2 BSA will lose $\simeq$ 100 ml of water per hour. Within 24 hours of the burn event colloids offer little advantage because the newly injured vasculature fails to retain even these large molecules. General guidelines for fluid replacement are given below.

Following fluid replacement *dopamine* may be required to maintain adequate cardiac output, blood pressure, and urine flow. Alpha agonists (e.g., norepinephrine) should be avoided because of their tendency to decrease nutritive blood flow to already injured skin.

Fluid Replacement Strategy

1. In the first 24 hours, give Ringer's solution or normal saline—½ of the deficit in first 8 hours and ½ in next 16 hours.
2. Colloid may be administered after first 24 hours as needed to maintain adequate central vascular pressure, colloid osmotic pressure, blood pressure, and urinary output (> 0.5–1.0 ml/kg/hr).
3. Supplemental free water (D5W) is usually required after the first 24 hours.

Airway Management

Airway complications are the *most common cause of early death* in burn patients. The history and physical examination provide clues to the extent of inhalational injury.

Clues to Inhalation Injury

1. Smoke inhalation in an enclosed space
2. Loss of consciousness
3. Nasal, oral, or facial burns
4. Carbonaceous sputum
5. Hoarseness or stridor

Burns and inhalation injuries cause respiratory complications through four basic mechanisms: (1) *inhalation of toxic fumes and gases*; (2) *airway obstruction*; (3) *increased metabolism and ventilation requirement*; and (4) *impairment of host defenses leading to infection.*

Minute ventilation may be extraordinarily high in large burns because of increased metabolism; a 50–60% burn may double caloric requirements and CO_2 production. Hyperpnea often raises concern for such complicating disorders as pneumonia, adult respiratory distress syndrome (ARDS), or pulmonary embolism.

Toxic Gases: Carbon Monoxide and Cyanide

One by-product of combustion, *carbon monoxide (CO)*, is the primary cause of death in almost 75% of fire fatalities. CO displaces the oxyhemoglobin dissociation curve leftward, resulting in impaired release of O_2 to the tissues. Inhaled CO also competes directly with oxygen for hemoglobin binding. Because the affinity of CO for hemoglobin is 250 times greater than that of oxygen, very low concentrations of inspired CO can rapidly produce high levels of (non-functional) carboxyhemoglobin (CO-Hgb).

The sensitivity of a patient to CO poisoning is influenced by underlying health. Patients with diseases of the central nervous system or heart are unusually susceptible. The clinical symptoms of CO poisoning are thos of *tissue hypoxia* and relate directly to the CO-Hgb level.

Symptoms in Carbon Monoxide Poisoning

Carboxy-hemoglobin Level	Symptoms
< 15%	Usually none
15–20%	Headache, confusion
20–40%	Disorientation, visual impairment, nausea
40–60%	Hallucinations, coma, shock
> 60%	Death

Two principles underpin treatment of CO poisoning: maximization of tissue O_2 delivery and use of high concentrations of O_2 to promote CO excretion. While breathing air, the elimination half-life (t½) of CO is 2–3 hours. When breathing pure O_2, however, t½ declines to 20–30 minutes. Because O_2 profoundly affects CO clearance, the most important therapy in patients with suspected CO poisoning is to immediately administer 100% oxygen. CO-Hgb levels exceeding 25% in normals or 15% in patients with ischemic heart disease should be treated aggressively. High fractions of inspired O_2 should be used until the CO-Hgb percentage falls below 10%. Hyperbaric O_2 can further speed removal of CO. However, hyperbaric chambers inhibit burn management and, after the first hour, offer little advantage over 100% oxygen at ambient pressure.

Closed space fires generate *cyanide* through the combustion of wood, silk, nylon, or polyurethane. Cyanide binds to tissue cytochrome enzymes, impairing normal O_2 utilization and causing lactic acidosis. Hyperbaric O_2 therapy is not useful in cyanide toxicity since the problem is in O_2 usage at the cellular level, not one of O_2 delivery. Tissue hypoxia due to CO or cyanide is usually evident immediately after exposure and should be suspected in burn patients with lactic acidosis whose tissue perfusion appears adequate. Arterial blood gases may demonstrate nearly a *normal PaO_2* but *decreased measured* (not calculated) *O_2 content* or *hemoglobin saturation*. Unlike CO poisoning, mixed venous O_2 saturations are inappropriately high in cyanide intoxication due to underutilization of delivered O_2.

Airway Obstruction

Depending on the fuel consumed, fires often produce toxic fumes and gases that cause inflammation of the airways. *Hot* gases or steam may rapidly produce upper airway obstruction and bronchospasm. *Laryngoscopy and bronchoscopy* are useful when evaluating the severity of airway edema and need for endotracheal intubation. Intubation should be performed if there is clinical evidence of airway obstruction or if laryngoscopy demonstrates supraglottic edema. Hypoxemia or diffuse radiographic infiltrates at the time of admission are poor prognostic signs indicating the need for early *intubation and mechanical ventilation*. In patients not requiring immediate intubation for airway obstruction or hypoxemia, aggressive respiratory therapy with bronchodilators and humidified oxygen may avert the need for mechanical ventilation. *Corticosteroids* are of no proven benefit in non-asthmatic patients with airway obstruction or toxic gas inhalation. Inhaled *racemic epinephrine* may be a useful temporizing measure in those with mild airway edema but should not delay intubation in patients with facial burns or symptomatic airway obstruction.

Bronchospasm and bronchorrhea commonly develop after inhalational injury to the lower airway. Although effective early on, bronchodilators are of less value late in the course of post-burn airway obstruction.

Heat-related tissue edema can progress for 24–48 hours. Patients with burns of the face or neck that appear inconsequential at the time of admission may quickly experience swelling that leads to life-threatening airway obstruction. Therefore, as a firm general rule, patients with second or third degree burns of the face or neck should be endotracheally intubated in the first hours of hospitalization to avoid airway obstruction. Failure to follow this principle will lead to situations in which massive tissue swelling precludes intubation. If intubation is required, a *large* diameter orotracheal tube should be placed to facilitate clearance of voluminous secretions. Prophylactic intubation should generally continue for at least 72 hours. Elevating the head of the bed to 30° during initial resuscitation may help to decrease airway edema. The rate of fluid administration should *not* be decreased in burns involving the airway; inadequate fluids may allow underperfusion and *worsening* of airway damage.

Chemicals carried in smoke also inflict inhalational injury. Some gases such as chlorine or sulfur dioxide combine with the water of upper airway secretions to form acids that irritate the *upper* airway, produce edema, and incite bronchospasm. Potent acids or aldehydes may gain access to the *lower* airways by binding to inhaled carbon particles. The resultant injury is very similar to acid aspiration presenting a diffuse bronchoconstriction, poor lung compliance, and ventilation/perfusion mismatching. Chemical lung injury is suggested by erythema below the level of the vocal cords or by scintigraphic demonstration of ventilation/perfusion mismatching.

The mucosal edema of chemical injury builds for 24–48 hours following exposure and severely impairs mucociliary transport. In addition, the inflammatory mediators and white cells released into the airways produce secretions, atelectasis, and ventilation/perfusion ($\dot{V}/\dot{Q}$) mismatching. Copious secretions, bronchospasm, airway obstruction, and ciliary damage warrant aggressive respiratory therapy. In severe inhalational injuries, the airway mucosa sloughs at about 72 hours and requires 7–14 days to regenerate. Bacterial superinfection and pneumonitis are common during this time.

Other Important Considerations

Major burns impair the ability to *conserve heat and maintain normal body temperature*. Therefore, after burn cleansing, wounds should be covered with clean warm coverings and body temperature monitored closely.

Ileus commonly follows major burns. Gastric distention or markedly diminished bowel sounds should prompt insertion of a nasogastric tube connected to suction.

After wound cleansing, a topical antibiotic should be applied to *limit skin colonization with bacteria*. Systemic antibiotics offer no demonstrated advantage in prophylaxis. Without confirmation of recent immunization, *tetanus toxoid* should be administered.

Pain relief, particularly in partial thickness burns, is critical to allow debridement, cleansing, and other therapeutic forms of patient manipulation. Full-thickness burns are frequently anesthetic so that patients often require little or no pain medication.

LATE COMPLICATIONS OF BURNS

The late complications of burns include: (1) infection; (2) gastrointestinal bleeding; (3) hypermetabolism; and (4) specific problems of local burn care.

Infection

Infection presents the greatest threat to life after the first 36 hours. Clearly, pneumonitis is an ever-present risk in the intubated patient, particularly when inhalation injury has compromised host defenses.

Devastating infection can also result from skin disruption. Massive numbers of bacteria may invade the burn wound and adjacent tissue. In the first 3–5 days following a burn, staphylococci are the most common invading organisms, but after 5 days, gram-negative rods predominate. Apart from standard methods of infection control, meticulous wound care, including the use of *topical antibiotics*, *early debridement and closure* of burn wounds, and use of *gown, mask, and gloves*, decrease the infection risk. Increased basal temperature renders the detection of wound infection difficult. Because the normal body temperature of burn patients may rise as high as 38.5°C as a result of hypermetabolism, fever to this degree does not necessarily warrant the institution of parenteral antibiotics. When burn wound sepsis is suspected, quantitative cultures of burned skin, subcutaneous tissue, and adjacent normal skin should be performed. Growth of $> 10^5$ organisms per gram of tissue or histologic evidence of invasion of adjacent unburned skin are highly suggestive of severe complicating infection. However, long before the results of these tests are available, antibiotics must be instituted on clinical grounds alone if high fever, leukocytosis, or other signs of sepsis are present.

Gastrointestinal Bleeding

Gastrointestinal (GI) bleeding due to stress (Curling) ulceration occurs commonly in burn patients. Effective prophylaxis uses antacids, histamine blockers, or sucralfate. Frequent pH testing of nasogastric (NG) aspirates (to raise gastric pH above 4.0.) is indicated to assure the adequacy of antacids or histamine blockers.

Hypermetabolism

Metabolic rate may double in patients with second and third degree burns exceeding 50% BSA. Indeed, extensive burns represent the single greatest sustained metabolic stress experienced by humans. Full expression of hypermetabolism may require 5–7 days.

Patients with major burns raise resting body temperature and dedicate a large fraction of energy consumption to the heat production that maintains the gradient with ambient temperature; therefore, establishing higher environmental temperature reduces caloric expenditure. *Aggressive nutritional support is required*, usually given parenterally to circumvent the high incidence of gastrointestinal malfunction. However, parenteral nutrition is usually withheld during the first 24–36 hours of hospitalization because of the complexities of fluid management in the period of initial resuscitation. In the initial phase of treatment the daily calorie requirement may be roughly estimated as 25 times the weight in kilograms plus 40 times the percentage of body surface area burned. Giving 60% of the estimated caloric requirement as glucose minimizes catabolic losses of nitrogen. Fat may be used as the source for the remaining 40% of nonprotein calories. Increased lipid clearance argues for raising the percentage of calories given as fat. Two grams of protein are usually given per kilogram of body weight. As in any patient, the transition from parenteral to enteral feeding should be made at the earliest possible time (see Chapter 15, Nutrition and Alimentation).

Burn Wound Care

Topical antibiotics are applied to the skin once or twice daily to limit wound colonization. Wounds should be cleaned and debrided before application of new antibiotic, a process often requiring narcotic analgesia. Several topical antibiotics are available, each with unique advantages, antibacterial spectrum, and complications (Table 35.2). If long-term topical antibiotics are needed, changing the agent used at 7–10 day intervals may prevent the overgrowth of resistant organisms. When sepsis is suspected empirical antibiotic regimens should cover *Pseudomonas aeruginosa* and staphlococci.

Mechanical Problems of the Burn Wound

Patients with circumferential burns of the trunk or extremity and those with burns of the face, hands, feet, or perineum unequivocally require hospital admission and immediate consultation by a burn specialist. Eschar frequently encases the trunk or extremities. These limiting shells may prevent the tissue expansion required to accommodate the massive edema that follows burn injury. Tissue edema reaches maximal severity 12–48 hours following burns and even occurs in non-burned tissue. Ischemia and/ or necrosis may result from the consequent rise in tissue pressure. Furthermore, eschar-related limitation of chest expansion may lead to respiratory failure. In the extremities, edema can be minimized by elevating the burned limb. Decreased capillary refill, cyanosis, parasthesia, and deep pain in tissues distal to the burn site dictate the need for escharotomy. A Doppler examination that demonstrates diminished pulse amplitude distal to the eschar confirms high tissue pressures and the risk of vascular compromise. In circumferential burns of the trunk, reduced thoracic compliance (noted during mechanical ventilation), disproportional tachypnea, or ventilatory distress suggests the need for escharotomy. Escharotomy is performed by incising devitalized wound tissue along the entire lateral and medial aspects of the trunk or affected limb. Once the healing process has begun, hydrotherapy debridement may become an important adjunct to the process.

NON-THERMAL BURN INJURIES

Chemical Injury

Copious irrigation with clear water comprises the primary initial treatment of chemical burns of all types. After flushing, chemical burns should be treated like thermal burns. Although alkaline and acidic chemicals injure tissue by altering its pH, strong neutralizing solutions should not be used because they may produce exothermic reactions, extending *thermal* damage. The adequacy of irrigation in pH-related chemical injury may be assessed by testing the area with litmus paper to assure neutral pH.

Table 35.2
Topical Antimicrobials

	Silver Sulfadiazine	Sodium Nitrate	Mafenide
Advantages	Painless Easily applied Wide spectrum	Painless Wide spectrum	Easily applied Good eschar penetration
Disadvantages	Poor eschar penetration Leukopenia	Poor eschar penetration Skin staining Leaches NaCl from tissue	Metabolic acidosis (carbonic anhydrase inhibitor) Rare aplastic crisis Narrow bacterial spectrum (GNR)*

*GNR, gram-negative rods.

Electrical Burns

Electrical burns inflicted by lightning or other high voltage source may produce extensive tissue damage with little external evidence of injury. Bone and muscle damage are frequent. Electrical injury may cause severe exit wounds at the hands, knees, or feet—sites frequently overlooked in the initial evaluation. (Such wounds are analogous to projectile injuries which produce small entrance but large exit wounds.) In all patients with electrical injury, an electrocardiogram should be performed to look for evidence of arrhythmias, myocardial injury, or conduction disturbance. Because of the high incidence of associated rhabdomyolosis, osmotic and loop diuretics in conjunction with sodium bicarbonate and volume loading may be indicated to avert renal failure.

SUGGESTED READINGS

1. Boswick, JA (ed): Burns. *Surg Clin N Am* 67(1), 1987.
2. Cahalane M, Demling RH: Early respiratory abnormalities from smoke inhalation. *JAMA* 251(6):771–773, 1984.
3. Demling RH: Burns. *N Engl J Med* 313(22):1389–1398, 1985.
4. Demling RH: Fluid resuscitation after major burns. *JAMA* 250(11):1438–1440, 1983.
5. Herndon DN, Curreri PW, Abston S, et al: Treatment of burns. *Curr Probl Surg* 24(6):341–397, 1987.
6. Luterman A, Dacso CC, Curreri PW: Infections in burn patients. *Am J Med* 81(Suppl 1A):45–52, 1986.
7. Sykes RA, Mani MM, Hiebert JM: Chemical burns: retrospective review. *J Burn Care Rehabil* 7(4):343–347, 1986.
8. Winter PM, Miller JN: Carbon monoxide poisoning. *JAMA* 236(13):1502–1504, 1976.

Appendix

Definitions and Normal Values

Conversion Factors

Temperature
  Fahrenheit to centigrade: $°C = (°F - 32) \times 5/9$.
  Centigrade to fahrenheit: $°F = (°C \times 9/5) + 32$.
Pressure
  1 mmHg = 1.36 cmH$_2$O (A pressure of 10 mmHg = 13.6 cmH$_2$O.)
  1 cm H$_2$O = 0.73 mmHg
Length
  1 inch (in) = 2.54 cm
  1 cm = 0.394 in
Weight
  1 pound (lb) = 0.454 kg
  1 kilogram (kg) = 2.2 lb
  1 grain (g) = 60 mg
Work
  1 joule = 1 watt·second
  1 joule = 0.1 kg·m
  1 joule = (10 cmH$_2$O)(1 liter)
Resistance
  1 hybrid (Wood) unit = 80 dyne·cm·sec^{-5}

Useful Renal Formulas and Normal Values[a]

Quantity	Formula	Normal
Estimated creatinine clearance (Cl$_{Cr}$)	$\dfrac{(140 - age)(wt\ in\ kg)}{72 \times serum\ [Cr]}$	> 100 ml/min
Renal failure index (RFI)	$\dfrac{Urine\ [Na^+] \times serum\ [Cr]}{Urine\ [Cr]}$	< 1 Pre-renal > 1 Intra-renal
Fractional excretion of sodium (FENa)	$\dfrac{(Urine\ [Na^+] \times serum\ [Cr])}{(Serum\ [Na^+] \times urine\ [Cr])} \times 100$	< 1 Pre-renal > 1 Intra-renal
Anion gap (AG)	$[Na^+] - ([Cl^-] + [HCO_3^-])$	8–12 mEq/l
Calculated osmolality (Osm)	$2 \times [Na^+] + [glucose]/18 + [BUN]/2.8$	285–295 mOsm/l
Calculated H$_2$O deficit (liters)	$0.6\ (wt\ in\ kg) \times ([Na^+] - 140)/140$	
Corrected [Ca^{2+}]	If albumin ↓ by 1 gm/dl [Ca^{2+}] ↓ by 0.8 mg/dl	
Colloid osmotic pressure (COP)	$1.4\ [globulin]^* + 5.5\ [albumin]^*$	24 ± 3 mmHg

[a]wt, weight; ↑, increased; ↓, decreased; *, (gm/dl).

Useful Circulatory Formulas and Normal Values[a]

Quantity	Formula	Normal
Mean arterial pressure (MAP)	$(P_{sys} + 2 P_{dia})/3$	> 70 mmHg
Heart rate max (HR_{max})	$220 - $ age	
Central venous pressure (CVP)		5–12 cmH$_2$O
Mean pulmonary artery pressure (P_{PA})		10–17 mmHg
Mean pulmonary capillary wedge (P_w)		5–12 mmHg
Cardiac output (CO)	HR $\times$ SV	> 5 l/min
Body surface area (BSA)	$0.202 \times wt_{kg}{}^{0.425} \times ht_m{}^{0.725}$	1.5–2.0 m^2
Stroke volume (SV)	CO/HR	> 60 ml
Cardiac index (CI)	CO/BSA	> 2.5 l/min/m^2
Systemic vascular resistance (SVR)	(MAP$-$CVP) $\times$ 80/CO	900–1200 dyne·sec·cm^{-5}
		11–15 Wood units
Pulmonary vascular resistance (PVR)	$(P_{\overline{PA}} - P_w) \times 80$/CO	150–250 dyne·sec·cm^{-5}
		2–3.1 Wood units
Ejection fraction (EF)	SV/end-diastolic volume	LV $> 65\%$, RV $> 50\%$
Circulating blood volume	$\simeq 70$ ml/kg	$\simeq 5000$ ml
Oxygen delivery	CO $\times$ CaO$_2$	$\simeq 700$ ml O$_2$/min/m^2

[a]LV, left ventricle; RV, right ventricle; wt, weight; ht, height; P_{sys}, systolic pressure; P_{dia}, diastolic pressure.

Useful Respiratory Formulas and Normal Values

Quantity	Formula	Normal
Tidal volume (V_T)	6–7 ml/kg	$\approx$ 500 ml
Vital capacity (VC)		65–70 ml/kg
Maximal inspiratory pressure (MIP)		> 75–100 cmH$_2$O
Deadspace (V_D)	$\approx$ ⅓ V_T	1 ml/pound or 0.45 ml/kg
Deadspace ratio (V_D/V_T)	$(PaCO_2 - P_ECO_2)/PaCO_2$	0.25–0.40
Minute ventilation ($\dot V_E$)		5–10 l/min
Maximal ventilatory volume (MVV)	$\approx$ 35 $\times$ FEV$_I$	
Peak flow	(height, age, sex dependent)	> 7 l/sec or > 425 l/min
Dynamic characteristic	$V_T / (P_{aw} - PEEP)$	Flow dependent
Static compliance (C_{stat})	$V_T / (P_{plat} - PEEP)$	80 ml/cmH$_2$O
Resistance to airflow (R_L)	$(P_{dyn} - P_{plat})/flow$	< 4 cmH$_2$O/l/sec
Alveolar partial pressure of O$_2$ (P_AO_2)	$(P_B - P_{H_2O}) \times FiO_2 - (PaCO_2) / 0.8$	> 100 mmHg
Arterial-alveolar difference (A-aDO$_2$)	$P_AO_2 - PaO_2$	< 10 mmHg @ FiO$_2$ = 0.21
Arterial PaO$_2$/FiO$_2$ ratio (P/F)	PaO_2/FiO_2	> 400
Arterial/alveolar ratio (a/A)	PaO_2/P_AO_2	> 0.9
Arterial O$_2$ tension (PaO$_2$)	100 − (age/3)	80–95 mmHg
Arterial O$_2$ saturation (SaO$_2$)		SaO$_2$ > 90%
Arterial CO$_2$ tension (PaCO$_2$)		37–43 mmHg
Mixed venous O$_2$ tension (P$\bar v$O$_2$)		$\approx$ 35–40 mmHg
Mixed venous O$_2$ saturation (S$\bar v$O$_2$)		> 70%
Mixed venous CO$_2$ tension (P$\bar v$CO$_2$)		$\approx$ 45 mmHg
Arterial O$_2$ content (CaO$_2$)	$(Hgb \times 1.34)SaO_2 + (PaO_2 \times .003)$	$\approx$ 20 ml/dl
Venous O$_2$ content (C$\bar v$O$_2$)	$(Hgb \times 1.34) S\bar vO_2 + (P\bar vO_2 \times .003)$	$\approx$ 15 ml/dl
Oxygen consumption ($\dot VO_2$)	$CO_I \times C(a\text{-}v)O_{2_{ml/dl}} \times 10$	$\approx$ 250 ml/min
Extraction ratio	$C(a\text{-}\bar v)O_2/CaO_2)$	$\approx$ 0.25
Pulmonary capillary O$_2$ content (CcO$_2$)	$(Hgb \times 1.34) + (P_AO_2 \times .003)$	$\approx$ 20 ml/dl
Shunt fraction (venous admixture) % ($\dot Q_S / \dot Q_T$)	$(CcO_2 - CaO_2)/(CcO_2 - C\bar vO_2) \times 100$	< 5%
Arterio-venous O$_2$ content difference C(a-$\bar v$)O$_2$	$CaO_2 - C\bar vO_2$	$\approx$ 5 ml/dl

Content of Common Intravenous Fluids

Type	Na$^+$	Cl$^-$	K$^+$	Ca^{2+}	Lactate	HCO$_3^-$	mOsm/l	kcal/l
	Electrolytes (mEq/l)						Calories and Osmolality	
D5W	0	0	0	0	0	0	252	170
D50W	0	0	0	0	0	0	2530	1700
½ NS	77	77	0	0	0	0	154	0
NS	154	154	0	0	0	0	308	0
Ringer's lactate	130	109	4	3	28	0	273	0
3% NaCl	513	513	0	0	0	0	1026	0
D5½NS	77	77	0	0	0	0	406	170
NaHCO$_3$	1000					1000	2000	0
20% Mannitol	0	0	0	0	0	0	1098	

Temperature Correction Factors for Blood pH and Gas Measurements
(Add to observed value)

°F	°C	pH	PCO₂ (%)	PO₂ (%)
110	43	−.09	+22	+35
107	41.5	−.07	+17	+27
106	41	−.06	+16	+25
105	40.5	−.05	+14	+22
104	40	−.04	+12	+19
103	39.5	−.04	+10	+16
102	39	−.03	+ 8	+13
101	38.5	−.02	+ 6	+10
100	38	−.01	+ 4	+ 7
98–99	**37**	**None**	**None**	**None**
97	36	+.01	− 4	− 7
96	35.5	+.02	− 6	−10
95	35	+.03	− 8	−13
94	34.5	+.04	−10	−16
93	34	+.04	−12	−19
92	33.5	+.05	−14	−22
91	33	+.06	−16	−25
90	32	+.07	−19	−30
88	31	+.09	−22	−35
86	30	+.10	−26	−39
84	29	+.12	−29	−43
82	28	+.13	−32	−47
80	26	+.15	−36	−53
75	24	+.19	−43	−60

Patient's temperature

INDEX

Dr Pearse – SHH pulmonary 4/6/93

ARDS

1. diffuse bil alveolar infiltrates
2. ↓ compliance
3. refractory hypoxemia - shunt
4. nl PCWP
5. acute resp distress ↑↑

Predicting factors for ARDs
in sepsis

1. ↓ plt count
2. von willebrand > 450.?u
   suggest → endothelial injury
   85% sensitivity for
   to dev. ARDS
3. hypotension

Etiologies
↓ pH ct

1. Sepsis syndrome – 40% of ARDS ~ 20-40% dev. ARDS
   of septic shock (esp c̄ shock & hypotension)
2. aspiration, gastric -35% of ARDS –
   – 50-70% of gastric aspiration → dev. ARDS
   – gastric acid ; ± food particles
   – blood - not very much.
3. trauma – multiple bone fx
4. must bld transfusions
5. pancreatitis,
6. near drowning
7. burns.
8. Drugs – ~~cocaine~~, narcotics, heroine, aspirin;
   ↑ tricyclic antidepressan ..
9. inhalational
10. fat embolism – <72 hours
    Tx steroids

72 hrs.

PATHOPHYSIOLOGY
- injury of pulm vasc endothelial cell
- exudative pulm edema ≃ blood a plasma → protein   3 vs ct=
- leak of protein rich fluid ↑ permeability

Mortality
depends   10% cant be oxygenated.

Death -most
due:- Nosocomial infections – lungs G(-) ((-) bld cultures)
                intra-abdominal -(+ bld cultures)
                    25% on autopsy c̄ abscess
⅓ Death 0 – 3 days post 2° inciting cause
⅔   3 – 2 wks → Nosocomial/ MOSF

Tx supportive –
not helpful : steroids, NSAIDs, PGE i, extracorporeal membrane oxygenation, naloxone

goals :
1. oxy. transport ↑ – Abo O₂ content x CO
2. FiO₂ nontoxic < 50-60 %, peep   Review of peep in ARDS
3. → ↓ shunt opens up collapse airways + alveoli   6 - 15 cm H₂O (80%)
   → activation of surfactant
   adverse effects: Barotrauma, ↓ CO, ↑ direct lung injury (over distention of lungs)
   4. ↓ pulm vaso- edema